The Infected Eye

Nora V. Laver • Charles S. Specht
Editors

The Infected Eye

Clinical Practice and Pathological Principles

Springer

Editors
Nora V. Laver
Tufts University School of Medicine
Tufts Medical Center
Boston, MA
USA

Charles S. Specht
Penn State College of Medicine
Penn State Health-Milton S. Hershey
Medical Center
Hershey, PA
USA

ISBN 978-3-319-42838-3 ISBN 978-3-319-42840-6 (eBook)
DOI 10.1007/978-3-319-42840-6

Library of Congress Control Number: 2016953483

Printed on acid-free paper

This Springer imprint is published by Springer Nature
The registered company is Springer International Publishing AG Switzerland
The registered company address is: Gewerbestrasse 11, 6330 Cham, Switzerland

Preface

In 2015, we were approached by Springer to develop a book on ocular infectious disease. On looking through texts available at the time, few were dedicated to the subject. What was lacking was a clinically accessible book that was intended for the practicing ophthalmologist, but that contained basic pathology information of value for the understanding of infectious processes in the eye and periocular tissues. Such a book need not be encyclopedic. It need not contain an atlas of ocular microbiology or include a manual of laboratory technique. It should, however, demonstrate useful clinical approaches to ocular infectious disease and describe key organisms with their effects on the eye.

To this end, contributing clinical authors were recruited from Tufts New England Eye Center and the Penn State Hershey Eye Center, and additional collaborators were included as these authors developed their chapters. The clinical sections are organized by anatomic site to cover periocular tissues and the ocular globe, with a separate chapter to address ocular infection in pediatric practice. A clinically oriented section on antimicrobial therapy and an introduction to specimen collection and the microbiology laboratory are included to support these clinical chapters. Tables and algorithms are employed throughout to enhance the clinical utility of this material.

Introductory chapters on epidemiology and the basics of pathological tissue reactions were written by the editors. Both NVL and CSS have extensive research and practice experience in ocular pathology. To provide a description of key organisms that serve as models for ocular infectious disease in parts of the world outside of North America and Western Europe, experts in the pathology of these diseases from the Joint Pathology Center, Washington, D.C., were invited to contribute a chapter on this topic. Again, illustrations and tables are used to make many of these concepts more accessible to the clinical audience.

As editors, the development of this book has provided both of us with its share of interesting experiences along the way. It has, moreover, been a satisfying and very educational process. We would like to thank all of our contributing authors, whose expertise in their respective fields made this work possible. We want to thank Alan Ball for his help and expertise in editing this work. Your dedication and willingness to assist us with this book is invaluable. Thanks to Dr. Nada Farhat for help with figure edits in Chap. 2. Nada, your work shows your amazing artistic abilities! Special thanks to Dr. Jay Duker, chairman of ophthalmology at Tufts Medical Center and the New England Eye Center, for his continued support and guidance.

We want to acknowledge our mentors Drs. Lorenz Zimmerman, Ahmed Hidayat, and Ian McLean from the former Armed Forces Institute of Pathology in Washington, D.C. Although they are no longer with us, their unparalleled dedication to ocular pathology taught us to love all aspects of pathology, in particular the eye.

We would also like to thank the development staff at Springer for their helpful advice and especially for their patience as the different sections of this work were prepared. And of course, the support and understanding of our spouses and families is acknowledged with affection and gratitude.

Ocular infectious disease comprises many sight-threatening conditions that can be prevented through education or treated with modern surgical or drug therapies. It is an important component of clinical ophthalmology. We are privileged to have had the opportunity to make this contribution.

Boston, MA, USA N.V. Laver, MD
Hershey, PA, USA C.S. Specht, MD

Contents

Contributors

Tayyeba K. Ali, MD Department of Ophthalmology, University of Arkansas for Medical Sciences, Little Rock, AR, USA

Jones Eye Institute, University of Arkansas for Medical Sciences, Little Rock, AR, USA

David W. Craft, PhD, D(ABMM) Department of Pathology, Penn State College of Medicine, Penn State Health-Milton S. Hershey Medical Center, Hershey, PA, USA

Wallace H. Greene, PhD, D(ABMM) Department of Pathology, Penn State College of Medicine, Penn State Health-Milton S. Hershey Medical Center, Hershey, PA, USA

Katrinka Heher, MD Ophthalmology-Oculoplastic Surgery, Tufts Medical Center-New England Eye Center, Boston, MA, USA

Mitesh Kapadia, MD, PhD Ophthalmology-Oculoplastic Surgery, Tufts Medical Center-New England Eye Center, Boston, MA, USA

Jihye Kim, PharmD, BCPS Department of Pharmacy, Penn State College of Medicine, Penn State Health-Milton S. Hershey Medical Center, Hershey, PA, USA

Mary Klassen-Fischer, MD Department of Defense, Joint Pathology Center, Silver Spring, MD, USA

Nora V. Laver, MD Ophthalmology and Pathology and Laboratory Medicine, Ocular Pathology Laboratory, Tufts Medical Center-New England Eye Center, Tufts University School of Medicine, Boston, MA, USA

Erica Liu, MD Ophthalmology, Tufts Medical Center-New England Eye Center, Boston, MA, USA

Ronald C. Neafie, MS Formerly Chief, Parasitic Diseases Pathology Branch Armed Forces Institute of Pathology, Washington, DC, USA

Seth M. Pantanelli, MD, MS Cornea and External Diseases, Department of Ophthalmology, Penn State College of Medicine, Penn State Health-Milton S. Hershey Medical Center, Hershey, PA, USA

Jennifer Renz, MD, MA Ophthalmology, Dartmouth-Hitchcock Medical Center, Lebanon, NH, USA

Tufts Medical Center-New England Eye Center, Boston, MA, USA

Guneet Sodhi, MD Ophthalmology, Eastern Virginia Medical School-Sentara Norfolk General Hospital Lions Center for Sight, Norfolk, VA, USA

Charles S. Specht, MD Departments of Pathology, Ophthalmology, Neurosurgery and Neurology, Penn State College of Medicine, Penn State Health-Milton S. Hershey Medical Center, Hershey, PA, USA

Mitchell B. Strominger, MD Pediatric Ophthalmology Service Director, Tufts Medical Center-New England Eye Center, Tufts University School of Medicine, Boston, MA, USA

Andre J. Witkin, MD Retina Service, Tufts Medical Center-New England Eye Center, Tufts University School of Medicine, Boston, MA, USA

Chapter 1
Epidemiology and Clinical Significance of Ocular Infection

Charles S. Specht and Nora V. Laver

Introduction

Homo sapiens has evolved as a diurnal species dependent on vision. Visual loss may represent a handicap ranging from minimal to severe and, despite the capability of humans to adapt, nevertheless manifests as a limitation to productivity and quality of life which challenges the individual. The numbers of people affected by vision-threatening infections render the implications large and social.

It is no surprise that the significance of blinding conditions may be felt most harshly where the population can least afford to deal with the problem. At the same time, sight-threatening infections occur worldwide across all ranges of socioeconomic conditions. An infection may be the primary cause of ocular tissue damage and visual loss, or it may arise as a secondary factor that complicates a wide spectrum of injury and disease processes.

In the world there exist differing classes of etiology for eye infections that vary with the level of economic development in any given region. This situation presents a unity of concern that demands a global understanding. This is illustrated in scenarios that include the improvement of surgical care available to the poor only to introduce the complications of infection to this population or, on the other hand,

C.S. Specht, MD (✉)
Departments of Pathology, Ophthalmology, Neurosurgery and Neurology, Penn State College of Medicine, Penn State Health-Milton S. Hershey Medical Center, Anatomic Pathology, MC H179 500 University Drive, P.O. Box 850, Hershey, PA 17033-0850, USA
e-mail: cspecht@hmc.psu.edu

N.V. Laver, MD
Ophthalmology and Pathology and Laboratory Medicine, Ocular Pathology Laboratory, Tufts Medical Center-New England Eye Center, Tufts University School of Medicine, 800 Washington Street, #6700, Boston, MA 02111, USA
e-mail: nlaver@tuftsmedicalcenter.org; laver.nora@gmail.com

N.V. Laver, C.S. Specht (eds.), *The Infected Eye*,
DOI 10.1007/978-3-319-42840-6_1

the exposure and spread of emerging infectious agents more widely and to new populations as increased economic development makes exotic travel feasible for larger numbers of individuals.

The extent and cost of blindness and vision impairment have been quantified and documented by the World Health Organization and other international agencies, and it is no small issue [1].

Overall, the most significant causes of visual loss worldwide are cataract, uncorrected refractive error, and age-related macular degeneration [2–9]. However, although factors other than infection account for a larger proportion of impaired vision and blindness, the fact that it is potentially treatable and preventable marks ocular infection for the attention of ophthalmic caregivers internationally. Moreover the toll such diseases take on regions that have the least economic development impels us to seek solutions at the level of the individual patient and through public health initiatives from which all patients and populations may benefit and learn.

As we review the present approaches to clinical understanding and treatment of eye infections, we will return to the concept that the nature of eye infection in a given region is associated with its level of economic development.

Infections in the Economically Developed World

In the more economically developed parts of the world, the nature of serious eye infection is often a function of the degree to which medical care has evolved and is available. In these areas, ocular infection largely presents as (1) a complication of surgical or nonsurgical trauma or of contact lens use; (2) as a secondary phenomenon in patients with degenerative changes, such as corneal ulcer associated with bullous keratopathy; or (3) in association with systemic disease as is seen with endogenous endophthalmitis in immune suppressed patients. Where medical practice makes extensive use of sophisticated (and costly) technological and pharmaceutical treatments, and as environmental factors that are associated with other classes of infection are either lacking or controlled, infections that arise as complications of these treatments have become the predominant concern.

The economies in more developed countries support the offering of many ophthalmic agents, such as compounded pharmaceuticals, that require sophisticated standards for safe manufacture [10]. Vision correction consumer products of convenience are widespread as well. In the case of products used directly by the patient, such as contact lenses and contact lens cleaning products, consistent compliance with recommended instructions for use is needed to prevent ocular infection [11–14]. With any of these products, lapses in sterile manufacturing methods or inappropriate use by physicians or patients can facilitate the development of ocular infection.

Every medical intervention has a complication rate that can be mitigated, but not eliminated, through conscientious attention to practice variables [15, 16]. The occurrence of endophthalmitis illustrates this point. Although a rare disorder on a population basis, endophthalmitis can cause considerable ocular morbidity with reduced visual acuity and blindness [15]. Most endophthalmitis is exogenous, either secondary to corneal ulceration, where common organisms include *Streptococcus*, *Staphylococcus*, and *Pseudomonas*, or associated with surgical or nonsurgical trauma [15, 17]. Ubiquitous cutaneous organisms such as *Streptococcus* and *Staphylococcus* are frequently involved in posttraumatic exogenous endophthalmitis, but gram-negative bacteria and pathogenic fungi that may be found in the environment can represent the sole infectious agent or may proliferate as a component of a mixed infection [15, 18–21].

Endophthalmitis that occurs as a complication of cataract extraction, vitrectomy, intravitreal injection of therapeutic drugs for retinal disorders, glaucoma bleb surgery, penetrating keratoplasty, and the use of keratoprostheses is a serious event whose frequency increases proportionately to the number of procedures performed. Reported examples that have occurred due to a lapse in sterile technique have been generally caused by commensal bacteria such as *Streptococcus* or *Staphylococcus*, whereas a larger variety of bacteria and fungi have been involved in cases where intraoperative irrigating solutions or medications used for intravitreal injection contained pathogenic organisms due to deficiencies in sterile manufacturing methods [15, 16, 19, 20, 22–30]. In a 2007 analysis of Medicare patients, the cost of treatment for endophthalmitis that occurs as a complication of cataract extraction was estimated at about 12,000 US dollars per affected patient [16].

Endogenous endophthalmitis, where infection is spread to the eye through sepsis or the circulation of infectious emboli, is less common than exogenous endophthalmitis [15]. It too, is a disease of "better health care." As this condition tends to arise in hospitalized patients with diabetes, systemic malignancy, various forms of immune deficiency, or cardiovascular diseases, these cases are most often reported from economically developed countries where more patients are treated for such disorders. Bacteria including streptococcal species, gram-negative bacilli, and anaerobes are often involved, but infection in this context can also arise from fungemia (most often due to *Candida*), and mixed infections can occur [15, 19, 21, 31, 32].

It should be noted that in economically developed regions, cases of nonsurgical ocular trauma receive primary treatment with microsurgical technique, and intravitreal or intravenous antibiotic therapy is used to prevent or treat endophthalmitis that may arise due to either surgical or nonsurgical ocular trauma; these practices serve to limit vision loss [15, 18]. Furthermore, endophthalmitis cases are rare compared with the overall number of ophthalmic surgical procedures performed in regions such as North America and Western Europe [15].

Infections in the Developing World

The contribution of ocular infection to the population burden of visual impairment varies considerably throughout the world [1–9]. The most important infectious cause of visual loss worldwide is trachoma due to infection with *Chlamydia trachomatis* [9]. Although declining due to international efforts that are dedicated to the eradication of this disease, significant endemic foci remain in Africa and Asia [3–5, 7–9].

An estimated 21 million people worldwide are affected by trachoma, of which about two million have visual loss. The disease occurs in poor remote areas of warm-weather countries in Asia, Africa, and the Pacific region; Egypt, Pakistan, Nigeria, and Ethiopia have the largest populations at risk for infection [33, 34]. There are no animal hosts for the human strains of *Chlamydia trachomatis* and so the infection is transmitted from person to person, with overcrowded living conditions and personal hygiene habits representing key risk factors in endemic areas. The primary cause of blindness is repeated episodes of conjunctival infection that leads to scarring with eventual development of lid entropion and trichiasis. The initial infection often occurs in childhood, and the prevalence of infection among children can be as high as 60 % in endemic areas [33]. Individuals infected with *Chlamydia trachomatis* can be successfully treated with antibiotics, and trichiasis can be treated with surgery. On a population basis, ocular morbidity can be reduced with educational efforts to improve personal hygiene (particularly proper face washing among children) and attention to sanitation that includes upgrading community water systems to hygienic standards.

The worldwide economic loss due to trachoma is estimated to be about 5.3 billion US dollars per year, a substantial burden in the very poor areas of the world where it is endemic [34]. An international effort led by the Global Alliance for the Elimination of Blinding Trachoma seeks to eliminate this disease as a major cause of blindness in endemic areas through widespread use of the SAFE strategy: surgery for trichiasis, mass distribution of antibiotics, educational efforts to increase facial cleanliness, and improved environmental sanitation [33, 34].

Ocular infection with a locally endemic organism can also have a relatively substantial effect in a single area of the world as is the case with onchocerciasis in endemic areas of sub-Saharan Africa. The incidence of this infection is also declining due to eradication efforts led by international agencies [8]. Onchocerciasis is caused by *Onchocerca volvulus*, a filarial parasite. Also known as river blindness, the parasitic pathogen is spread by riparian black flies of the genus *Simulium* [35]. The filariae primarily infect the skin but can spread throughout the body, with an associated inflammatory reaction and fibrosis that cause the clinical manifestations of the disease. The skin lesions are intensely pruritic and are a major source of morbidity. Infection of the eye can manifest as punctate keratitis, sclerosing keratitis, iridocyclitis, chorioretinitis, and papillitis [35–37]. Central nervous system involvement can also occur with the development of seizures [35]. Onchocerciasis is endemic in much of sub-Saharan Africa, where more than 99 % of cases occur. More limited endemic areas are found in Latin America and Yemen. Overall, cutaneous, ocular, or systemic lesions of this disease affect about 37 million people [35, 36]. Onchocerciasis can be limited through control of the *Simulium* black fly vector in endemic areas, and *Onchocerca volvulus* can be treated with antibiotics. An international effort, the African Program for Onchocerciasis Control, has been fighting this disease since the early 1990s with mass distribution of antibiotics donated by the pharmaceutical industry [35–39]. The economic burden of onchocerciasis includes the cost of treatment and vector control and losses from reduced individual productivity due to visual loss and the syndrome of intense pruritus. These effects can hamper economic development in the poor rural areas that are most affected by onchocerciasis [38–40]. The African Program for Onchocerciasis Control has had success in many places, but endemic regions remain. Successful eradication efforts will require the continued cooperation and coordination of donor countries, international aid agencies, and the governments of the affected countries [39, 40].

Thus, in contrast to the infections seen in the developed part of the world, those of the developing world occur as a primary disorder associated with environmental factors and a limited ability to address environmental issues such as substandard public water supplies and sanitary systems that compound the causative or contributory effects of warm-weather conditions; a high prevalence of bacteria, fungi, viruses, or parasitic organisms in the environment; and a large local population of arthropod vector species. These conditions foster the development of infections such as keratitis due to bacteria or fungi (more common in warm climates), conjunctivitis and trichiasis due to trachoma (associated with crowding and substandard sanitation), and onchocerciasis (an arthropod-borne filarial disease).

Given these causative or aggravating factors, the prevalence of many ocular infections in less developed countries can be substantially impacted by educational efforts, changes in public policy toward essential services, and mass distribution of therapeutic medications. These efforts are important, as morbidity due to visual loss can cause significant loss of individual productivity, and the cost of medical care for these patients can represent a crippling expense in an economically disadvantaged area.

Keratitis and corneal ulceration are relatively common in less developed countries, especially those that have a tropical or subtropical climate in Asia or Africa. Bacterial organisms such as *Staphylococcus*, *Streptococcus*, and *Pseudomonas* are frequent corneal pathogens in these warm-weather environments, and the number of mycotic infections such as those caused by *Fusarium* species is higher than that seen at temperate latitudes [13, 41, 42]. Herpes simplex seroprevalence is high in countries such as Tanzania, where greater than 90 % of the adult population is affected, and so herpes simplex keratitis and its secondary complications are also relatively common [43]. The cost of keratitis and corneal ulcer can be high relative to per capita income in developing countries; one study from southern India put the average cost for medical care in these cases at nearly 57 US dollars in an area where the average per capita income is about 30 US dollars per month [42]. That figure does not include the effects of lost work time and future visual morbidity on the economic well-being of these patients.

In recent years the ophthalmic effects of emerging infectious diseases including rickettsial diseases, West Nile virus, Rift Valley fever, dengue fever, chikungunya, and influenza A (H1N1) have been recognized [44]. These conditions tend to cause uveitis or retinitis as their primary ocular lesion. Although several of these uncommon infections are more frequently found in less developed countries, they are not restricted to these areas; West Nile virus and several rickettsioses are endemic in large areas of North America, and the H1N1 strain was the most common cause of influenza worldwide in 2009. The spread of such conditions is facilitated by the relative ease of travel in the modern world. Still other less common viruses (herpes virus 6 [HHV-6], parechovirus, and parvovirus B19) may be implicated in the development of uveitis [44]. One result of the 2015 Ebola virus epidemic in Africa was the recognition of uveitis that can occur during the convalescent phase of this illness; Marburg virus, a related pathogen, can also cause uveitis [45]. Infections such as this do not cause significant ocular morbidity on a population basis, but the possibility of their involvement should be considered as part of the differential diagnosis for retinitis or uveitis in endemic areas. The presence of these ocular pathogens highlights the ever evolving clinical spectrum of ocular infectious disease. While the complication of uveitis among Ebola survivors is minor in view of the fact that the disease kills half its victims, it illustrates that a variety of infectious diseases may have known or unsuspected ocular involvement and, more importantly, that diseases that yesterday were confined to a limited corner of the globe can, quite suddenly, threaten other parts of the world. Today, we are confronted with the Zika virus. While only conjunctivitis had been previously reported as an ophthalmological finding in adults with this disorder, experience with the 2015–2016 outbreak in Brazil indicates that infants of infected mothers can show retinopathic changes and optic nerve abnormalities [46, 47]. The potential for the occurrence and spread of such perilous infections underscores the need for worldwide efforts to remain vigilant for them.

Infections Relevant Worldwide

The major ocular infections prevalent in more developed countries can and do occur in less economically developed regions of the world primarily in the context of medical care that is provided in some larger urban hospitals. However, for much of the population in these societies, the cost of care, as well as residence in a rural area far from a major city, means less access to medical treatment. Under these conditions, there is less possibility of infection due to a complication of surgical therapy. Obviously, patients who do not have the opportunity for treatment of their cataract, glaucoma, and retinal diseases will sustain visual loss in greater numbers than their counterparts who have access to ophthalmic care in clinics and hospitals, but they will have fewer infections resulting from surgery. Ocular infection identified as secondary to other primary disease processes, as is seen with orbital cellulitis or endogenous endophthalmitis, is also less likely.

Ocular surface infections are reported in both developed and less developed regions, although the pathogens involved and the mechanisms of infection vary by environment. In general, pathogens that flourish in warm climates, in environments with inadequate public sanitation or water supplies, or in association with the ready availability of arthropod vector species are more common in tropical and subtropical areas and less common in regions such as North America or Western Europe.

The incidence of *Acanthamoeba* keratitis presents a curious example, however. Although the causative organisms survive more readily in a tropical or subtropical environment, the overall number of individuals with *Acanthamoeba* keratitis in a given population is strongly influenced by the rate of contact lens use [11, 12]. Hence rates of *Acanthamoeba* keratitis are relatively high in more developed countries where contact lens use is more common, although rates of infection tend to increase during the warm months of the year [11].

Contact lenses are commonly used to correct refractive error in more developed countries. If worn through the night or improperly cleaned, these devices can be associated with degradation of corneal barrier functions and keratitis due to infection with bacteria, fungi, or *Acanthamoeba*. Lapses in sterile manufacturing methods for contact lens cleaning solutions have led to outbreaks of infectious keratitis; fungal organisms such as *Fusarium* have been implicated [11–14, 21]. If contact lens wear were to become more common among the poorer populations of the world, incidence of the same problems might soar, particularly if the availability increased without an accompanying provision for education in proper use.

Epidemic keratoconjunctivitis caused by adenovirus infection appears as outbreaks where children or the elderly congregate and share items that can carry infected ocular secretions [48]. Thus schools, day care centers, and assisted living facilities may be involved. Although self-limited, this condition can lead to considerable morbidity through absence from school and disruption in the daily care and comfort of the elderly.

Herpes simplex infection is ubiquitous throughout the world, with seroprevalence in the adult population of over 50 % in the USA and over 75 % in Germany. Herpes simplex keratitis (HSK) may present as an acute or recrudescent infection in any country and affects about 30 people per 100,000 in North America and Western Europe. Ocular morbidity arises from ulceration during primary herpetic infection, corneal scarring associated with recrudescent infection, and the development of secondary infection with other organisms that include bacterial pathogens. In more developed countries, HSK is treated with antiviral medications, steroids, and corrective corneal surgery [43].

Infectious scleritis can develop as a complication of ophthalmic surgical procedures such as pterygium excision, vitrectomy, or scleral buckle procedures. Bacteria (such as *Pseudomonas*, *Staphylococcus*, and *Streptococcus*) and fungi such as *Fusarium* are common pathogens [49]. Orbital cellulitis in patients with a history of paranasal sinusitis or orbital trauma has most often been reported in more economically developed areas where medical imaging studies are commonly done, but occurrence in some less developed countries has been described [50–53]. Orbital cellulitis is often caused by *Staphylococcus*, *Streptococcus*, or *Haemophilus*; fungal organisms are occasionally involved. Such infections can lead to visual loss and there is the potential for life-threatening extension through the cavernous sinus to the brain. Early treatment with systemic antibiotics is often needed and surgical correction of abscesses within the orbit, skull base, or brain may be required. The potential for increased visual and neurological morbidity and the use of costly therapeutic modalities in these cases can be a significant burden in less developed areas [52, 53].

In economically developed countries, immune suppression with resulting opportunistic infection of the eye due to HIV infection is less common in the current era of highly active antiretroviral therapy (HAART). However, cases may still present to the ophthalmology clinic in endemic communities of North America and Western Europe. These patients have an increased risk for secondary ocular infection with cytomegalovirus, toxoplasmosis, or syphilis, and either the HIV organism itself or antiretroviral therapy may cause retinal changes that lead to visual impairment [54]. In less developed regions where treatment of HIV infection with HAART may not be available, this type of immune suppression can lead to an increased prevalence of ocular infectious disease [55]. In recent years it has been recognized that HIV infection can be a predisposing factor in the development of ocular surface squamous neoplasia (OSSN) [54–56]. The presence of HIV infection may facilitate ocular surface infection with human papillomavirus (HPV) and may thus contribute to the number of patients with OSSN in parts of Africa that have a relatively high prevalence of HIV infection [56].

Conclusion

Whether a condition that arises in a relatively small number of susceptible patients, a preventable complication of contact lens use or of ophthalmic surgical procedures in more developed countries, or a source of large-scale visual loss on a population basis that leads to significant economic burden in a less developed region of the world, the consideration and exclusion of infection is a key part of clinical assessment and therapeutic decision-making in ophthalmology. Pathogenic organisms can nearly always be classified with modern laboratory methods, providing an opportunity for rational therapy. This can lead to recovery of some or all of a patient's vision if the pathogen is identified early in the course of the disease. There are few more effective exercises in medicine where clinical acumen can be used to formulate a treatment plan that will cure or significantly ameliorate a disease, with substantial benefit to the patient. Increased awareness and caregiver response to infections that affect the eye will benefit the world population and support its progress.

References

1. World Health Organization. Blindness. http://www.who.int/topics/blindness/en/. Accessed 6 Jan 2016.
2. Furtado JM, Lansingh VC, Carter MJ, Milanese MF, Peña BN, Ghersi HA, et al. Causes of blindness and visual impairment in Latin America. Surv Ophthalmol. 2012;57:149–77. doi:10.1016/j.survophthal.2011.07.002.
3. Khairallah M, Kahloun R, Flaxman SR, Jonas JB, Keeffe J, Leasher J, et al. Prevalence and causes of vision loss in North Africa and the Middle East: 1990–2010. Br J Ophthalmol. 2014;98:605–11. doi:10.1136/bjophthalmol-2013-304068.

4. Jonas JB, George R, Asokan R, Flaxman SR, Keeffe J, Leasher J, et al. Prevalence and causes of vision loss in Central and South Asia: 1990–2010. Br J Ophthalmol. 2014;98:592–8. doi:10.1136/bjophthalmol-2013-303998.
5. Wong TY, Zheng Y, Jonas JB, Flaxman SR, Keeffe J, Leasher J, et al. Prevalence and causes of vision loss in East Asia: 1990–2010. Br J Ophthalmol. 2014;98:599–604. doi:10.1136/bjophthalmol-2013-304047.
6. Bourne RRA, Jonas JB, Flaxman SR, Keeffe J, Leasher J, Naidoo K, et al. Prevalence and causes of vision loss in high-income countries and in Eastern and Central Europe: 1990–2010. Br J Ophthalmol. 2014;98:629–38. doi:10.1136/bjophthalmol-2013-304033.
7. Keeffe J, Taylor HR, Fotis K, Pesudovs K, Flaxman SR, Jonas JB, et al. Prevalence and causes of vision loss in Southeast Asia and Oceania: 1990–2010. Br J Ophthalmol. 2014;98:586–91. doi:10.1136/bjophthalmol-2013-304050.
8. Naidoo K, Gichuhi S, Basáñez M-G, Flaxman SR, Jonas JB, Keeffe J, et al. Prevalence and causes of vision loss in sub-Saharan Africa: 1990–2010. Br J Ophthalmol. 2014;98:612–8. doi:10.1136/bjophthalmol-2013-304081.
9. Bourne RRA, Stevens GA, White RA, Smith JL, Flaxman SR, Price H, et al. Causes of vision loss worldwide, 1990–2010: a systematic analysis. Lancet Glob Health. 2013;1:e339–49. doi:10.1016/S2214-109X(13)70113-X.
10. Staes C, Jacobs J, Mayer J, Allen J. Description of outbreaks of healthcare associated infections related to compounding pharmacies, 2000–2012. Am J Health Syst Pharm. 2013;70:1301–12. doi:10.2146/ajhp130049.
11. Ibrahim YW, Boase DL, Cree IA. Factors affecting the epidemiology of Acanthamoeba keratitis. Ophthalmic Epidemiol. 2007;14:53–60. doi:10.1080/09286580600920281.
12. Lorenzo-Morales J, Martín-Navarro CM, López-Arencibia A, Arnalich-Montiel F, Piñero JE, Valladares B. Acanthamoeba keratitis: an emerging disease gathering importance worldwide? Trends Parasitol. 2013;29:181–7. doi:10.1016/j.pt.2013.01.006.
13. Thomas PA, Kaliamurthy J. Mycotic keratitis: epidemiology, diagnosis and management. Clin Microbiol Infect. 2013;19:210–20. doi:10.1111/1469-0691.12126.
14. Stapleton F, Carnt N. Contact lens-related microbial keratitis: how have epidemiology and genetics helped us with pathogenesis and prophylaxis. Eye. 2012;26:185–93. doi:10.1038/eye.2011.288.
15. Durand ML. Endophthalmitis. Clin Microbiol Infect. 2013;19:227–34. doi:10.1111/1469-0691.12118.
16. Schmier JK, Halpern MT, Covert DW, Lau EC, Robin AL. Evaluation of Medicare costs of endophthalmitis among patients after cataract surgery. Ophthalmology. 2007;114:1094–9. doi:10.1016/j.ophtha.2006.08.050.
17. O'Neill EC, Yeoh J, Fabinyi DCA, Cassidy D, Vajpayee RB, Allen P, et al. Risk factors, microbial profiles and prognosis of microbial keratitis-associated endophthalmitis in high-risk eyes. Graefes Arch Clin Exp Ophthalmol. 2014;252:1457–62. doi:10.1007/s00417-014-2732-1.
18. Ahmed Y, Schimel AM, Pathengay A, Colyer MH, Flynn Jr HW. Endophthalmitis following open-globe injuries. Eye. 2012;26:212–7. doi:10.1038/eye.2011.313.
19. Keynan Y, Finkelman Y, Lagacé-Wiens P. The microbiology of endophthalmitis: global trends and a local perspective. Eur J Clin Microbiol Infect Dis. 2012;31:2879–86. doi:10.1007/s10096-012-1659-x.
20. Sadaka A, Durand ML, Gilmore MS. Bacterial endophthalmitis in the age of outpatient intravitreal therapies and cataract surgeries: host-microbe interactions in intraocular infection. Prog Retin Eye Res. 2012;31:316–31. doi:10.1016/j.preteyeres.2012.03.004.
21. Kalkanci A, Ozdek S. Ocular fungal infections. Curr Eye Res. 2011;36:179–89. doi:10.3109/02713683.2010.533810.
22. Packer M, Chang DF, Dewey SH, Little BC, Mamalis N, Oetting TA, et al. Prevention, diagnosis, and management of acute postoperative bacterial endophthalmitis. J Cataract Refract Surg. 2011;37:1699–714. doi:10.1016/j.jcrs.2011.06.018.

23. Pathengay A, Flynn Jr HW, Isom RF, Miller D. Endophthalmitis outbreaks following cataract surgery: causative organisms, etiologies, and visual acuity outcomes. J Cataract Refract Surg. 2012;38:1278–82. doi:10.1016/j.jcrs.2012.04.021.
24. Cornut P-L, Thuret G, Creuzot-Garcher C, Maurin M, Pechinot A, Bron A, et al. Relationship between baseline clinical data and microbiologic spectrum in 100 patients with acute postcataract endophthalmitis. Retina. 2012;32:549–57. doi:10.1097/IAE.0b013e3182205996.
25. Park JC, Ramasamy B, Shaw S, Ling RHL, Prasad S. A prospective and nationwide study investigating endophthalmitis following pars plana vitrectomy: clinical presentation, microbiology, management and outcome. Br J Ophthalmol. 2014;98:1080–6. doi:10.1136/bjophthalmol-2013-304486.
26. Fileta JB, Scott IU, Flynn Jr HW. Meta-analysis of infectious endophthalmitis after intravitreal injection of anti-vascular endothelial growth factor agents. Ophthalmic Surg Lasers Imaging Retina. 2014;45:143–9. doi:10.3928/23258160-20140306-08.
27. Alwitry A, King AJ. Surveillance of late-onset bleb leak, blebitis and bleb-related endophthalmitis - a UK incidence study. Graefes Arch Clin Exp Ophthalmol. 2012;250:1231–6. doi:10.1007/s00417-011-1920-5.
28. Chen JY, Jones MN, Srinivasan S, Neal TJ, Armitage WJ, Kaye SB. Endophthalmitis after penetrating keratoplasty. Ophthalmology. 2015;122:25–30. doi:10.1016/j.ophtha.2014.07.038.
29. Behlau I, Martin KV, Martin JN, Naumova EN, Cadorette JJ, Sforza JT, et al. Infectious endophthalmitis in Boston keratoprosthesis: incidence and prevention. Acta Ophthalmol. 2014;92:e546–55. doi:10.1111/aos.12309.
30. Robert M-C, Moussally K, Harissi-Dagher M. Review of endophthalmitis following Boston keratoprosthesis type 1. Br J Ophthalmol. 2012;96:776–80. doi:10.1136/bjophthalmol-2011-301263.
31. Vaziri K, Pershing S, Albini TA, Moshfeghi DM, Moshfeghi AA. Risk factors predictive of endogenous endophthalmitis among hospitalized patients with hematogenous infections in the United States. Am J Ophthalmol. 2015;159:498–504. doi:10.1016/j.ajo.2014.11.032.
32. Jackson TL, Paraskevopoulos T, Georgalas I. Systematic review of 342 cases of endogenous bacterial endophthalmitis. Surv Ophthalmol. 2014;59:627–35. doi:10.1016/j.survophthal.2014.06.002.
33. Taylor HR, Burton MJ, Haddad D, West S, Wright H. Trachoma. Lancet. 2014;384:2142–52. http://dx.doi.org/10.1016/S0140-6736(13)62182-0.
34. Rajak SN, Collin JRO, Burton MJ. Trachomatous trichiasis and its management in endemic countries. Surv Ophthalmol. 2012;57:105–35. doi:10.1016/j.survophthal.2011.08.002.
35. Crump A, Morel CM, Omura S. The onchocerciasis chronicle: from the beginning to the end? Trends Parasitol. 2012;28:280–8. http://dx.doi.org/10.1016/j.pt.2012.04.005.
36. Taylor MJ, Hoerauf A, Bockarie M. Lymphatic filariasis and onchocerciasis. Lancet. 2010;376:1175–85. doi:10.1016/S0140-6736(10)60586-7.
37. Banla M, Tchalim S, Karabou PK, Gantin RG, Agba AI, Kére-Banla A, et al. Sustainable control of onchocerciasis: ocular pathology in onchocerciasis patients treated annually with ivermectin for 23 years: a cohort study. PLoS One. 2014;9, e98411. doi:10.1371/journal.pone.0098411.
38. Coffeng LE, Stolk WA, Zouré HGM, Veerman JL, Agblewonu KB, Murdoch ME, et al. African Programme for Onchocerciasis Control 1995–2015: model-estimated health impact and cost. PLoS Negl Trop Dis. 2013;7, e2032. doi:10.1371/journal.pntd.0002032.
39. Keating J, Yukich JO, Mollenkopf S, Tediosi F. Lymphatic filariasis and onchocerciasis prevention, treatment, and control costs across diverse settings: a systematic review. Acta Trop. 2014;135:86–95. doi:10.1016/j.actatropica.2014.03.017.
40. Bockarie MJ, Kelly-Hope LA, Rebollo M, Molyneux DH. Preventive chemotherapy as a strategy for elimination of neglected tropical parasitic diseases: endgame challenges. Phil Trans R Soc B. 2013;368:20120144. doi:10.1098/rstb.2012.0144.
41. Shah A, Sachdev A, Coggon D, Hossain P. Geographic variations in microbial keratitis: an analysis of the peer-reviewed literature. Br J Ophthalmol. 2011;95:762–7. doi:10.1136/bjo.2009.169607.
42. Prajna VN, Nirmalan PK, Saravanan S, Srinivasan M. Economic analysis of corneal ulcers in south India. Cornea. 2007;26:119–22.

43. Rowe AM, St. Leger AJ, Jeon S, Dhaliwal DK, Knickelbein JE, Hendricks RL. Herpes keratitis. Prog Retin Eye Res. 2013;32:88–101. doi:10.1016/j.preteyeres.2012.08.002.
44. Khairallah M, Kahloun R. Ocular manifestations of emerging infectious diseases. Curr Opin Ophthalmol. 2013;24:574–80. doi:10.1097/ICU.0b013e3283654e09.
45. Varkey JB, Shantha JG, Crozier I, Kraft CS, Lyon GM, Mehta AK, et al. Persistence of Ebola virus in ocular fluid during convalescence. N Engl J Med. 2015;372:2423–7. doi:10.1056/NEJMoa1500306.
46. Duffy MR, Chen TH, Hancock WT, Powers AM, Kool JL, Lanciotti RS, et al. Zika virus outbreak on Yap Island, Federated States of Micronesia. N Engl J Med. 2009;360:2536–43. doi:10.1056/NEJMoa0805715.
47. de Paula Freitas B, de Oliveira Dias JR, Prazeres J, Sacramento GA, Ko AI, Maia M, et al. Ocular findings in infants with microcephaly associated with presumed Zika virus congenital infection in Salvador, Brazil. JAMA Ophthalmol. 9 Feb 2016. doi:10.1001/jamaophthalmol.2016.0267.
48. Meyer-Rüsenberg B, Loderstädt U, Richard G, Kaulfers P-M, Gesser C. Epidemic keratoconjunctivitis-the current situation and recommendations for prevention and treatment. Dtsch Arztebl Int. 2011;108:475–80. doi:10.3238/arztebl.2011.0475.
49. Hodson KL, Galor A, Karp CL, Davis JL, Albini TA, Perez VL, et al. Epidemiology and visual outcomes in patients with infectious scleritis. Cornea. 2013;32:466–72. doi:10.1097/ICO.0b013e318259c952.
50. Murphy C, Livingstone I, Foot B, Murgatroyd H, MacEwen CJ. Orbital cellulitis in Scotland: current incidence, aetiology, management and outcomes. Br J Ophthalmol. 2014;98:1575–8. doi:10.1136/bjophthalmol-2014-305222.
51. Chaudhry IA, Shamsi FA, Elzaridi E, Al-Rashed W, Al-Amri A, Al-Anezi F, et al. Outcome of treated orbital cellulitis in a tertiary eye care center in the Middle East. Ophthalmology. 2007;114:345–54. doi:10.1016/j.ophtha.2006.07.059.
52. Uy HS, Tuaño PMC. Preseptal and orbital cellulitis in a developing country. Orbit. 2007;26:33–7. doi:10.1080/01676830600671474.
53. Onakpoya OH, Adeoye AO, Akinpelu OV. Cost-related antibiotic dosage omissions-challenge for orbital cellulitis management in resource poor communities. Orbit. 2009;28:147–52. doi:10.1080/01676830902919811.
54. Butler NJ, Thorne JE. Current status of HIV infection and ocular disease. Curr Opin Ophthalmol. 2012;23:517–22. doi:10.1097/ICU.0b013e328358ba85.
55. Schaftenaar E, van Gorp ECM, Meenken C, Osterhaus ADME, Remeijer L, Struthers HE, et al. Ocular infections in sub-Saharan Africa in the context of high HIV prevalence. Trop Med Int Health. 2014;19:1003–14. doi:10.1111/tmi.12350.
56. Carreira H, Coutinho F, Carrilho C, Lunet N. HIV and HPV infections and ocular surface squamous neoplasia: systematic review and meta-analysis. Br J Cancer. 2013;109:1981–8. doi:10.1038/bjc.2013.539.

Chapter 2
Pathogenic Properties of Infectious Organisms and Tissue Reactions

Nora V. Laver and Charles S. Specht

Introduction

Despite historical dramatic progress in their prevention and treatment, infectious diseases remain a major cause of morbidity and mortality for millions of people around the globe. Infections must be considered in the etiologic differential diagnosis of symptoms affecting any ocular tissue. The major types of infectious agents that cause disease, with examples of specific microbes causing ocular infection, are described in this chapter. A discussion on the human immune system and host defense mechanisms will allow the reader to better understand the different types of inflammation and the cells involved in the process.

Infection involves complicated interactions between microbes and hosts, and in most cases, a pathogenic process consisting of several steps is required for an infection to develop. A competent host has a complex array of physical and immunological defenses to prevent infection, and invading pathogens adapt mechanisms to overcome these progressive impediments. The various modes of invasion among bacteria, viruses, fungi, and parasites share some similarities but in detail are unique for each class of organism.

N.V. Laver, MD (✉)
Ophthalmology and Pathology and Laboratory Medicine, Ocular Pathology Laboratory, New England Eye Center, Tufts Medical Center and Tufts University School of Medicine, 800 Washington Street, #6700, Boston, MA 02111, USA
e-mail: nlaver@tuftsmedicalcenter.org; laver.nora@gmail.com

C.S. Specht, MD
Departments of Pathology, Ophthalmology, Neurosurgery and Neurology, Penn State College of Medicine, Penn State Health-Milton S. Hershey Medical Center, Anatomic Pathology, MC H179 500 University Drive, P.O. Box 850, Hershey, PA 17033-0850, USA
e-mail: cspecht@hmc.psu.edu

N.V. Laver, C.S. Specht (eds.), *The Infected Eye*,
DOI 10.1007/978-3-319-42840-6_2

Understanding how these agents infect the host and cause damage to tissue, and the host responses to specific infections, is the key to better diagnosis and treatment of ocular infections.

Classification of Infectious Organisms

Ocular infections can be classified by their most common clinical presentation (such as endogenous endophthalmitis), by microbiological characteristics (Table 2.1), or by epidemiologic characteristics (means of transmission and reservoir of the organism, e.g., food-borne infections) [1]. There are a wide range of infectious agents that vary in size from 27-kD nucleic acid-free prions to the 20-nm poliovirus to 10-m tapeworms [2]. They can be classified within five major categories: bacteria, viruses, fungi, parasites, and prions (Table 2.1).

Bacteria are characterized by a peptidoglycan-rich cell membrane and the lack of a membrane-bound nucleus. There are two forms of cell wall structures: a thick wall surrounding the cell membrane that retains crystal violet stain (gram-positive bacteria) or a thin cell wall sandwiched between two phospholipid bilayer membranes (gram-negative bacteria). Bacteria are classified by gram staining (positive or negative), shape (cocci or bacilli), and need for oxygen (aerobic or anaerobic)

Table 2.1 Microbiological classification of infectious organisms

Classification	Organism	Examples
Bacterial	**Gram positive**	
	Cocci	*Staphylococcus aureus* *Staphylococcus epidermidis* *Streptococcus pneumoniae* *Streptococcus pyogenes*
	Bacilli	*Propionibacterium acnes* *Corynebacterium diphtheria* *Clostridium perfringens* *Clostridium septicum*
	Gram negative	
	Coccobacilli	*Moraxella lacunata* *Neisseria gonorrhoeae*
	Bacilli	*Haemophilus influenza* *Pseudomonas aeruginosa* *Chlamydia trachomatis* *Bartonella henselae*
	Mycobacteria	*Mycobacterium tuberculosis* *Mycobacterium leprae* *Mycobacterium bovis* *Mycobacterium avium* *Mycobacterium intracellulare*
	Spirochetes	*Treponema pallidum* *Borrelia burgdorferi*

Table 2.1 (continued)

Classification	Organism	Examples
Viral	**DNA viruses**	
	Enveloped	Poxviruses (vaccinia, molluscum contagiosum) Herpesviruses Herpes simplex Varicella zoster Epstein-Barr virus Cytomegalovirus
	Nonenveloped	Adenovirus Papillomavirus
	RNA viruses	
	Enveloped	Influenza A and B Paramyxoviruses (measles, mumps) Rubella
	Nonenveloped	Picornavirus (echovirus, enterovirus, coxsackievirus, poliovirus)
Fungal	Yeast	*Candida* spp. *Cryptococcus neoformans*
	Mold	*Aspergillus* spp. *Penicillium* spp. *Cephalosporium* spp. *Fusarium* spp. *Mucoraceae* spp.
	Dimorph	*Blastomyces dermatitis* *Coccidioides immitis* *Histoplasma capsulatum* *Sporothrix schenckii*
	Other	Microsporidia
Parasitic	Protozoa	*Acanthamoeba* spp. (*polyphaga*, *castellanii*) *Leishmania donovani* *Toxoplasma gondii*
	Nematodes	*Onchocerca volvulus* *Loa loa*
	Helminths	*Toxocara canis* *Wuchereria bancrofti*
Prion	Prion protein	Creutzfeldt-Jakob disease

(Table 2.1). Most bacteria synthesize their own DNA, RNA, and proteins, but they depend on the host for favorable growth conditions [3].

Bacteria can cause endophthalmitis post cataract surgery [4]; this is almost always due to gram-positive cocci (Fig. 2.1). Coagulase-negative staphylococci are a major pathogen, causing up to 70 % of culture-positive cases. *Staphylococcus aureus* (10 %), streptococci (9 %), and other gram-positive cocci and gram-negative bacilli account for the remaining cases.

Viruses are obligate intracellular organisms that depend on the host cell's metabolic machinery for their replication. They consist of a nucleic acid genome

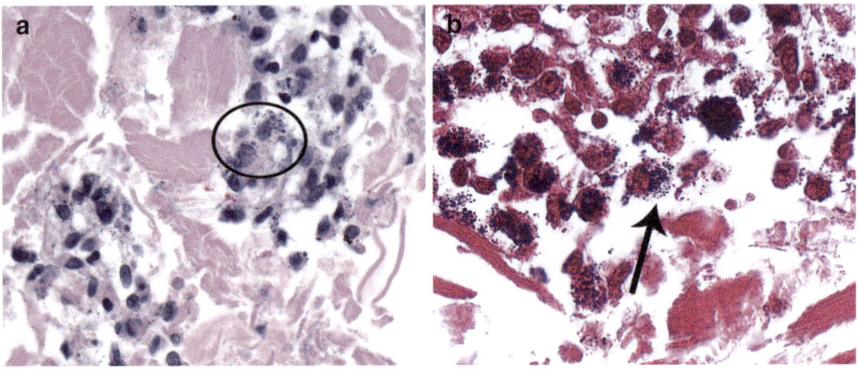

Fig. 2.1 (**a**) Vitrectomy cellblock preparation of a 58-year-old male with gram-positive bacterial endophthalmitis due to *Staphylococcus aureus* and retained lens fragments. A *circle* highlights the inflammatory cells present (H&E, ×40). (**b**) Gram-positive bacteria (gram stain, ×40, *arrow* points to gram-positive cocci)

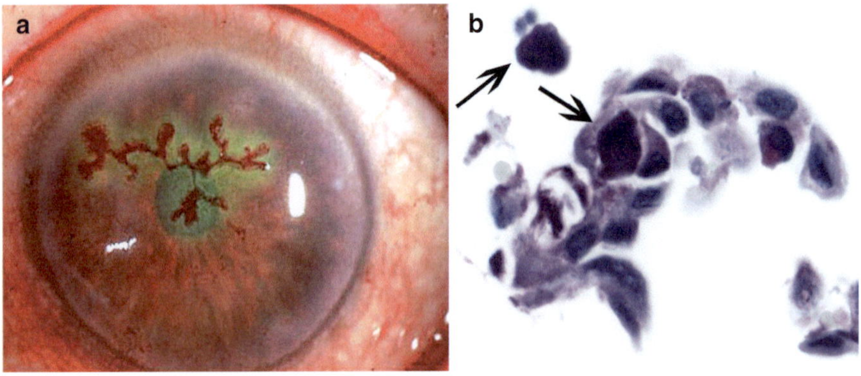

Fig. 2.2 (**a**) Recurrent herpes simplex keratitis infection in a 45-year-old female. Multiple corneal dendritic ulcers are present following a primary infection. (**b**) Corneal scrape cytology specimen showing herpes virus intranuclear inclusions (*arrows*) in infected cells (PAS stain, ×40)

surrounded by a protein coat or capsid that is sometimes encased in a lipid membrane. They are classified by their nucleic acid genome ("DNA" or "RNA" viruses), the shape of the capsid (icosahedral or helical), the presence or absence of a lipid envelope, their mode of replication, the preferred cell type for replication, and the type of pathology. Acute retinal necrosis is a rapidly necrotizing retinitis caused by herpesviruses that mainly affects immunocompetent patients [5]. *Herpes simplex* virus (HSV) or *varicella zoster* virus (VZV) is the culprit in nearly all cases (Table 2.1). This infection causes major destruction of retinal tissue with dramatic damage to vision. About 15 % of people with chronic ocular herpes simplex lose some vision (Fig. 2.2).

Fungi possess thick chitin-containing cell walls and ergosterol-containing cell membranes. Fungi can grow either as rounded yeast cells or as slender filamentous hyphae. Hyphae may be septate (with cell walls separating individual cells) or aseptate. Some pathogenic fungi show thermal dimorphism, that is, they grow as hyphal forms at room temperature but as yeast forms at body temperature (Table 2.1).

Fungi may cause superficial or deep infections. Superficial infections involve the skin, hair, and nails [6]. Certain fungal species invade the subcutaneous tissue, causing abscesses or granulomas (an example is sporotrichosis). Deep fungal infections can spread systemically and invade vital organs in immunocompromised hosts, but usually heal or remain latent in immunocompetent individuals.

Some deep fungal species are limited to a particular geographic region (such as *Coccidioides* in the Southwestern United States and *Histoplasma* in the Ohio River Valley). By contrast, opportunistic fungi (such as *Candida*, *Aspergillus*, *Mucor*, and *Cryptococcus*) are ubiquitous organisms that either colonize individuals or are encountered from environmental sources (Fig. 2.3). In immunodeficient individuals, opportunistic fungi give rise to life-threatening infections characterized by tissue necrosis, hemorrhage, and vascular occlusion, with little or no inflammatory response [7].

Parasitic infections are caused by unicellular protozoa or multicellular helminths (worms) [8]. Various types of parasitic protozoa replicate extracellularly (such as *Acanthamoeba* spp.) or within the cells of a tissue (such as *Toxoplasma gondii*). For example, *Acanthamoeba* spp. are ubiquitous as free-living organisms in the environment, but favor warm wet conditions; ocular infection most often arises as keratitis associated with contact lens use [9] (Fig. 2.4). Ingestion of *Toxoplasma gondii* may occur either during contact with oocyst-shedding kittens or by eating cyst-ridden, undercooked meat. These intracellular parasites can thus gain access to internal organs and the bloodstream; infection of the eye can develop as endogenous endophthalmitis [10].

Parasitic worms, or helminths, are highly differentiated multicellular organisms. Helminths at adult or larval stages may involve human ocular tissues by infection of external structures (such as eyelids, conjunctival sacs, subconjunctival tissue, or lacrimal glands) (Fig. 2.5) or through intraocular infection that can involve the anterior segment structures or more posterior tissues (vitreous, retina, and optic nerve). Several parasitic helminths show tropism for the eyes and related tissues as they migrate through the host body during their immature stages. This is the case of ascarids (such as *Toxocara canis*) and strongyloids (such as *Angiostrongylus cantonensis*) which cause ocular larva migrans, and the larvae of *Trichinella spiralis* that can infect extraocular muscles. Human ocular infestations by zoonotic helminths may also be caused by the parasitic adult stages as in the case of *Thelazia* (eye worm infestation) and filarioid species including those belonging to the genera *Dirofilaria* and *Onchocerca* [11].

Prions are composed of an abnormal form of a host protein known as prion protein (PrP) that is normally found in neurons [12]. Diseases occur when the PrP undergoes a conformational change that promotes conversion of normal PrP to the abnormal form. Accumulation of abnormal PrP intracellularly leads to neuronal damage and spongiform pathologic changes in the brain. The most common cause of prion disease is Creutzfeldt-Jakob disease (CJD). CJD can affect the retina and cause changes in the electroretinogram [13].

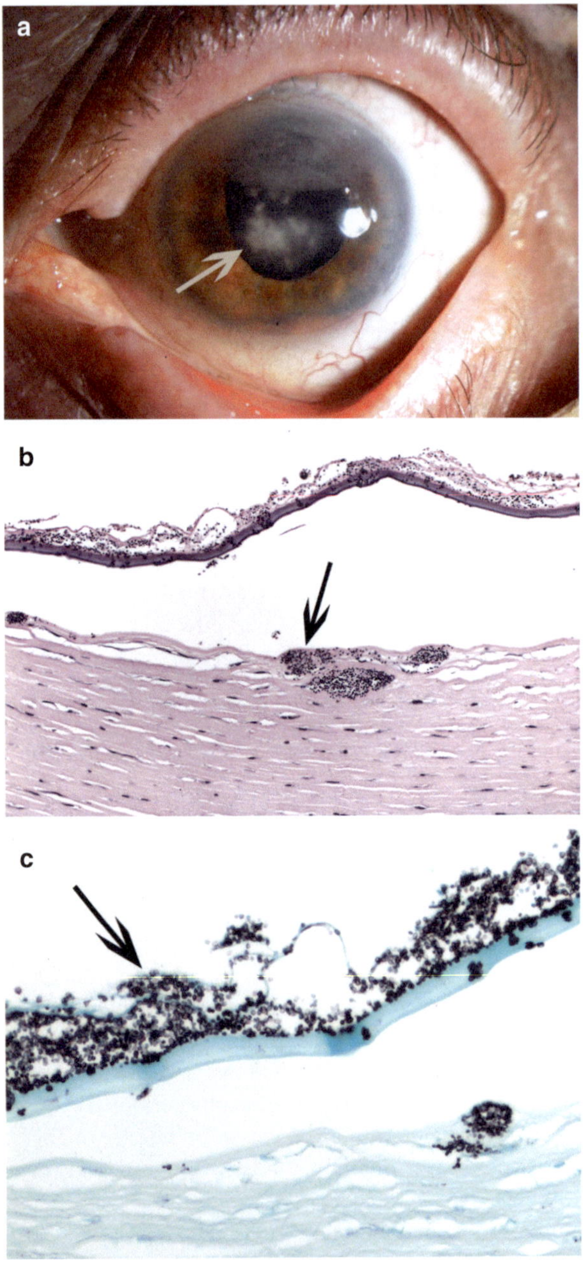

Fig. 2.3 (**a**) Corneal fungal infection and with subsequent endophthalmitis due to *Candida parapsilosis* in an 89-year-old male post cataract surgery (*arrow*). (**b**) *Candida parapsilosis* keratitis present in the deep corneal stroma (*arrow*), at the level of Descemet's membrane, the endothelial layer, and the anterior chamber (H&E, ×10). (**c**) *Candida parapsilosis* (*arrow*) keratitis present at the level of Descemet's membrane (GMS stain, ×10)

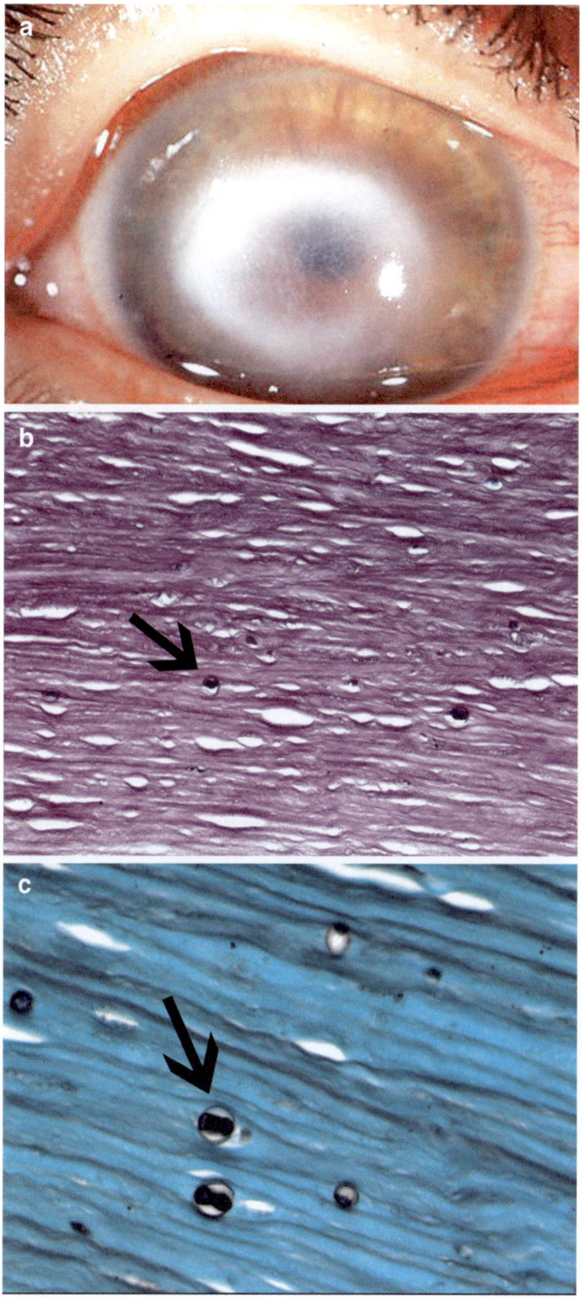

Fig. 2.4 (**a**) Corneal *Acanthamoeba polyphaga* infection in a 30-year-old female contact lens user. (**b**) Corneal stroma showing amebic cysts (*arrow*) and almost no inflammation present (PAS stain, ×40). (**c**) Amebic cysts (*arrow*) seen with GMS stain (GMS, ×40)

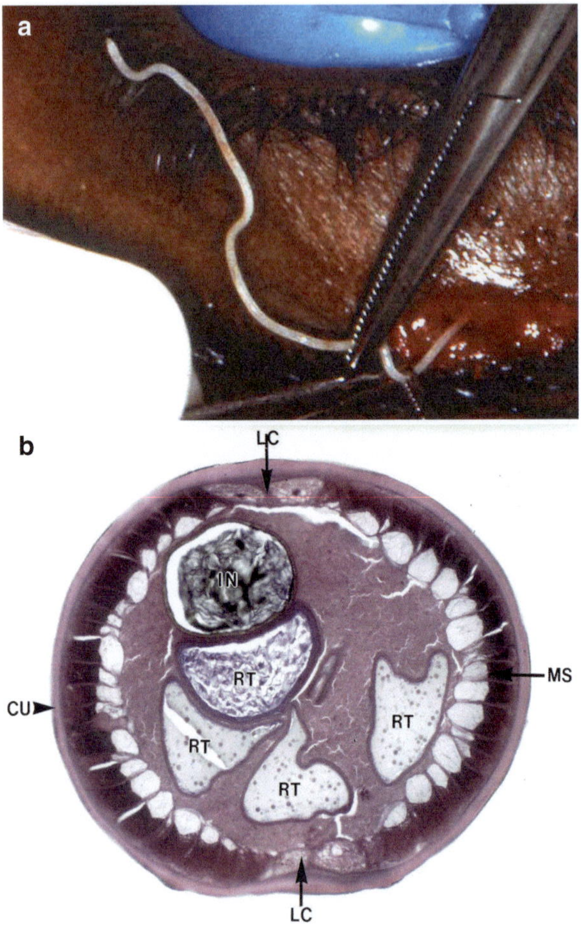

Fig. 2.5 (**a**) Right upper eyelid undulating worm being removed via a lid crease incision in a 27-year-old female from Cameroon. (**b**) Transverse section through an adult nongravid female *Loa loa*. There are a cuticle (*CU*), muscle (*MS*), lateral chords (*LC*), intestine (*IN*), and reproductive tubes (*RT*) (Movat stain, ×50)

The Immune System and Host Defense Against Infections

We live in a world teaming with pathogenic organisms that can potentially do great harm if allowed to infect the body unchecked. The human immune system is composed of a diverse array of cells that protect the individual from infectious organisms. Cells of the immune system include lymphocytes, mononuclear phagocytes, macrophages, and dendritic cells. There are two distinct but interrelated systems that play a role in the recognition of pathogens and foreign molecules: a highly specific one (adaptive immunity) and a more general immune response (innate immunity) [14].

There is overwhelming evidence that clonal expansion of antigen-specific T-lymphocytes (T-cells) and B-lymphocytes (B-cells) is necessary for the generation of an efficient, long-lasting immune response custom-tailored to each invading organism. This antigen-specific response is known as *adaptive immunity*. Although the adaptive immune response can effectively eliminate most pathogens, it takes at least 5–7 days for appropriate lymphocyte clones to be selected and then to expand and differentiate into effector cells. In contrast, the average bacterial generation time is in the order of 20 min. Scientists therefore reasoned that there must be another form of immunity (*innate immunity*) that is responsible for controlling the proliferation of invading pathogens until an efficient lymphocyte response can be generated. Since invertebrates such as jellyfish and fruit flies lack adaptive immune responses and rely only on innate immunity to survive in the environment, this innate response is highly conserved through evolution. Pattern recognition receptors (such as toll-like receptors) that are constitutively expressed on endothelial cells and on leukocytes such as dendritic cells, macrophages, granulocytes, and natural killer (NK) cells are involved in the innate immune response.

During an infection, the innate immune response plays a major role in establishing acute inflammation as a response to various bacteria and viruses [15, 16]. As an example, this system detects lipopolysaccharide, a molecule found in gram-negative bacteria. Even very small amounts of lipopolysaccharide are recognized by lipopolysaccharide-binding protein (CD14) and toll-like receptor 4, proteins that serve as pattern recognition receptors on leukocytes. When gram-negative bacteria breach a mucosal barrier, the presence of lipopolysaccharide prompts macrophages to produce cytokines (such as TNF-α, IL-1, IL-23, and others) to attract and activate inflammatory cells and enzymes that enhance the clearance of microbes (Table 2.2).

The cells that regulate and carry out most of the major effector functions of the adaptive immune response are lymphocytes (T-cells and B-cells) [17]. Lymphocytes provide the specificity of this response through antigen-specific surface receptors; after clearing the pathogen, the cells develop a long-term "memory" of the exposure that can be quickly mobilized upon reexposure. Cellular immunity, comprising T-cells, macrophages, and natural killer cells, primarily recognize and combat pathogens that proliferate intracellularly, including most viruses and bacteria. T-cells are activated by macrophages and B-cells, which present foreign antigens to the T-cell receptor. Activated T-cells have several ways to fight infection. Cytotoxic T-cells may directly attack and lyse host cells that express foreign antigens. Helper T-cells stimulate the proliferation of B-cells and the production of immunoglobulins. Antigen-presenting cells and T-cells communicate with each other by signaling with an array of cytokines and thus coordinate the immune system to respond in a specific fashion. T-cells elaborate cytokines that directly inhibit the growth of pathogens or stimulate killing by host macrophages and cytotoxic cells. The immune system has also developed cells that downregulate immune responses. An example of this is the Treg cells, a subgroup of CD4+T-cells that prevent autoimmune responses by other T-cells.

Table 2.2 Comparison between innate and adaptive immunity

	Innate	Adaptive
Cells expressing receptors	Macrophages, granulocytes, NK cells, dendritic cells	T-cells, B-cells
Type of receptor	Toll-like, NOD, collectin	T-cell receptor, immunoglobulin
Receptors conserved through evolution	Yes	No
Receptor specificity	Identical for each pathogen	Unique for each pathogen
Percentage of cells expressing a given receptor	100 %	0.0001 %
Amount of time before effector cells respond to pathogen	Immediate	Days
Receptors encoded in germline DNA	Yes	No

Mechanisms of Microbial Pathogenesis

Pathogens cause infections through different processes that can be classified into several stages: microbial encounter with and entry into the host, microbial growth after entry, avoidance of innate host defenses, tissue invasion and tropism, tissue damage, and transmission to new hosts [18–20].

Microbial Entry Sites

The most common sites of microbial entry are mucosal surfaces and the skin. Other portals of entry include sites of injury (cuts, bites, burns, trauma) along with injection via natural (i.e., vector-borne) or artificial (i.e., needlestick) routes. As a mucosal surface, the conjunctiva can serve as an entry point for pathogens into the eye. During entry into the host, microbes rely on specific factors that are needed for persistence and growth in a tissue. For example, protozoan parasites such as *Plasmodium* undergo morphogenic changes that permit transmission to mammalian hosts during insect feeding for blood meals. Plasmodia are injected as infective sporozoites from the salivary glands of mosquitos as they feed.

Microbial Adherence and Host Receptors

Once in a host, most microbes must anchor themselves to a tissue or tissue factor; the exceptions are organisms that enter the bloodstream directly and multiply there (an example is bacterial sepsis). Specific ligands or adhesins for host receptors comprise a wide range of surface structures that anchor the microbe to a tissue and promote cellular entry. Many of these proteins also elicit host responses critical to the pathogenic process. Microbes generally produce multiple adhesins that are specific for multiple host receptors. These adhesins are often redundant, serologically variable and capable of synergy with other microbial factors to promote microbial sticking to host tissues (Table 2.3) [20, 21]. Some microbes also absorb host proteins into their surface and utilize natural host protein receptor for microbial binding and entry into target cells.

All viral pathogens must bind to host cells, enter them, and replicate within them. Viral coat proteins serve as ligands for cellular entry. For example, the gB and gC proteins on herpes simplex virus bind to heparan sulfate (Table 2.3); this adherence is not essential for entry but rather serves to concentrate virions close to the cell surface. This is followed by attachment to cells mediated by the viral gD protein. Herpes simplex virus can use a number of cell receptors for entry including the herpesvirus entry mediator, members of the immunoglobulin superfamily, nectin-1 and nectin-2, and modified heparan sulfate [18, 22].

Gram-negative and gram-positive bacteria commonly attach to host cells and tissues using surface structures called pili. *E. coli* mediate adherence to specific target surfaces with mannose-binding type 1 containing pili that bind to integral membrane glycoproteins. Specific streptococcal proteins bind to human extracellular matrix proteins such as fibrin, fibronectin, fibrinogen, laminin, and collagen. Fibronectin appears to be a commonly used receptor for various pathogens [18, 19, 21].

Table 2.3 Examples of microbial ligand-receptor interaction

Microorganism	Type of microbial ligand	Host receptor
Viral pathogens		
Herpes simplex virus	Glycoprotein C	Heparan sulfate
Coxsackievirus	Viral coat proteins	CAR and major histocompatibility class I antigens
Bacterial pathogens		
Escherichia coli	Pili	Ceramides/mannose and digalactosyl residues
Streptococcus pyogenes	Hyaluronic acid capsule	CD44
Mycobacterium tuberculosis	Absorbed C3bi	CR3; DC-SIGN
Fungal pathogens		
Blastomyces dermatitidis	WI-1	Possibly matrix proteins and integrins
Candida albicans	Int1p	Extracellular matrix proteins
Protozoal pathogens		
Leishmania	Gp63 glycoprotein	Fibronectin and complement receptors on macrophages

Modified from Pier [18]

Fungal adhesins mediate the colonization of epithelial surfaces. The product of the *Candida albicans* INT1 gene bears similarity to mammalian integrins that bind to extracellular matrix proteins. These adhesins are expressed under stress and are crucial for pathogenesis of fungal infections. Parasites use complicated surface glycoproteins as adhesins, some of which are lectins. Leishmanial promastigotes use a major surface glycoprotein, gp63, to enter human macrophages. This glycoprotein promotes complement binding, which allows the parasite to use complement receptors for entry into macrophages [18].

Microbial Growth and Avoidance of Innate Host Defenses

Pathogenic microbes establish themselves and proliferate once on a mucosal or skin site before causing symptomatic infection [18, 23]. Viruses proliferate in several ways. The nucleic acids from these organisms may be directly translated into viral proteins (positive-strand RNA viruses), transcribed from a negative strand of RNA into complementary mRNA (negative-strand RNA viruses) or transcribed into a complementary strand of DNA (retroviruses). In the case of DNA viruses, the viral DNA is transcribed directly into mRNA, either within the nucleus or cytoplasm of a host cell. Bacteria in comparison must acquire specific nutrients or synthesize them from precursors in host tissues in order to proliferate.

Host tissues have a variety of innate defense mechanisms to eliminate microbes. The skin is acidic and is bathed in fatty acids that are toxic to many microbes. Mucosal surfaces are covered by a thick mucus layer that entraps microbes and facilitates their elimination. Pathogens have to survive host endocytic, phagocytic, and inflammatory responses and host genetic factors that determine the degree to which a pathogen can survive and grow [23].

Tissue Damage and Disease

Pathogenic microbes establish infection and damage tissues by three mechanisms: (1) through contact or entry into host cells to directly cause cell death; (2) through release of toxins that kill cells at a distance, release of enzymes that degrade tissue components, or direct damage to blood vessels with resulting ischemic necrosis; or (3) through elicitation of a host immune response that, though directed against the invader, causes additional tissue damage [19, 20].

Bacterial infection with injury to the host depends on the ability to adhere to host cells, invade host cells or tissue, and deliver toxins. Pathogenic bacteria have virulence genes that encode proteins for these properties. Bacterial toxins are classified as endotoxins (components of the bacteria cell) and exotoxins (proteins secreted by bacteria). Bacterial endotoxin is a lipopolysaccharide (LPS) that is a large component of the outer membrane of gram-negative bacteria. The response to bacterial lipopolysaccharide can be both beneficial and harmful to the host. Small amounts of LPS can act as an early trigger for the helpful activation of cytokines and chemokines of the innate immune system. At higher concentrations, however, LPS can induce excessive levels of immune cytokines. This can result in septic shock and disseminated intravascular coagulation. Exotoxins are secreted proteins that cause cellular injury and disease. Staphylococci, streptococci, and *P. aeruginosa* produce various toxins that cause disease; these include toxic shock syndrome toxin 1and erythrogenic toxic exotoxins AST and U. Several bacterial exotoxins have adenosine diphosphate (ADP)-ribosyltransferase activity that enables the inactivation of specific cellular proteins. Loss or inactivation of this virulence system greatly reduces the capacity of a bacterial pathogen to cause disease [3].

Plasmids and bacteriophages are mobile genetic elements that spread between bacteria and can encode tissue-damaging toxins or enzymes that facilitate antibiotic resistance. Communities of bacteria can form biofilms, a viscous layer of extracellular polysaccharide that adheres to host tissues or devices and in which organisms can survive.

When pathogens invade host tissues, they must avoid major host defenses that are mediated by complement opsonins, molecules that are deposited onto bacterial cell complement, and phagocytic cells. Bacteria avoid these defenses through their cell-surface polysaccharides. These molecules can prevent the activation and deposition of surface opsonins (opsonization) that enhances phagocytosis by macrophages, or they can limit the access of phagocytic cells to the opsonized bacteria.

Viruses can damage host cells directly by entering them and replicating at the host's expense. Viruses possess specific cell-surface proteins that bind to host cell-surface proteins. Once inside host cells, viruses can damage or kill the cells by direct cytopathic effects, by antiviral immune responses, or by transforming the infected cells into benign or malignant tumors (oncogenic viruses) [3, 22]. Some viruses kill cells by preventing synthesis of host macromolecules like host cell DNA, RNA, or proteins. Viral proteins on the surface of the host cells may be antigenic, and the immune response can lead to tissue injury. Different oncogenic viruses can stimulate cell growth and survival by a variety of mechanisms (insertional mutagenesis, anti-apoptosis, virus-encoded oncogenes, and others).

Types of Inflammation

Inflammation is divided into acute and chronic patterns (Table 2.4) [24]. Acute inflammation is rapid in onset (seconds or minutes) and is of relatively short duration, lasting for minutes, several hours, or a few days; its main characteristics are the exudation of fluid and plasma proteins (edema) and the emigration of leukocytes, predominantly neutrophils. It is related to histamine release from mast cells and

Table 2.4 Differences between acute and chronic inflammation

	Acute inflammation	Chronic inflammation
Clinical onset	Rapid (hours to days)	Slow (days, weeks, or longer)
Clinical course	Usually resolves within days or weeks with complete healing	Lasts longer; can persist or progress
Histological onset	Rapid (minutes to hours)	Slow (days, weeks)
Characteristic histology	Tissue necrosis Vascular changes Fluid and cell exudation Neutrophil infiltration followed by macrophages	Lymphocytes, plasma cells, and macrophages Granulomata may form Can be simultaneous with repair and regeneration
Typical etiologies	Gram-positive and gram-negative bacteria	Fungi, mycobacteria, parasites
Immune response	Innate	Adaptive

factors released from plasma (kinins, plasmin, complement, and clotting systems). Chronic inflammation is of longer duration and is associated histologically with infiltrates of lymphocytes and macrophages, proliferation of blood vessels, fibrosis, and tissue necrosis. Many factors modify the course and morphologic appearance of both acute and chronic inflammation.

Acute Inflammation

Following tissue injury, leukocytes travel through the bloodstream and traffic to the site of the lesion to participate in acute inflammation [25, 26]. This process is particularly amazing when one considers that leukocytes are born in the bone marrow and are able to navigate through thousands of miles of blood vessels to localize specifically at a site that may be only a few millimeters in size. A complex leukocyte navigation system has developed through evolution. In order for a leukocyte to traffic to damaged tissue, it must first travel through the bloodstream to the blood vessels supplying the damaged tissue, bind to the endothelium, and cross three physical barriers: (a) the endothelial cells, (b) the endothelial basement membrane, and (c) the pericytes or smooth muscle surrounding the vessel [26]. Leukocyte trafficking to a site of acute inflammation involves a number of discrete steps that must occur in a specific sequence. If any one of the steps is interrupted, leukocytes are inhibited from trafficking to a tissue. Interestingly, each step in this sequence involves specific adhesion molecules or mediators. Leukocytes that traffic to damaged tissue following injury include granulocytes (neutrophils, eosinophils, and basophils), monocytes (macrophages), and lymphocytes. Mast cells are resident leukocytes that are present in tissues prior to the onset of inflammation. In addition to leukocytes, blood platelets also participate in acute inflammation.

Neutrophils are the first leukocytes to arrive at a site of acute inflammation, as early as minutes following an injury [25, 27, 28]. Like all leukocytes, neutrophils arise from a common stem cell precursor in the bone marrow. There are two distinct pools of neutrophils of approximately equal size in the blood. The circulating pool consists of cells in the laminar blood flow; these neutrophils are not in contact with the vessel wall. Cells in this pool circulate widely and rapidly and have a half-life of 4–6 h. In contrast, cells in the marginated pool adhere loosely to the endothelial surfaces of vascular lumens through interactions with adhesion molecules called selectins. Cells in the marginated pool roll along the surface of the blood vessel looking for damaged areas of the endothelial surface or injured tissue.

Neutrophils can move rapidly from the circulating pool to the marginated pool and vice versa in response to various stimuli. When neutrophils roll into an area of tissue damage, they are activated by interaction with soluble mediators known as chemokines and enter the tissue to participate in the inflammatory process (Fig. 2.6) [29]. Neutrophils are one-way cells (like all granulocytes); they migrate from the bone marrow to the blood and then to tissue for the remainder of their life span. These cells can survive in tissue for up to 2 days, after which they undergo apoptosis.

By electron microscopy, neutrophils contain two distinct subsets of cytoplasmic granules: primary granules and secondary granules. Myeloperoxidase and lysozyme, as well as a number of proteases and acid hydrolases, are found in the primary granules. Major constituents of the secondary granules include lysozyme, lactoferrin, and collagenase.

A major function of neutrophils is to eliminate invading bacteria. When a neutrophil encounters a bacterium that has been coated (opsonized) with fibronectin, antibody, or complement C3b, the organism is engulfed by an invagination of the cytoplasmic membrane called a phagosome; shortly thereafter, the phagosome fuses with a cytoplasmic granule, thus forming a phagolysosome and initiating the process of bacterial killing. Bacteria may be killed using either oxygen-dependent (oxygen radical or myeloperoxidase-halide systems) or oxygen-independent mechanisms.

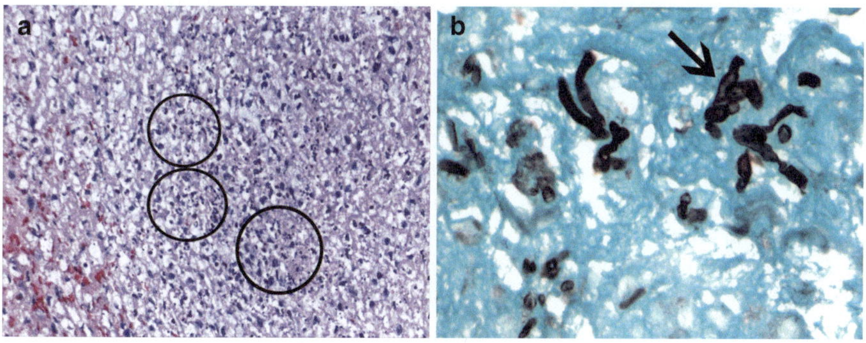

Fig. 2.6 (**a**) Orbital tissue biopsy of a 65-year-old immunocompetent Chinese female. Acute inflammation with tissue necrosis due to *Aspergillus fumigatus* orbital and sinus infection (H&E, ×10). Acute inflammation is highlighted in circles (**b**) GMS stain of Aspergillus spp. (*arrow*) (GMS stain, ×40)

Eosinophils are most commonly associated with diseases that are allergic (asthma) or immunologic in origin, but may be found in practically any leukocyte infiltrate. Most notably, eosinophils are abundant in diseases involving helminth parasites and are recognized as potent parasite killers. During periods of increased demand (parasitic infestation) [30], the maturation time of eosinophils in the bone marrow is shortened, and increased numbers of these cells are released into the bloodstream. This causes the relative percentage of eosinophils in the blood to increase, sometimes reaching 30–40 % of the total number of leukocytes. On microscopic examination of normal mucosal tissues, it is not unusual to see eosinophils in the submucosa. Eosinophil granules contain many enzymes and bactericidal proteins; the most abundant component is called major basic protein. Major basic protein binds avidly with numerous molecules due to its strong positive charge; it is extremely toxic to parasites, as well as to cells of the host.

Mast cells are derived from a common stem cell precursor in the bone marrow. Two distinct mast cell subsets have been identified: mucosal mast cells (most numerous within the submucosa of the conjunctiva) and connective tissue mast cells (present in orbital inflammatory lesions). Mast cells store preformed histamine, heparin, and various proteases within numerous intracytoplasmic granules and have many Fc receptors on their surfaces that avidly bind IgE. Patients with allergies typically have abundant IgE in their serum that is specific for a particular antigen, and this IgE can bind to the mast cell Fc receptors. Mast cells also have receptors for complement C5a. When antigen binds to IgE that is attached to the mast cell Fc receptors, or serum C5a binds to mast cell C5a receptors, a complex series of intracellular signals results in fusion of the intracytoplasmic granules with the plasma membrane and subsequent release of granule contents. This causes vasodilation and edema in the tissue that contains the mast cells [31].

Monocytes and macrophages are derived from the same stem cell precursor in the bone marrow as granulocytes. Monocytes emerge from the bone marrow and circulate in the peripheral blood. When they move into tissues, they mature and are called macrophages. Under the influence of chemotactic stimuli, IFN-γ (interferon gamma), and bacterial endotoxins, resident tissue macrophages are activated and proliferate, while circulating monocytes are recruited and differentiate into tissue macrophages. The most important contribution these cells make to acute inflammation is to serve as a primary source of the pro-inflammatory cytokines TNF-α and IL-1 [32]. Blood monocyte granules contain serine proteinases, and macrophages contain cysteine proteinases. The activity of these enzymes is central to the tissue destruction in chronic inflammation.

Lymphocytes undergo a complex maturation process after leaving the bone marrow. They are key cells in humoral and cell-mediated immune responses. There are multiple subtypes: B-cell, T-cell, cytotoxic natural killer (NK) cell, and null cell. Lymphocytes can contribute cytokines such as TNF-α and IL-17, which promote endothelial activation and leukocyte trafficking at the site of acute inflammation. B-cells produce immunoglobulins (Ig) that are present on the cell membrane (surface Ig). Each individual B-cell manufactures only one type of Ig – IgA, IgG, IgM,

IgD, or IgE. IgM is produced the first time that a B-cell has contact with an immunogen; IgG is produced upon recall of an immunogen [24].

During embryogenesis, T-cells pass through the thymus and are grouped into a special pool of lymphocytes. Approximately 70 % of lymphocytes in normal blood and lymph nodes are T-cells. T-cell receptors (TCR) that recognize specific antigens are present on the surface of T-cells, and nearly all T-cells are positive for surface CD3. Subsets of these CD3-positive T-lymphocytes, called regulatory cells, modulate the immune response by interacting with B-cells through lymphokine signaling to produce or suppress Ig production. CD4-positive T-cells are known as "helper cells"; these lymphocytes assist in antigen processing and work with macrophages to stimulate the immune response. CD8-positive T-cells are known as "suppressor cells" and can have a cytotoxic effect.

Plasma cells are a specialized differentiation of the B-lymphocyte; these cells produce immunoglobulin that can accumulate within the cytoplasm (cytoplasmic Ig). Plasma cells develop when a stimulated B-lymphocyte produces a specific Ig response to a presenting antigen [24]. One important contribution to acute inflammation is the production of antigen-specific IgE by plasma cells. IgE subsequently can bind to Fc receptors on the cell surface of mast cells, basophils, and eosinophils.

Dendritic cells have many long cytoplasmic processes that aid in capturing antigenic material and then presenting it to lymphocytes. Those located in epithelia are known as Langerhans cells; those in lymphoid follicles are known as follicular dendritic cells. These cells have surface Fc and C3b receptors to facilitate the uptake of opsonized bacteria; they contain cytoplasmic myeloperoxidase and can produce oxygen free radicals to kill the engulfed pathogens [24]. As part of the innate immune system, they express pathogen recognition receptors (toll-like receptors, mannose receptors, NOD receptors, and others) on their plasma membranes. Dendritic cells also produce the pro-inflammatory cytokines TNF-α and IL-1 after pathogen recognition and present antigen to T-cells.

Chronic Inflammation

The most frequent cause of chronic inflammation is infection [33]. The pathogens cause cell and tissue necrosis and engender inflammatory, immune, and reparative responses. According to their type and localization, pathogens elicit different immune responses, and different immune mechanisms generate different forms of immunopathology. Chronic inflammation is a long-lasting or permanent form of inflammation in which an organ or tissue is infiltrated by characteristic inflammatory cells; this is frequently associated with elements of regeneration and repair such as fibroblasts and reactive vascular changes.

Chronic inflammation can follow or be admixed with acute inflammation or can arise de novo in a previously unaffected organ or tissue. Chronic inflammation can begin insidiously, as a low-grade, smoldering, often asymptomatic response.

This type of chronic inflammation is the cause of tissue damage in some of the most common and disabling human diseases, such as tuberculosis [24]. With few exceptions, chronic inflammation indicates that an adaptive immune response (cellular or humoral) against foreign or self-antigens is present. In essence, chronic inflammation is the pathology – *immunopathology* – that results from an ongoing immune response.

In contrast to acute inflammation, which is manifested by vascular changes, edema, and a predominantly neutrophilic infiltrate, chronic inflammation is characterized by infiltration with mononuclear cells (macrophages, lymphocytes, and plasma cells) and tissue destruction that is caused by the persistent offending agent or by the inflammatory cells (Fig. 2.7). Tissue healing occurs by connective tissue replacement of damaged tissue, with proliferation of small blood vessels (angiogenesis) and fibrosis.

Macrophages (also called histiocytes) are central to chronic inflammation. They derive from blood monocytes, which, in turn, originate from myeloid stem cell precursors in the bone marrow. Monocyte extravasation into tissues is governed by a variety of adhesion molecules and tissue-specific chemokine/chemokine receptor pairs. Macrophages are normally widely distributed throughout the body, where

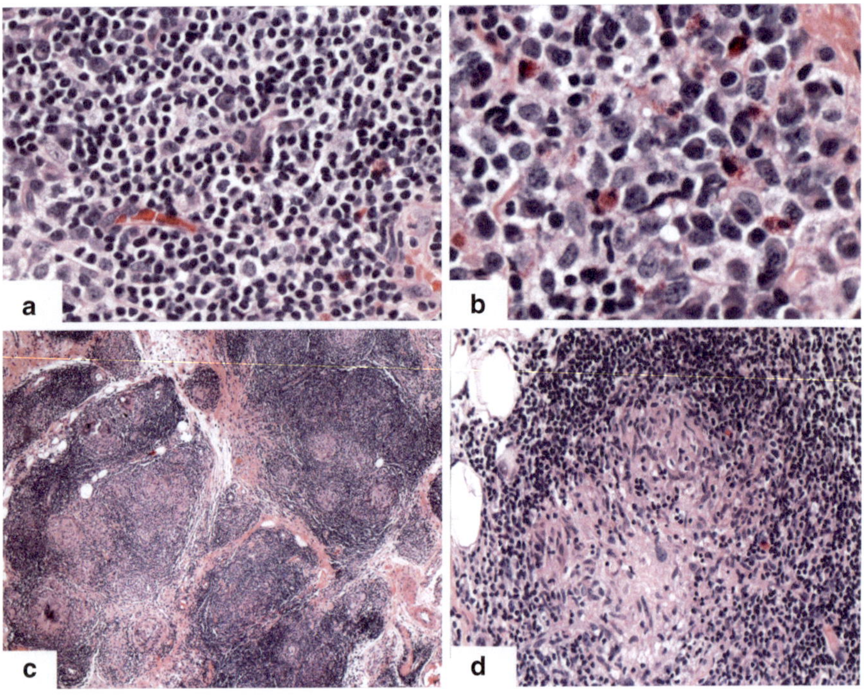

Fig. 2.7 (**a**) Chronic inflammation composed of lymphocytes, macrophages, plasma cells, and eosinophils in orbital pseudotumor (H&E, ×40). (**b**) Higher magnification of chronic inflammation in orbital pseudotumor (H&E, ×60). (**c**) Chronic non-necrotizing granulomatous inflammation in orbital sarcoidosis (H&E ×4). (**d**) Orbital sarcoid granuloma (H&E, ×20)

they constitute the mononuclear phagocyte system. They function as sentinel cells that monitor the presence of, and react to, foreign antigens. Kupffer cells in the liver and microglia in the brain are examples of the mononuclear phagocyte system.

Macrophages play a critical role in response to invading pathogens as well as in sterile inflammation such as wound healing or removal of necrotic tissue. Macrophages become activated, which increases their metabolic activity, secretion, size, and motility, and are endowed with multiple functions [17]. To a lesser extent than dendritic cells, macrophages make use of pattern recognition receptors to sense invading pathogens, which results in activation and upregulation of MHC class II and costimulatory molecule expression. Macrophages are dedicated phagocytes that are capable of killing intracellular pathogens through oxygen-dependent and oxygen-independent mechanisms.

Macrophages and dendritic cells present antigenic peptides to T-cells, linking innate immunity with adaptive immunity. Th1-type (T helper cell type 1) T-cells then further activate macrophages by secreting interferon gamma (IFN-γ). Such pro-inflammatory macrophages are termed M1 macrophages [34]. On occasion, excessive release of lysosomal enzymes or reactive oxygen species release from M1 macrophages can exacerbate tissue destruction. In contrast, in the context of a Th2-type (T helper cell type 2) immune response such as that generated for helminth parasites, IL-4 and IL-13 stimulate macrophages to secrete anti-inflammatory cytokines that include IL-10 and TGF-β. These anti-inflammatory macrophages are called M2 macrophages. They express distinct phenotypic markers and actively participate in tissue repair.

Granulomatous inflammation is a distinctive pattern of chronic inflammatory reaction that is characterized by focal accumulations of activated macrophages. These macrophages can develop an epithelial-like (epithelioid) appearance (discrete granuloma); such a granuloma may be surrounded by lymphocytes and occasionally plasma cells (Fig. 2.7). Granulomatous inflammation is encountered in a limited number of infectious and some noninfectious conditions. Tuberculosis is the prototype of the infectious granulomatous disease, but cat-scratch disease, leprosy, brucellosis, syphilis, and some mycotic infections also elicit this type of inflammatory response. Numerous eosinophils may be present in association with the granulomatous response to helminthic parasites. Noninfectious granulomatous reactions can arise in patients with immune disorders (such as sarcoidosis or sympathetic uveitis), systemic connective tissue disease (such as rheumatoid arthritis or Crohn's disease), and as a response to irritation by a foreign body (such as suture granuloma, lipid granuloma, or ruptured epidermoid cyst). The recognition of granulomatous inflammation in a biopsy specimen is important because of the limited number of possible conditions that can cause it and the significance of these conditions to the patient's health and well-being.

Another feature that may be seen in the chronic inflammatory reaction to some helminths, fungi, and bacteria, as well as to some inert substances like suture, is the Splendore-Hoeppli phenomenon [30]. This is composed of chronic inflammation with a necrotized, often refractile, eosinophilic center, surrounded by a ring of epithelioid cells, giant cells, and eosinophils. The Splendore-Hoeppli phenomenon is thought to represent a localized antigen-antibody reaction in a sensitized host (Fig. 2.8).

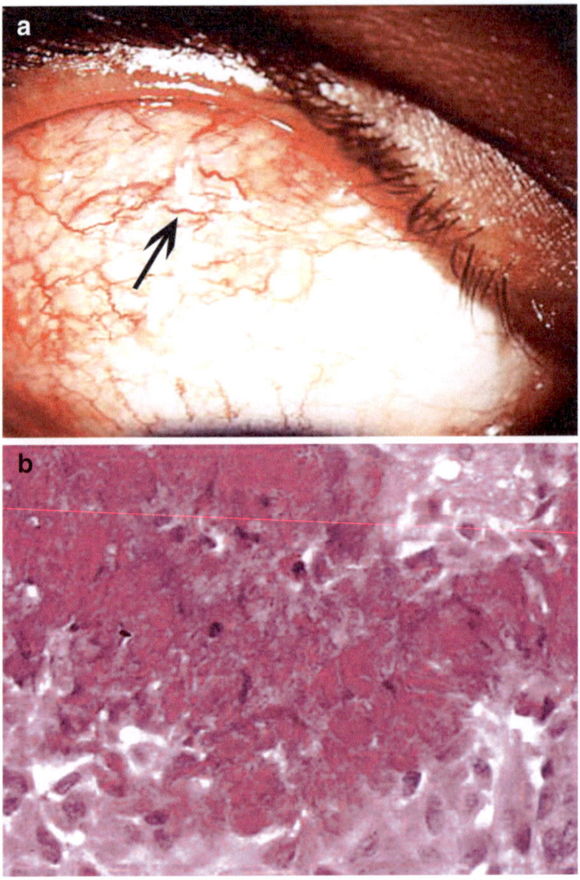

Fig. 2.8 (**a**) Multiple conjunctival nodules present in a 26-year-old male from Saudi Arabia (*arrow*). (**b**) Histologic sections show Splendore-Hoeppli phenomenon characterized by chronic inflammation with a necrotized, eosinophilic center with eosinophils (PAS stain, ×20)

Tissue Repair Post Inflammation: Inflammatory Sequelae

As the necrotic tissue is removed by macrophages and inflammation subsides, the affected area is first invaded by proliferating blood vessels (neoangiogenesis). The resulting highly vascularized and edematous tissue is called granulation tissue. Fibroblasts brought in by the new vessels begin to proliferate and produce new matrix components. As more and more collagen fibers are laid down and cross-linked, the granulation tissue becomes more dense and gradually transforms into a scar. Scars are then subject to extensive and prolonged remodeling which results in increased strength. In this way, although the tissue cannot be made normal again, a site of severe injury and inflammation can be repaired and brought back to functional usefulness [35].

Like all other tissues, the eye responds to injury with inflammation. The repair process may be the same, but the consequences are often of greater concern since the fibroblastic response and scarring may lead to impairment of vision. As such, control of the inflammatory response to infection can be as important in ophthalmology as elimination of the inciting pathogen. For example, the highly regularized structure of stromal collagen fibers with tightly defined interfiber spacing parameters determines the transparency of the cornea. Any fibroblastic healing of the cornea leads to scarring and loss of transparency due to disruption of the stromal collagen fibers, with loss of vision. Depending on the pathogen, corneal infections are sometimes managed with immunosuppressive therapy (steroids) in conjunction with antibiotics.

Orbital cellulitis or abscess (due to bacterial or fungal infection that generally arises in the paranasal sinuses) can lead to fibrosis with resulting diplopia, optic nerve dysfunction, or proptosis. The conjunctival and corneal surface epithelium often responds to exposure injury (as can occur with proptosis) by changing function of the surface cells to make protective keratin (squamous metaplasia).

Concerning the sequelae of intraocular infection, each anatomic component has a pattern of reaction to injury. In all cases, these responses lead to decreased visual acuity. The lens responds to injury by metaplasia and migration of the lens epithelial cells, leading to cataract. The injured ciliary body can generate proliferative cells that form a cyclitic membrane. Acute suppurative injury to the vitreous or retina leads to dissolution of the neural structures, which are unable to regenerate themselves. The retina and the optic nerve respond to injury by proliferation of glial cells to heal the damaged zone. Gliosis is equivalent to fibrosis in the rest of the body. The retinal pigment epithelium (RPE) cells can become necrotic (leaving a punched-out depigmented lesion), they may participate in fibrous tissue scarring, or they may induce osseous metaplasia in the choroid (as seen in the bone formation of phthisis).

Conclusion

There is an impressive history of progress made by science, medicine, and society as a whole to combat infections, yet infectious diseases continue to pose new problems. We are threatened by the appearance of new diseases such as Ebola virus and by the reemergence of old ones such as tuberculosis and infection with *Streptococcus pyogenes*. Pathogens have an impressive adaptability and diversity. Environmental changes, rapid global travel, population movements, and medicine itself through its use of antibiotics and immunosuppressive agents all increase the impact of infections. Pathogenic microbes will continue to develop new responses to our strategies to control them, presenting an unending and dynamic challenge for ophthalmologists in diagnosing and treating infections.

References

1. Nelson KE. Epidemiology of infectious disease: general principles. In: Nelson KE, Williams CM, editors. Infectious disease epidemiology. Theory and practice. 2nd ed. Boston: Jones and Barlett; 2007. p. 25–61.
2. Bennett JE, Dolin R, Blaser MJ. Mandell, Douglas and Bennett's principles and practice of infectious diseases. 8th ed. Philadelphia: Elsevier Saunders; 2015.
3. McAdam AJ, Milner DA, Sharpe AH. Infectious diseases. In: Kumar V, Abbas AK, editors. Robbins and Cotran pathologic basis of disease. 9th ed. Philadelphia: Elsevier Saunders; 2015.
4. Miller JJ, Scott IU, Flynn Jr HW, Smiddy WE, Newton J, Miller D. Acute-onset endophthalmitis after cataract surgery (2000–2004): incidence, clinical settings, and visual acuity outcomes after treatment. Am J Ophthalmol. 2005;139:983–7.
5. Iwashashi-Shima C, Azumi A, Ohguro N, Okada AA, Kaburaki T, Goto H, Sonoda K-H, Namba K, Mizuki N, Mochizuki M. Acute retinal necrosis: factors associated with anatomic and visual outcomes. Jpn J Ophthalmol. 2013;57:98–103.
6. Edwards Jr JE. Diagnosis and treatment of fungal infections. In: Kasper LK, Fauci AS, editors. Harrison's infectious diseases. New York: McGraw-Hill; 2010. p. 1000–3.
7. Oude Lashof AML, Rothova A, Sobel JD, Ruhnke M, Pappas PG, Viscoli C, Schlamm HT, Oborska IT, Rex JH, Kullberg BJ. Ocular manifestations of candidemia. Clin Infect Dis. 2011;53(3):262–8.
8. Reed SL, Davis CE. Laboratory diagnosis of parasitic infections. In: Kasper LK, Fauci AS, editors. Harrison's infectious diseases. New York: McGraw-Hill; 2010. p. 1042–9.
9. Yoder JS, Verani J, Heidman N, Hoppe-Bauer J, Alfonso EC, Miller D, Jones DB, Bruckner D, Langston R, Jeng BH, Joslin CE, Tu E, Colby K, Vetter E, Ritterband D, Mathers W, Kowalski RP, Acharya NR, Limaye AP, Leiter C, Roy S, Lorick S, Roberts J, Beach MJ. *Acanthamoeba* keratitis: the persistence of cases following a multistate outbreak. Ophthalmic Epidemiol. 2012;19(4):221–5.
10. Khairallah M, Kahloun R, Ben Yahia S, Jelliti B. Clinical, tomographic, and angiographic findings in patients with acute toxoplasmic retinochoroiditis and associated serous retinal detachment. Ocul Immunol Inflamm. 2011;19(5):307–10.
11. Otranto D, Eberhard ML. Zoonotic helminthes affecting the human eye. Parasites Vectors. 2011;4:41.
12. Kovacs GG, Budka H. Prion diseases: from protein to cell pathology. Am J Pathol. 2008;172:555.
13. Hamaguchi T, Noguchi-Shinohara M, Nakamura Y, Sato T, Kitamoto T, Mizusawa H, Yamada M. Ophthalmic surgery in prion diseases. Emerg Infect Dis. 2007;13(1):162–4.
14. Janeway Jr CA, Travers P, Walport M, et al. Immunobiology: the immune system in health and disease, Principles of innate and adaptive immunity. 5th ed. New York: Garland Science; 2001.
15. Janeway Cam Medzhitov R. Innate immune recognition. Annu Rev Immunol. 2002;20: 197–216.
16. Dieffenbach CW, Tramont EC. Innate (general or nonspecific) host defense mechanisms. In: Mandell, Douglas and Bennett's, editors. Principle and practice of infectious diseases. 8th ed. Philadelphia: Saunders; 2015. p. 26–33.
17. Hohl TM. Cell-mediated defense against infection. In: Mandell, Douglas and Bennett's, editors. Principle and practice of infectious diseases. 8th ed. Philadelphia: Saunders; 2015. p. 50–69.
18. Pier GB. Molecular mechanisms of microbial pathogenesis. In: Kasper LK, Fauci AS, editors. Harrison's infectious diseases. New York: McGraw-Hill; 2010. p. 9–19.
19. Madoff L, Kasper DL. Introduction to infectious diseases: host pathogen interactions. In: Kasper LK, Fauci AS, editors. Harrison's infectious diseases. New York: McGraw-Hill; 2010. p. 2–9.
20. Relman, DA, Falkow S. A molecular perspective of microbial pathogenicity. In: Mandell, Douglas and Bennett's, editors. Principle and practice of infectious diseases. 8th ed. Philadelphia: Saunders; 2015. p. 1–10.

21. Honda K, Littman DR. The microbiome in infectious disease and inflammation. Annu Rev Immunol. 2012;30:759–95.
22. Wang F, Kieff E. Medical virology. In: Kasper LK, Fauci AS, editors. Harrison's infectious diseases. New York: McGraw-Hill; 2010. p. 706–17.
23. Finlay BB, McFadden G. Anti-immunology: evasion of the host immune system by bacterial and viral pathogens. Cell. 2006;124:767.
24. Ward P. Acute and chronic inflammation. In: Sherhan CN, Ward P, Gilroy DW, editors. Fundamentals of inflammation. Cambridge: Cambridge University Press; 2010. p. 1–16.
25. Borregaard N. Neutrophils, from marrow to microbes. Immunity. 2010;33:657–70.
26. Springer TA. Traffic signals for lymphocyte recirculation and leukocyte emigration: the multi-step paradigm. Cell. 1994;76:301–14.
27. Nathan C. Neutrophils and immunity: challenges and opportunities. Nat Rev Immunol. 2006;6(March):173–82.
28. Witko-Sarsat V, Rieu P, Descamps-Latscha B, Lesavre P, Halbwachs-Mecarelli L. Neutrophils: molecules, functions and pathophysiological aspects. Lab Invest. 2000;80(5):617–53.
29. Mantovani A, Cassatella MA, Costantini C, Jaillon S. Neutrophils in the activation and regulation of innate and adaptive immunity. Nat Rev Immunol. 2011;11:519–31.
30. Klion AD, Nutman TB. The role of eosinophils in host defense against helminth parasites. J Allergy Clin Immunol. 2004;113(1):30–7.
31. Theoharides TC, Alysandratos KD, Angelidou A, Delivanis DA, Sismanopoulos N, Zhang B, Asadi S, Vasiadi M, Weng Z, Miniati A, Kalogeromitros D. Mast cells and inflammation. Biochim Biophys Acta. 2012;1822(1):21–33.
32. Fujiwara N, Kobayashi K. Macrophages in inflammation. Cur Drug Targets – Inflamm Allergy. 2005;4(3):281–6.
33. Aderem A. Phagocytosis and the inflammatory response. J Infect Dis. 2003;187:S340–5.
34. DeLeo FR, Nauseef WM. Granulocytic phagocytes. In: Mandell, Douglas and Bennett's, editors. Principle and practice of infectious diseases. 8th ed. Philadelphia: Saunders; 2015. p. 78–92.
35. Godwin JW, Brockes JP. Regeneration, tissue injury and the immune response. J Anat. 2006;209(4):423–32.

Chapter 3
Ocular Infection Worldwide

Mary Klassen-Fischer and Ronald C. Neafie

Introduction

One of the first steps in diagnosing an ocular infection is to question the patient about his travel history. Consideration must be given to the infections that are endemic in the parts of the world to which the patient has traveled or has lived (Table 3.1). Knowing what parts of the eye are affected by these infections is also useful (Table 3.2). A more detailed list of ocular conditions is presented in Table 3.3. In the following text, a representative viral, bacterial, fungal, protozoan, and helminthic infection is described in greater detail.

Hemorrhagic Fevers

Dengue, Ebola, and other hemorrhagic fever viruses may affect the eye. Familiarity with the incubation periods of endemic viruses may be useful in excluding them as etiologies for acute eye disease in returning travelers (Table 3.4).

Dengue is a very common viral disease with endemic locations throughout the world [8]. There is a wide range of symptoms ranging from mild febrile illness to life-threatening hemorrhagic shock [9]. Retro-orbital pain is a common symptom;

The views expressed in this chapter are those of the authors and do not reflect the official policy of the Department of the Army, Navy or Air Force, Department of Defense, or US Government.

M. Klassen-Fischer, MD (✉)
Department of Defense, Joint Pathology Center,
606 Stephen Sitter Avenue, Silver Spring, MD 20910, USA
e-mail: mary.k.klassen-fischer.civ@mail.mil

R.C. Neafie, MS
Formerly Chief, Parasitic Diseases Pathology Branch Armed Forces Institute of Pathology,
Washington, DC, USA

N.V. Laver, C.S. Specht (eds.), *The Infected Eye*,
DOI 10.1007/978-3-319-42840-6_3

Table 3.1 Geographic distribution of endemic infections that affect the eye

Africa:	**Asia:**	**Europe:**
Dengue[a]	Dengue[a]	Powassan encephalitis
Ebola[a]	Powassan encephalitis	Hemorrhagic fevers[a]
Rift Valley fever	Rift Valley fever	Lyme disease
Other hemorrhagic fevers[a]	Other hemorrhagic fevers[a]	Leishmaniasis
Yellow fever	Leprosy	Cysticercosis
Leprosy	Trachoma[a]	–
Trachoma[a]	Rhinosporidiosis	**Oceania**:
Rhinosporidiosis	Leishmaniasis	Dengue[a]
African trypanosomiasis	Malaria	Trachoma[a]
Leishmaniasis	Parastrongyliasis (angiostrongyliasis)	Bancroftian filariasis
Malaria	Sparganosis	Parastrongyliasis (angiostrongyliasis)
Cysticercosis	Cysticercosis	Paragonimiasis
Dracunculiasis	Malayan filariasis	–
Loiasis	Bancroftian filariasis	**South America**:
Mansonelliasis	Thelaziasis	Dengue[a]
Onchocerciasis[a]	Paragonimiasis	Other hemorrhagic fevers[a]
Bancroftian filariasis	Schistosomiasis	Yellow fever
Paragonimiasis	–	Leprosy
Schistosomiasis	**Central America**:	Trachoma[a]
Pentastomiasis	Dengue[a]	Coccidioidomycosis[a]
–	Leprosy	Rhinosporidiosis
North America:	Trachoma[a]	American trypanosomiasis[a]
Dengue[a]	Coccidioidomycosis[a]	Leishmaniasis
Powassan encephalitis	American trypanosomiasis[a]	Malaria
Lyme disease	Leishmaniasis	Mansonelliasis
Coccidioidomycosis[a]	Malaria	Onchocerciasis[a]
North American blastomycosis	Cysticercosis	Bancroftian filariasis
Thelaziasis	Onchocerciasis[a]	Paragonimiasis
Paragonimiasis	Bancroftian filariasis	Schistosomiasis
Pentastomiasis	Paragonimiasis	–

[a]Described in the text

Table 3.2 Parts of the eye affected by endemic infections

Eyelids:	**Conjunctiva**:	**Retina**:
African trypanosomiasis	Bancroftian filariasis	Bancroftian filariasis
American trypanosomiasis[a]	Coccidioidomycosis[a]	Coccidioidomycosis[a]
Coccidioidomycosis[a]	Cysticercosis	Cysticercosis
Dengue[a]	Dengue[a]	Leprosy
Dracunculiasis	Dracunculiasis	Loiasis
Leishmaniasis	Ebola[a]	Malaria

Table 3.2 (continued)

Eyelids:	**Conjunctiva**:	**Retina**:
Leprosy	Leishmaniasis	Onchocerciasis[a]
Onchocerciasis[a]	Loiasis	Parastrongyliasis (angiostrongyliasis)
Schistosomiasis	Lyme disease	Rift Valley fever
Sparganosis	Malaria	–
–	Malayan filariasis	**Orbit**:
Cornea:	Mansonelliasis	Coccidioidomycosis[a]
African trypanosomiasis	North American blastomycosis	Cysticercosis
Leishmaniasis	Onchocerciasis[a]	Loiasis
Leprosy	Other hemorrhagic fevers[a]	Lyme disease
Lyme disease	Parastrongyliasis (angiostrongyliasis)	Malaria
Onchocerciasis[a]	Pentastomiasis	Mansonelliasis
Thelaziasis	Rhinosporidiosis	Onchocerciasis[a]
–	Rift Valley fever	Powassan encephalitis
–	Schistosomiasis	Sparganosis
–	Thelaziasis	–
–	Trachoma[a]	–
	Yellow fever	–

[a]Described in the text

Table 3.3 Sites and types of ocular lesions caused by endemic infectious agents

Infectious disease	Category	Ocular site[a]	Type of lesions
African trypanosomiasis	Protozoan	Li Cor I Ch	Eyelid swelling, keratitis, iritis, choroiditis
American trypanosomiasis	Protozoan	Li	Eyelid swelling (Figs. 3.5a, b)
Bancroftian filariasis	Helminth	U	Conjunctivitis, granulomatous iridocyclitis, subretinal inflammation
Coccidioidomycosis	Fungus	Li Con U Ch R Op	Conjunctivitis, eyelid lesions, chorioretinal lesions, uveitis, secondary glaucoma, optic neuritis, retinal detachment (Figs. 3.4a, b)
Cysticercosis	Helminth	Li Con Ch V R Op	Chorioretinitis, retinal detachment, cataract
Dengue	Virus	Li Con U R Op	Retrobulbar pain, conjunctival congestion, eyelid swelling (Fig. 3.1b)
Dracunculiasis	Helminth	Li Con Or	Granulomatous inflammation of eyelids, conjunctiva, orbit (Figs. 3.8a, b)
Ebola	Virus	Con U	Hemorrhagic conjunctivitis, uveitis
Leishmaniasis	Protozoan	Li Con Cor	Eyelid, conjunctival or corneal ulcers or nodules (Fig. 3.9)

(continued)

Table 3.3 (continued)

Infectious disease	Category	Ocular site[a]	Type of lesions
Leprosy	Bacteria	Li La Cor U Le I Sc R	Lagophthalmos, corneal anesthesia, exposure keratitis, scleritis, iridocyclitis, low intraocular pressure, cataract (Fig. 3.11)
Loiasis	Helminth	Con Ch V R Or	Bulbar conjunctivitis, choroiditis, retinal hemorrhage, granuloma of orbit (Fig. 3.10)
Lyme disease	Bacteria	Con Cor U V Op M	Conjunctivitis, keratitis, uveitis, vitritis, optic neuropathy, defects of pupillary function, ocular motor nerve palsies, supranuclear disorders of ocular motility
Malaria	Protozoan	Con R Op	Retinal hemorrhage, subconjunctival hemorrhage, papilledema (Fig. 3.12)
Malayan filariasis	Helminth	Con U	Bulbar conjunctivitis, uveitis
Mansonelliasis	Helminth	Con Or	Nodules of conjunctiva, periorbital fat (Figs. 3.13a, b)
North American blastomycosis	Fungus	Con U I Ch V	Conjunctivitis, anterior uveitis, secondary glaucoma, endophthalmitis, iritis, iridocyclitis, choroidal lesions
Onchocerciasis	Helminth	Li Con Cor I R Op Or	Eyelid nodule, keratitis, iridocyclitis, cataract, retinopathy, optic nerve atrophy, orbital nodule (Fig. 3.7a, b)
Other hemorrhagic fevers (e.g. Ebola, others)	Virus	Con U	Conjunctival hemorrhage, uveitis (Fig. 3.1a)
Parastrongyliasis (angiostrongyliasis)	Helminth	Con A	Anterior uveitis, episcleritis, raised intraocular pressure, macular edema, pigment dispersion, retinal detachment (Fig. 3.14)
Pentastomiasis	Arthropod	Con A I	Conjunctivitis, conjunctival nodule, iridocyclitis (Figs. 3.15a, b)
Powassan encephalitis	Virus	M	Diplopia, ophthalmoplegia
Rhinosporidiosis	Fungus	Con	Conjunctivitis (Fig. 3.16)
Rift Valley fever	Virus	Con U R	Conjunctivitis, uveitis, retinitis
Schistosomiasis	Helminth	Li Con La Ch	Eyelid edema, subconjunctival, lacrimal gland or choroid nodules (Fig. 3.17)
Sparganosis	Helminth	Li Con A Or	Inflammatory nodule of eyelid, conjunctiva, anterior chamber, orbit
Thelaziasis	Helminth	Con Cor	Conjunctivitis, keratitis
Trachoma	Bacteria	Con Cor Li	Conjunctivitis, conjunctival scarring (Figs. 3.2a–c and 3.3a, b)
Yellow fever	Virus	Con	Conjunctivitis, conjunctival hemorrhage

[a]*Key*: *A* anterior chamber, *Ch* choroid, *Con* conjunctiva, *Cor* cornea, *I* iris, *La* lacrimal duct, *Le* lens, *Li* eyelid, *M* extraocular muscles, *Op* optic nerve, *Or* orbit, *R* retina, *Sc* sclera, *U* uvea, *V* vitreous

however, other ocular manifestations are rare [10]. Symptoms may include blurred vision, scotomas, metamorphopsia, and floaters. On ophthalmic examination, subconjunctival, vitreous, and retinal hemorrhages; posterior uveitis; optic neuritis; and maculopathy such as foveolitis, hemorrhage, and edema may be observed (Fig. 3.1a).

Two types of conjunctivitis occur in patients with Ebola virus infection: nonhemorrhagic and hemorrhagic [2]. Early bilateral nonhemorrhagic, asymptomatic, and nonicteric conjunctivitis occurs frequently and may appear 6–7 days before Ebola is suspected. Unlike Ebola, the conjunctivitis associated with Lassa fever is severe with periorbital swelling and pain. Hemorrhagic conjunctivitis occurs later and is a poor prognostic indicator. One to 2 months later, up to 20 % of patients convalescing from Ebola develop uveitis with ocular pain, photophobia, hyperlacrimation, and loss of visual acuity. Similar uveitis has been reported in patients who recovered from Marburg disease [11].

Table 3.4 Maximum incubation periods of endemic viruses that affect the eye

Virus	Maximum incubation period (days)	Reference
Dengue	15	[1]
Ebola	21	[2]
Lassa	21	[3]
Marburg	21	[4]
Powassan encephalitis	28	[5]
Yellow fever	9	[6]
Rift Valley	6	[7]

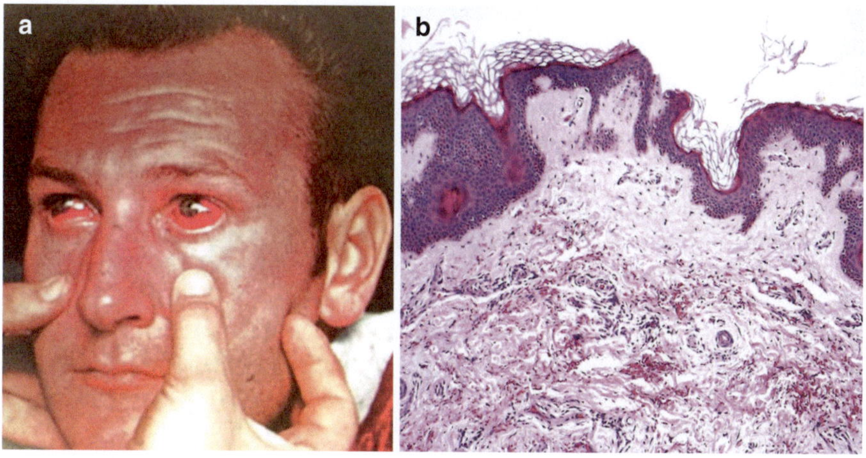

Fig. 3.1 (**a**) An example of conjunctival hemorrhage in a patient with hemorrhagic fever is seen in this man with Korean hemorrhagic fever (all figures courtesy of the Armed Forces Institute of Pathology). (b) The skin of a patient with dengue hemorrhagic fever shows vascular permeability with hemorrhage in the dermis (H&E, original magnification ×30)

Cytologic or histologic examination of ocular specimens is rarely performed on patients with hemorrhagic fever. Skin biopsies from patients with dengue may show hemorrhage (Fig. 3.1b), endothelial cell swelling in small vessels, perivascular edema, and mononuclear cell infiltrates [1]. No diagnostic viral cytopathic changes such as nuclear or cytoplasmic inclusions are seen in pathologic specimens.

Trachoma

Trachoma is an infection of the eye by *Chlamydia trachomatis* serotypes A, B, Ba, and C, which are endemic in resource-limited areas in Africa, the Middle East, Asia, Latin America, Pacific Islands, and Australia. *Chlamydia trachomatis* is transmitted by direct contact, fomites, and flies. Trachoma occurs in two phases: active trachoma largely in young children and cicatricial disease in adults. Acute infection causes mild, self-limited follicular conjunctivitis that is often asymptomatic (Fig. 3.2a). Some patients have mucopurulent discharge. On ophthalmic examination, 0.5–2 mm, white or pale yellow follicles are present on the superior tarsal conjunctiva. Pinpoint red papillae may also be present and can enlarge and coalesce. Follicles leave pathognomonic shallow Herbert's pits at the limbus. Adults with acute infection are less likely to have follicles but may have papillae, especially in the case of secondary infection by other bacteria. Repeated infections cause eyelid scarring that leads to entropion and trichiasis, which in turn cause corneal edema, ulceration, and scarring (Fig. 3.2b). Corneal scarring from trachoma (Fig. 3.2c) is the most common infectious cause of blindness [12].

Chlamydiae exist in two forms: intracellular reticulate bodies and extracellular elementary bodies, which have a cellular envelope similar to that of Gram-negative bacteria [13]. Reticulate bodies, which are 0.5–1.9 μm in diameter, replicate within a vacuole to form an inclusion that may be visible on cytologic or histologic slides prepared from ocular scrapings or biopsies, respectively [14].

In Giemsa-stained conjunctival scrapings, inclusions appear as dark purple masses in the cytoplasm of epithelial cells. Acridine orange or iodine stains may be used as an alternative to Giemsa.

Conjunctival biopsies from patients with acute infection show a marked inflammatory cell infiltrate and hyperplastic conjunctival epithelium. The inflammatory infiltrate is organized into follicles of B lymphocytes within a diffuse infiltrate of T- and B lymphocytes, macrophages, plasma cells, and neutrophils [15]. Chlamydial intracellular inclusion bodies can be seen within epithelial cells in sections stained with hematoxylin and eosin (H&E; Fig. 3.3a) and Warthin-Starry (Fig. 3.3b). Collagen deposition may also be detected but to a lesser extent than that seen in conjunctival scarring [16].

Biopsies from patients with conjunctival scarring show atrophic epithelium, subepithelial scarring, chronic inflammation, and meibomian gland atrophy [17]. The conjunctival epithelium may be only one cell thick with loss of goblet cells. A collagenous scar along the conjunctival basement membrane replaces the normally

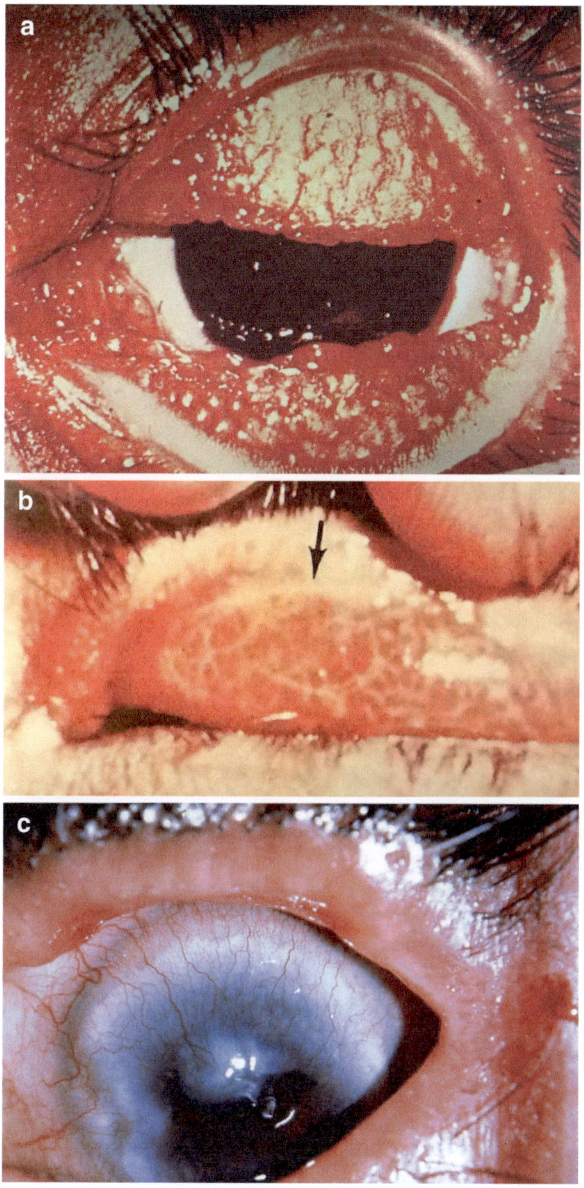

Fig. 3.2 (**a**) Follicular conjunctivitis due to trachoma (*Chlamydia trachomatis* infection). (**b**) Eyelid scarring (*arrow*) due to trachoma. (**c**) Corneal scarring due to trachoma

loose subepithelial stroma. Unlike acute trachoma, the inflammatory infiltrate in scarred conjunctivae consists predominantly of T cells [18]. In one study, cystically dilated glands containing concretions of inspissated secretions and cell debris were seen [19].

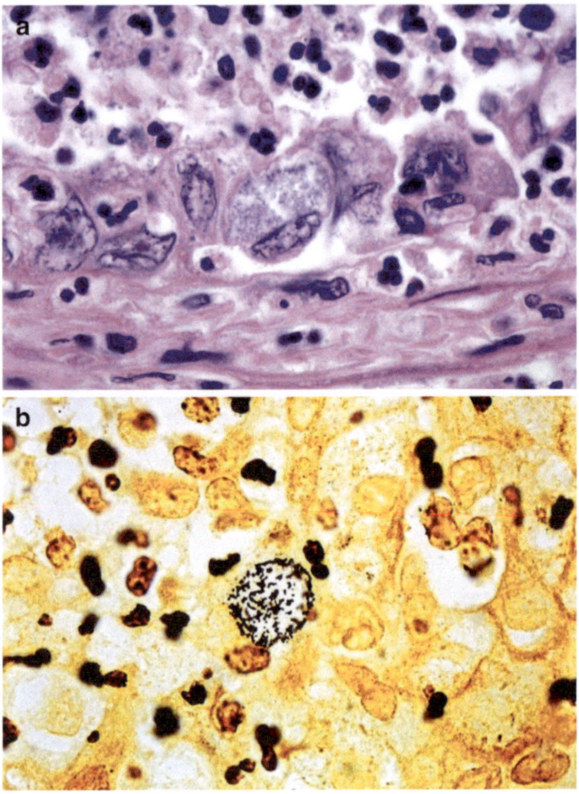

Fig. 3.3 (**a**) *Chlamydia trachomatis* organisms resemble fine grains of sand within a vacuolated cell in the epithelium in H&E-stained sections (original magnification ×330). (**b**) Numerous silvered *Chlamydia trachomatis* elementary bodies in a vacuolated cell (Warthin-Starry, original magnification ×330)

Follicles at the corneal limbus resolve leaving Herbert's pits and a vascular pannus [20]. Corneal buttons examined histopathologically show vascularity of all layers [21].

Coccidioidomycosis

Coccidioidomycosis is an infection by *Coccidioides immitis* or *Coccidioides posadasii* fungi that are endemic in the Sonoran Desert of Arizona, New Mexico, and Mexico; the San Joaquin Valley of California; and parts of West Texas, Central America, and Argentina. Ocular involvement is rare but should be considered in patients with eye disease who have been to one of the endemic areas [22]. Various ocular findings have been described, including eyelid and conjunctiva granulomas (Fig. 3.4a), phlyctenular conjunctivitis, recurrent uveitis, iritis, bilateral multifocal choroiditis, choroidal neovascularization with scarring, vitritis, retinal lesions, serous retinal detachment, optic neuritis, and secondary glaucoma [23–27].

Specimens acquired from aqueous or vitreous aspiration may show diagnostic fungal spherules. Biopsies of the eyelid skin, conjunctiva, choroid, or retina may show granulomas and fungal spherules, although early infection may be nongranulomatous [28, 29]. *Coccidioides* species usually present as spherules containing endospores that stain with H&E (Fig. 3.4b), although periodic acid-Schiff or Grocott methenamine silver stains help to highlight the walls of the spherules and the endospores. Spherules appear in various stages of growth and development. The mature spherules are usually 30–60 μm in diameter. Endospores are 2–5 μm in diameter. Some spherules may rupture releasing endospores. The spherules may have thick walls, and not all spherules will contain endospores.

American Trypanosomiasis

Chagas disease is caused by the protozoan parasite *Trypanosoma cruzi*, which is endemic in parts of Mexico and Central and South America. Rare infections are acquired in southern United States. The vectors are triatomid bugs, or "kissing bugs," which are a type of reduviid bug that live in thatch and in the cracks of trees and houses. At night the bug bites a sleeping human and defecates while taking a blood meal. Trypomastigotes, the infective stage of the parasite, are excreted in the bug's feces and introduced into the bite or nearby mucosa, especially the conjunctiva. Swelling at the site of a bite is called a chagoma. A periorbital bite may cause the characteristic Romaña sign (Fig. 3.5a): intense unilateral palpebral swelling, periorbital and facial edema, and conjunctivitis [30].

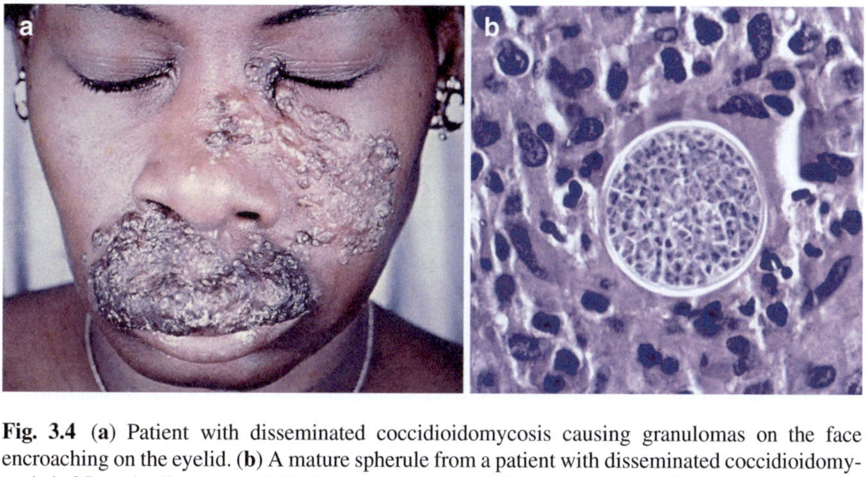

Fig. 3.4 (**a**) Patient with disseminated coccidioidomycosis causing granulomas on the face encroaching on the eyelid. (**b**) A mature spherule from a patient with disseminated coccidioidomycosis is 35 μm in diameter and filled with endospores (H&E, original magnification ×250)

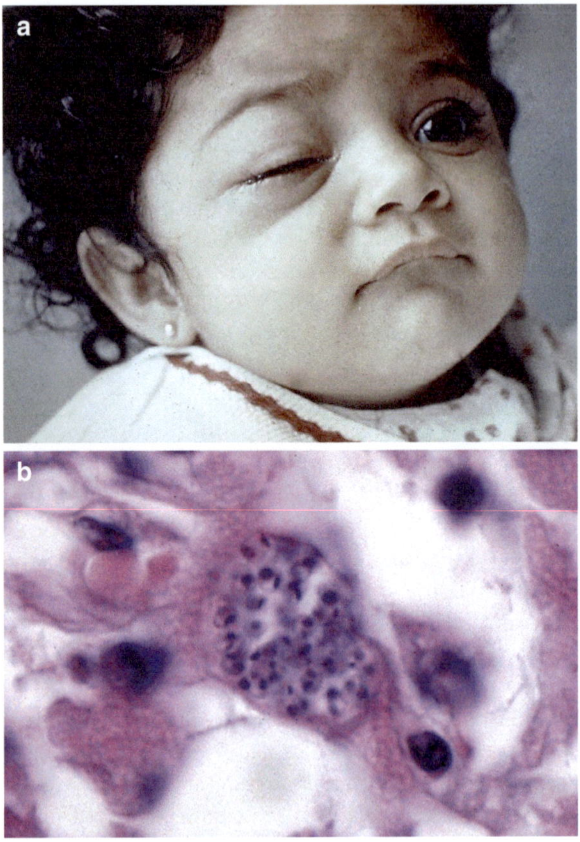

Fig. 3.5 (**a**) A patient with characteristic unilateral palpebral swelling (Romaña sign) due to Chagas disease (American trypanosomiasis). (**b**) Acute chagasic myocarditis with a cluster of amastigotes in a myofiber. Amastigotes are spherical, 2–4 μm in diameter, and have a nucleus and rod-shaped kinetoplast (H&E, original magnification ×300)

Trypomastigotes at the inoculation site transform into amastigotes and multiply within histiocytes. Amastigotes released from these histiocytes may invade other cells or transform into trypomastigotes, which disseminate through blood to invade different tissues especially the heart, central nervous system, and smooth and striated muscle. Patients with Chagas disease may present with ocular findings due to autonomic nervous system disease, for example, greater pupil diameter, irregularity of the pupil border, altered response to dilating agents, or decreased ability to maintain intraocular pressure with changes in posture [31, 32].

Diagnostic techniques for Chagas disease include microscopic identification of the parasite in peripheral blood smears. In peripheral blood smears stained with Giemsa, trypomastigotes are often C or U shaped 16–22 μm in length with a large central nucleus; a narrow undulating membrane; a large, spherical kinetoplast at the posterior end; and a long free flagellum at the anterior end. Trypomastigotes may also be seen in wet mount preparations of chagomas. Eyelid lesions are not often biopsied. Histologic sections of the skin show a mixed dermal and subcutaneous inflammatory infiltrate. When amastigotes are seen in histologic sections (such as in the brain or muscle biopsies), they are 2–4 μm in diameter with a spherical nucleus and a rod-shaped kinetoplast (Fig. 3.5b). Both the nucleus and the kinetoplast will not be present in the same plane of sectioning on every amastigote.

Onchocerciasis

Eye lesions resulting from infection by *Onchocerca volvulus* (onchocerciasis or river blindness) are prevalent in parts of West and Central Africa and Central America. The vectors are *Simulium* species blackflies that bite humans and transmit larvae. African *Simulium damnosum* blackflies tend to bite the lower part of the body, while *Simulium ochraceum* blackflies in Central America tend to bite the upper part of the body. The adult worms develop in subcutaneous tissues where they become encased in fibrous tissue to form nodules called "onchocercomas." The fertilized female releases microfilariae that migrate through the dermis.

Microfilariae from the periorbital skin or conjunctiva may infiltrate every part of the eye except the lens. Ocular lesions due to microfilariae include subepithelial punctate keratitis, iridocyclitis, chorioretinitis, and optic atrophy. Viable microfilariae in the cornea may not provoke an inflammatory response; however, dying larvae cause punctate keratitis with minute opacities. Iridocyclitis may result as an inflammatory response to onchocercal antigens diffusing from microfilariae in the cornea. Intense or recurrent infection results in sclerosing keratitis or cataract formation (Fig. 3.6a). Chorioretinitis due to invasion of the posterior segment by microfilariae is a frequent cause of visual impairment in advanced onchocerciasis [33]. Some patients develop a virtually pathognomonic retinal lesion (Fig. 3.6b) consisting of atrophy of the retinal pigment epithelium and diffuse chorioretinal scarring [34]. Some patients with posterior segment infection develop optic atrophy due to retinal changes or direct invasion of the optic nerve [35].

Onchocercomas of the anterior orbit are rare. Onchocercomas on the upper part of the body are more likely to produce microfilariae that reach the eye area than those on the lower part of the body.

Light microscopic examination of infected tissue shows microfilariae migrating through collagen (Fig. 3.7a). Inflammatory reactions occur in response to necrotic microfilariae and onchocercal antigens especially following treatment with microfilaricides such as diethylcarbamazine. In sclerosing keratitis, there is a fibrovascular

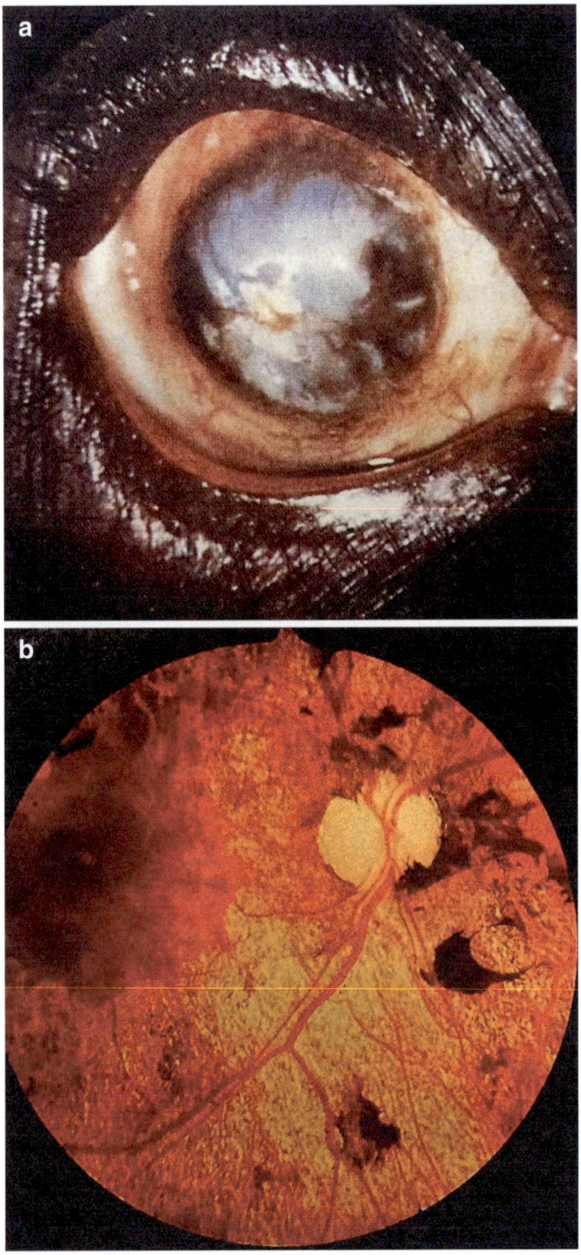

Fig. 3.6 (**a**) Advanced sclerosing keratitis of onchocerciasis. (**b**) Chorioretinal changes due to onchocerciasis (Ridley fundus) and optic atrophy

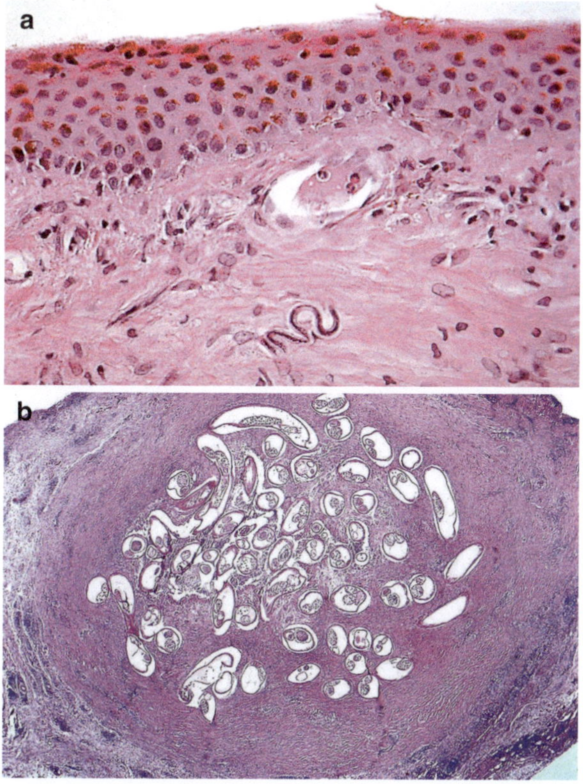

Fig. 3.7 (**a**) Anterior end of *Onchocerca volvulus* microfilaria in collagen. The microfilaria is 5 μm wide and has a long cephalic space (Giemsa, original magnification ×1080). (**b**) Onchocercal nodule, removed from subcutaneous tissue of an African, containing numerous sections of coiled adult female and male worms (H&E, original magnification ×5)

pannus with chronic inflammation [36]. Viable and degenerating microfilariae and chronic inflammatory cells have been described in the choroid and retina [33]. In pigmentary retinopathy, there is hyperplasia and degeneration of the retinal pigment epithelium and chronic inflammation [35].

The microfilariae are 220–360 μm in length and 5–9 μm in width but are only 5 μm wide in tissue sections. They have a striated cuticle, a long cephalic space, and a sharply pointed tail and are sheathless.

In an onchocercoma or onchocercal nodule (Fig. 3.7b), multiple adult male and female worms cut at various angles are usually present and are surrounded by an acute inflammatory reaction that over time becomes a foreign body-type giant cell

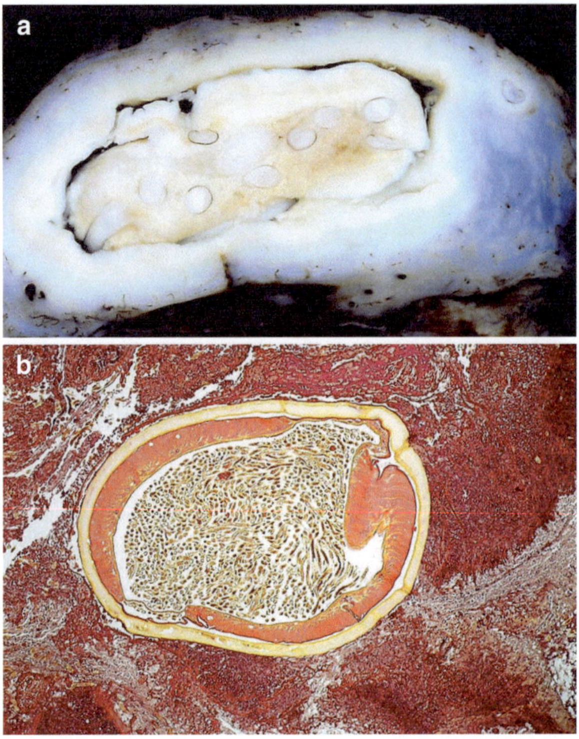

Fig. 3.8 (**a**) Dracunculiasis of the eyelid lesion of a 3-year-old Nigerian boy. Multiple cross sections of the worm are evident within a fibrinopurulent exudate (unstained gross specimen). (**b**) Adult gravid female *Dracunculus medinensis* in eyelid lesion shown in **a**. The worm is 1 mm in diameter, has two prominent bands of smooth muscle, and is filled with rhabditoid larvae (Movat, original magnification ×18)

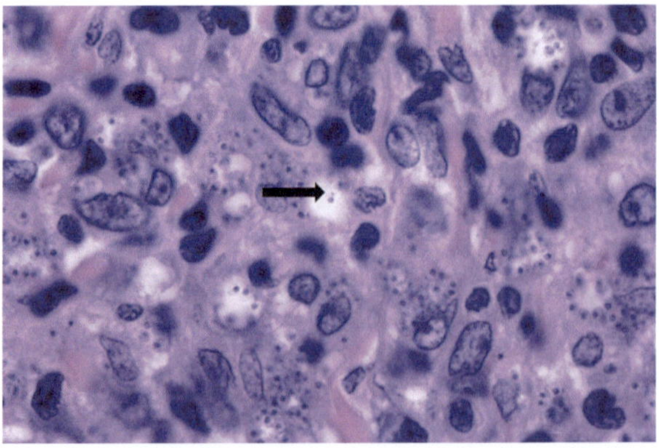

Fig. 3.9 Section of the skin contains many amastigotes of *Leishmania* spp. within histiocytes. Amastigotes are 2–3 μm in diameter and have a round nucleus and a rod-shaped kinetoplast (*arrow*; H&E, original magnification ×300)

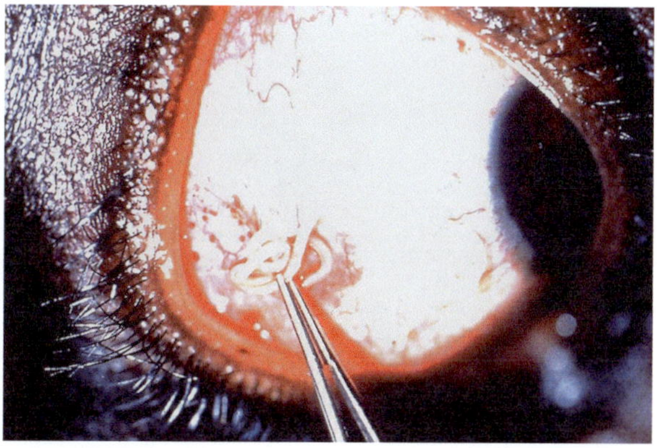

Fig. 3.10 Extraction of *Loa loa* from the conjunctiva

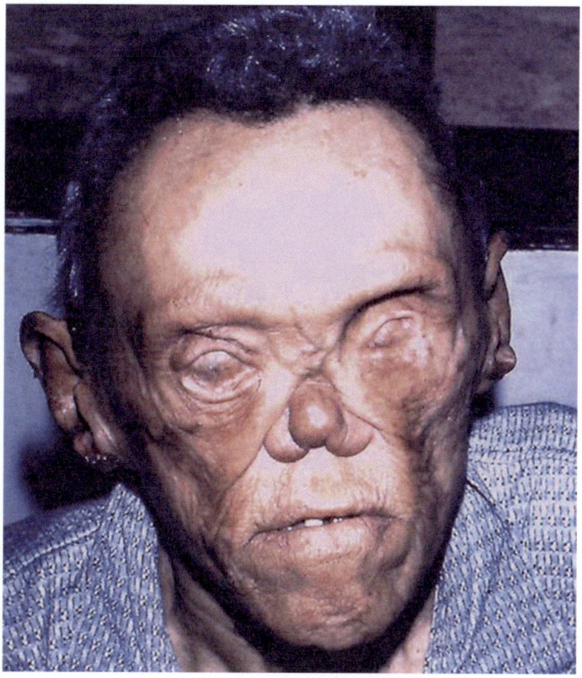

Fig. 3.11 In leprosy (*Mycobacterium leprae* infection), lagophthalmos and corneal anesthesia may lead to exposure keratitis and corneal scarring

reaction with fibrosis [37]. Male worms are up to 200 μm in diameter and have a cuticle with prominent annulations and a single reproductive tube. Female worms are up to 450 μm in diameter and have a cuticle with regularly spaced transverse ridges and usually two reproductive tubes. Microfilariae are frequently observed within onchocercomas, especially those with suppuration.

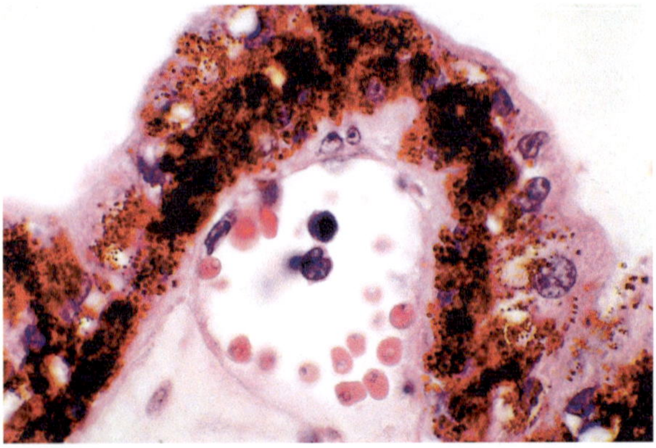

Fig. 3.12 Plasmodium falciparum trophozoites in virtually every erythrocyte in capillary of ciliary process from a 53-year-old traveler to Kenya and Tanzania who died of chloroquine-resistant malaria. Ocular complications of malaria are usually the result of hemorrhage, although not evident in this photo (H&E, original magnification ×250)

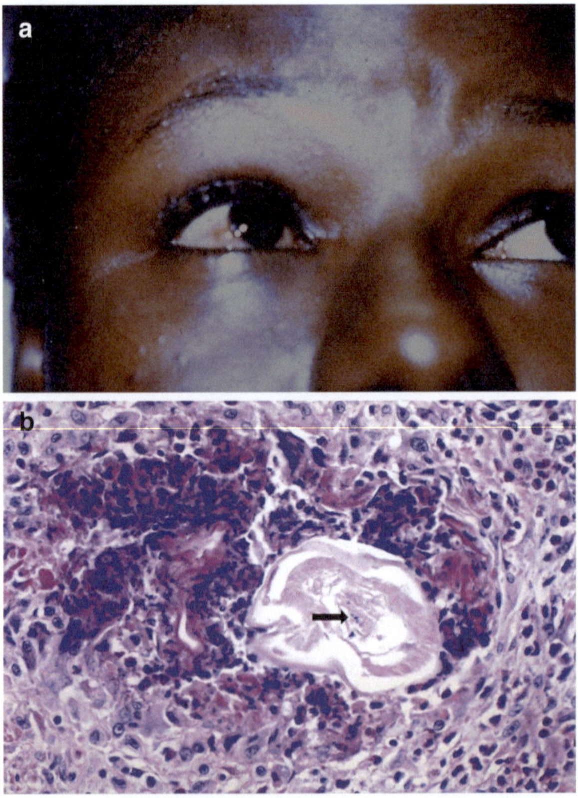

Fig. 3.13 (**a**) Bung-eye due to adult *Mansonella perstans* infection in a Ugandan man. (**b**) Adult gravid female *Mansonella perstans* within necrotizing granuloma of conjunctiva in a Sudanese man (Bung-eye). The worm is 100 μm in diameter and contains 2–3 μm wide microfilariae (*arrow*) in the uterus (H&E, original magnification ×100)

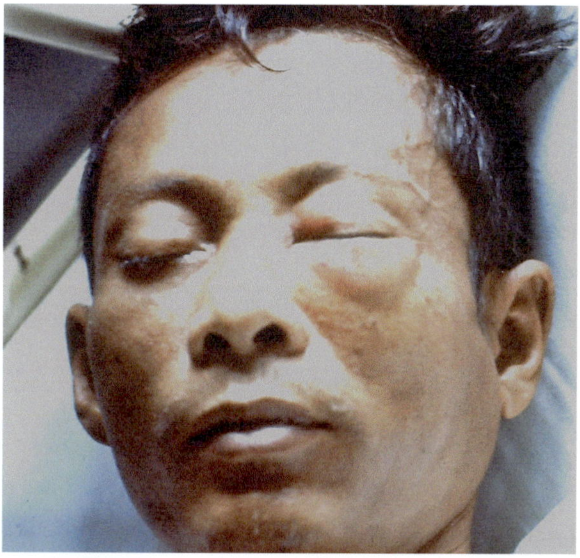

Fig. 3.14 Ocular *Parastrongylus* (*Angiostrongylus*) *cantonensis* infection in a Thai patient

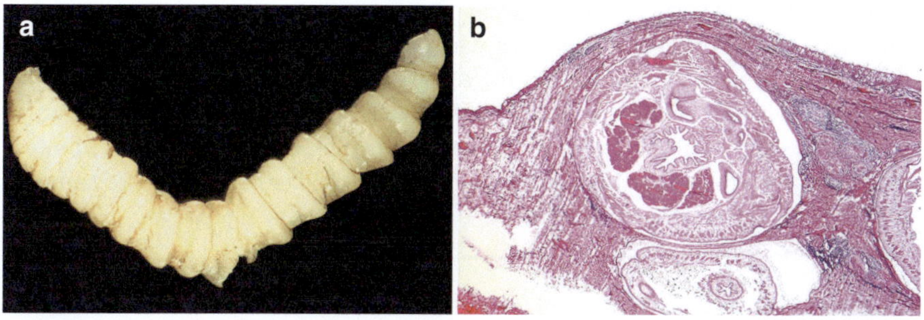

Fig. 3.15 (**a**) Pentastome removed from the conjunctiva of a 44-year-old man from the Central African Republic. The third-stage larval *Armillifer armillatus* is white and 2 cm long and appears pseudosegmented (unstained gross specimen). (**b**) Section of pentastome in conjunctiva. The third-stage larval *Armillifer armillatus* has striated muscle, an intestine, and acidophilic glands (H&E, original magnification ×7)

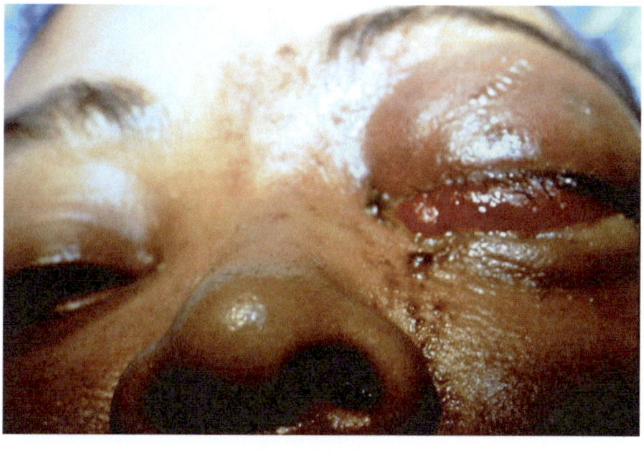

Fig. 3.16 Conjunctivitis due to *Rhinosporidium seeberi* infection

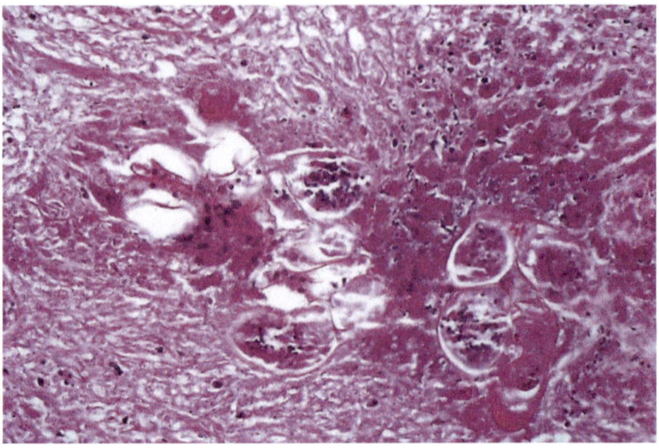

Fig. 3.17 *Schistosoma haematobium* eggs in a necrotic focus of lacrimal gland from an 11-year-old boy from Sierra Leone. Terminal spines are not evident in this photo (H&E, original magnification ×72)

Conclusion

Ocular infectious disease is found around the world, and many of the bacteria, fungi, viruses, and parasites that can cause eye lesions are absent or rare in North America and Western Europe. Such infections can present as keratoconjunctivitis, uveitis, or endophthalmitis. For ophthalmologists who practice in an endemic area, an understanding of the pathogens native to the region is important. For ophthalmologists who practice in non-endemic areas of North America or Western Europe, an awareness of these organisms and an appreciation for the typical clinical features of infection are important when evaluating a patient who has traveled widely or lived abroad.

References

1. Henchal EA, Putnak JR. The dengue viruses. Clin Microbiol Rev. 1990;3:376–96.
2. Vingolo EM, Messano GA, Fragiotta S, Spadea L, Petti S. Ocular manifestations of Ebola virus disease: an ophthalmologist's guide to prevent infection and panic. Biomed Res Int. 2015;2015:487073.
3. Yun NE, Walker DH. Pathogenesis of Lassa fever. Viruses. 2012;4:2031–48.
4. Brauburger K, Hume AJ, Mühlberger E, Olejnik J. Forty-five years of Marburg virus research. Viruses. 2012;4:1878–927.
5. Birge J, Sonnesyn S. Powassan virus encephalitis, Minnesota. USA Emerg Infect Dis. 2012;18:1669–71.
6. Johansson MA, Arana-Vizcarrondo N, Biggerstaff BJ, Staples JE. Incubation periods of yellow fever virus. Am J Trop Med Hyg. 2010;83:183–8.
7. Ikegami T, Makino S. The pathogenesis of Rift Valley fever. Viruses. 2011;3:493–519.
8. Bhatt S, Gething PW, Brady OJ, Messina JP, Farlow AW, Moyes CL, et al. The global distribution and burden of dengue. Nature. 2013;496:504–7.
9. Teixeira MG, Barreto ML. Diagnosis and management of dengue. BMJ. 2009;339:b4338.
10. Ng AW, Teoh SC. Dengue eye disease. Surv Ophthalmol. 2015;60:106–14.
11. Gear JSS, Cassel GA, Gear AJ. Outbreak of Marburg virus disease in Johannesburg. BMJ. 1975;4:489–93.

12. Pascolini D, Mariotti SP. Global estimates of visual impairment: 2010. Br J Ophthalmol. 2012;96:614–8.
13. Solomon AW, Peeling RW, Foster A, Mabey DC. Diagnosis and assessment of trachoma. Clin Microbiol Rev. 2004;17:982–1011.
14. Hadfield TL, Lamy Y, Wear DJ. Demonstration of *Chlamydia trachomatis* in inguinal lymphadenitis of lymphogranuloma venereum: a light microscopy, electron microscopy and polymerase chain reaction study. Mod Pathol. 1995;8:924–9.
15. el-Asrar AM, Van den Oord JJ, Geboes K, Missotten L, Emarah MH, Desmet V. Immunopathology of trachomatous conjunctivitis. Br J Ophthalmol. 1989;73:276–82.
16. Abu el-Asrar AM, Geboes K, al-Kharashi SA, al-Mosallam AA, Tabbara KF, al-Rajhi AA, et al. An immunohistochemical study of collagens in trachoma and vernal keratoconjunctivitis. Eye (Lond). 1998;12:1001–6.
17. al-Rajhi AA, Hidayat A, Nasr A, al-Faran M. The histopathology and the mechanism of entropion in patients with trachoma. Ophthalmology. 1993;100:1293–6.
18. Reacher MH, Pe'er J, Rapoza PA, Whittum-Hudson JA, Taylor HR. T cells and trachoma. Their role in cicatricial disease. Ophthalmology. 1991;98:334–41.
19. Abrahams C, Ballard RC, Sutte EE. The pathology of trachoma in a black South African population: light microscopical, histochemical and electron microscopical findings. S Afr Med J. 1979;55:1115–8.
20. Dawson CR, Juster R, Marx R, Daghfous MT, Ben DA. Limbal disease in trachoma and other ocular chlamydial infections: risk factors for corneal vascularisation. Eye (Lond). 1989;3:204–9.
21. Biswell R. Keratoplasty and trachoma in the southwestern American Indian. Arch Ophthalmol. 1969;81:791–6.
22. Rodenbiker HT, Ganley JP. Ocular coccidioidomycosis. Surv Ophthalmol. 1980;24:263–90.
23. Boyden BS, Yee DS. Bilateral coccidioidal choroiditis: a clinicopathologic case report. Trans Am Acad Ophthalmol Otolaryngol. 1971;75:1006–10.
24. Olavarria R, Fajardo LF. Ophthalmic coccidioidomycosis: case report and review. Arch Pathol. 1971;92:191–5.
25. Rainin EA, Little HL. Ocular coccidioidomycosis: a clinicopathologic case report. Trans Am Acad Ophthalmol Otolaryngol. 1972;76:645–51.
26. Lamer L, Paquin F, Lorange G, Bayardelle P, Ojeimi G. Macular coccidioidomycosis. Can J Ophthalmol. 1982;17:121–3.
27. Moorthy RS, Rao NA, Sidikaro Y, Foos RY. Coccidioidomycosis iridocyclitis. Ophthalmology. 1994;101:1923–8.
28. Cunningham Jr ET, Seiff SR, Berger TG, Lizotte PE, Howes Jr EL, Horton JC. Intraocular coccidioidomycosis diagnosed by skin biopsy. Arch Ophthalmol. 1998;116:674–7.
29. Glasgow BJ, Brown HH, Foos RY. Miliary retinitis in coccidioidomycosis. Am J Ophthalmol. 1987;104:24–7.
30. Tanowitz HB, Kirchhoff LV, Simon D, Morris SA, Weiss LM, Wittner M. Chagas' disease. Clin Microbiol Rev. 1992;5:400–19.
31. Prata JA, Prata Jr JA, de Castro CN, Macedo V, Prata A. The pupil in the chronic phase of Chagas disease and the reaction to pilocarpine and phenylephrine. Rev Soc Bras Med Trop. 1996;29:567–70.
32. Luna JD, Sonzini EE, Díaz HD, Iosa, DJ, Juárez, CP. Anomalous intraocular pressure changes in Chagas' disease elicited by postural test. Int Ophthalmol. 1996–1997;20:329–32.
33. Neumann E, Gunders AE. Pathogenesis of the posterior segment lesion of ocular onchocerciasis. Am J Ophthalmol. 1973;75:82–9.
34. Bird AC, Anderson J, Fugslang H. Morphology of posterior segment lesions of the eye in patients with onchocerciasis. Br J Ophthalmol. 1976;60:2–20.
35. Paul EV, Zimmerman LE. Some observations on the ocular pathology of onchocerciasis. Hum Pathol. 1970;1:581–94.
36. Garner A. Pathology of ocular onchocerciasis. Trans R Soc Trop Med Hyg. 1976;70:374–7.
37. Garner A. Pathology of pseudotumours of the orbit: a review. J Clin Pathol. 1973;26:639–48.

Chapter 4
Conjunctivitis

Tayyeba K. Ali and Seth M. Pantanelli

Introduction

"Pink eye" is one of the most common complaints seen by doctors and a source of frequent referral to ophthalmology. Infectious conjunctivitis is one of the leading components of the pink-eye differential. Nevertheless, redness is not the only way microbial disease of the conjunctiva manifests. The conjunctiva is a mucous membrane that lines the sclera and is composed of two layers: epithelium and submucosal substantia propria. When these layers become inflamed or infected, it manifests as conjunctivitis. Physiologically speaking, conjunctivitis is a vascular dilation accompanied by cellular infiltration and exudation. Proper eyelid closure, meibomian gland function, and ocular surface health are required to keep the conjunctiva moist and healthy. Disorders that affect these parameters, such as Bell's palsy, meibomian gland dysfunction, and cicatrizing disease, can lead to compromised conjunctival health and microbial infections.

While most infectious conjunctivitis is self-limiting, sequelae of microbial disease include membrane/pseudomembrane formation, cicatrization, and extension of the disease to the cornea and lacrimal system, as the epithelium that covers the conjunctiva is contiguous with the corneal epithelium and also extends to the

The authors of this article have no financial disclosures.

T.K. Ali, MD (✉)
Department of Ophthalmology, University of Arkansas for Medical Sciences,
Little Rock, AR 72205, USA

Jones Eye Institute, University of Arkansas for Medical Sciences,
4301 W. Markham Street, Little Rock, AR 72205, USA
e-mail: tkali@uams.edu

S.M. Pantanelli, MD, MS
Cornea and External Diseases, Department of Ophthalmology, Penn State College of
Medicine, Penn State Health-Milton S. Hershey Medical Center, Hershey, PA 17033, USA

N.V. Laver, C.S. Specht (eds.), *The Infected Eye*,
DOI 10.1007/978-3-319-42840-6_4

lacrimal apparatus and glands [1]. Additionally, post-infectious cicatrizing conjunctivitis holds significant morbidity, and common causes include trachoma, diphtheria, and streptococcal infection [2–4]. In the United States, the leading post-infectious sources are adenovirus and herpes simplex [5, 6].

Clinicians should be aware of the various presentations of conjunctivitis, particularly the factors that are common in infectious processes. The disease can be classified by laterality, onset of activity, morphology, discharge, and associated systemic illnesses. Taking a thorough history is key, followed by a focused physical examination in order to make a quick, accurate diagnosis and provide the most appropriate therapy.

Most cases of infectious conjunctivitis can be treated conservatively; nevertheless, it is imperative not to miss visually threatening or systemic disease. Morphology that is commonly associated with infectious etiologies includes papillary or follicular reactions, secondary to bacteria or to *Chlamydia* and viruses, respectively. The substantia propria has a superficial adenoid cell layer that contains lymphoid tissue. This layer is where follicles form. The deeper fibrous layer is composed of connective tissue, where fibroblasts, macrophages, mast cells, and polymorphonuclear cells are present in healthy tissue [1]. Other factors to consider are rapidity of onset, type of discharge, history of sick contacts, and presence of systemic illness.

Epidemiology of Conjunctivitis

While the numbers are likely higher today, older studies show that 1 % of annual primary care visits in the United States are related to conjunctivitis and 70 % of patients with conjunctivitis present to general practitioner offices or urgent care facilities [7]. Despite the fact that most cases of infectious conjunctivitis are self-limiting, it imposes a significant social and financial burden. Estimates suggest that four to six million people are affected annually in the United States [8], with an average of $705 million spent on direct and indirect costs related to the illness [9]. These numbers are conservative and only take into account office visits, not cases secondary to atypical causes of disease, such as conjunctivitis neonatorum.

Host Defenses (Table 4.1)

The eye's natural defense against pathogen invasion is multitiered and listed in Table 4.1. Initially, the physical barrier of the orbital rim and eyebrows keeps foreign material away from the ocular surface. This is followed by protection from the eyelashes and blink response, which work to keep smaller particles away from the surface of the eye. An additional mechanical tool includes the tear film, which washes away pathogens. The tear film is composed of many antimicrobial components, including lysozyme, beta-lysin, lactoferrin, immunoglobulins (primarily IgA), complement, and cathelicidin [10–15], which decrease colonization of

Table 4.1 Host defenses

Orbital rim
Eyelids
Eyebrows/eyelashes
Blink reflex
Tear film
Lysozyme
Beta-lysin
Lactoferrin
Immunoglobulins (IgA)
Complement
Cathelicidin
Goblet cell mucus
Conjunctiva-associated lymphoid tissue (CALT)
Low temperature
Ocular microbiota

microbes by killing the pathogens and preventing adhesion to the ocular surface. Mucus from goblet cells traps bacteria [10]. Furthermore, the ocular microbiota, composed of inherent and indigenous bacteria, prevents more pathogenic microbes from colonizing the surface [16, 17]. Conjunctiva-associated lymphoid tissue along with Toll-like receptors that regulate the adaptive immune response provides further protection [17]. Finally, the temperature of the ocular surface is not advantageous for microbial growth [17].

Risk Factors (Table 4.2)

Intrinsic

Any specific abnormality in the series of host defenses listed above can lead to microbial infection of the conjunctiva. While exposure from eyelid dysfunction or an absent Bell's phenomenon can often lead to corneal pathology, these factors also cause conjunctival drying and secondary infection. Severe meibomian gland dysfunction, abnormal tear film, and an altered microbiota can also be underlying factors that lead to further problems.

Extrinsic

Worldwide, a leading cause of preventable blindness is trachoma, which spreads from direct contact from ocular or nasal secretions, fomites, or via flies [18]. The most common type of infectious conjunctivitis in the United States is adenoviral conjunctivitis, and this occurs secondary to direct inoculation by ocular or nasal secretions, similar to the common cold. Less commonly, infectious organisms

Table 4.2 Risk factors

Intrinsic	Extrinsic
Abnormal lid anatomy	Direct inoculation
Lid retraction	Adenoviral
Lagophthalmos	Common bacterial
Abnormal blink reflex	Trachoma
Abnormal tear film	Transvaginal
Mucin layer	Sexual contact
Vit A deficiency	HSV/VZV
Aqueous layer	Trauma
Rheumatoid	Prior ocular surgery
Sjögren	Contaminated topical medications
Lipid layer	
Rosacea	
MGD	
CCC	
Altered microbiota	
Systemic	
NLDO	
Infection	

Abbreviations: *MGD* meibomian gland dysfunction, *CCC* chronic cicatrizing conjunctivitis, *NLDO* nasolacrimal duct obstruction

similar to trachoma and also sexually transmitted diseases can spread to the conjunctiva of neonates through transvaginal or perivaginal exposure during delivery [19].

Infection with herpes-family viruses typically manifests as a keratitis or sclerokeratitis but can present as blepharoconjunctivitis and should be kept in the differential for cases that are not self-limiting or that get worse on steroid eye drops. Trauma, previous eye surgery, and contaminated topical medications can all lead to spread of pathogenic bacteria. Common risk factors are listed in Table 4.2.

History and Clinical Examination

Numerous algorithms have been constructed to help guide the diagnosis of conjunctivitis. A detailed history is imperative to make a timely and accurate diagnosis. Often the physical examination will simply confirm the leading diagnosis and allow for appropriate therapy to be implemented quickly.

Questions important to ask on a history are: time of onset (hyperacute, acute, or chronic), laterality, presence of sick contacts, previous episodes, systemic diseases, and other risk factors. Hyperacute onset is typically defined by rapidity of onset and extent of disease. In adults, this would be <48 h after inoculation and with copious, hyperpurulent discharge, which generally represents gonorrheal disease. In neonates, conjunctivitis within the first 48 h of birth is usually toxic, whereas conjunctivitis due

Table 4.3 Differential for chronic, noninfectious conjunctivitis

Vernal keratoconjunctivitis
Atopic keratoconjunctivitis
Secondary giant papillary conjunctivitis
Foreign body
Sebaceous cell carcinoma
Floppy eyelid syndrome
Superior limbic keratoconjunctivitis
Toxic keratoconjunctivitis
Mucus-fishing syndrome
Keratoconjunctivitis sicca
Ligneous conjunctivitis
Stevens–Johnson syndrome
Ocular cicatricial pemphigoid
Sarcoidosis
Lymphoma

to *Neisseria gonorrhoeae* typically presents between days 2 and 5. In the general population, if onset of symptoms is less than 2 weeks, the likely etiology will be viral or nongonococcal bacterial. Up to 75 % of acute conjunctivitis has been attributed to viral infection [20]. Chronic conjunctivitis has an extensive, noninfectious differential and is listed in Table 4.3. Infection may be secondary to local spread from a dacryocystitis or canaliculitis. Chronic infection may be secondary to *Moraxella catarrhalis*, *Chlamydia* species, *Borrelia burgdorferi* (Lyme disease), molluscum contagiosum, or Parinaud's oculoglandular syndrome. Diagnoses based on onset of symptoms and then further subdivided based on morphology are listed in Fig. 4.1.

Laterality is the next question to probe, as adenoviral conjunctivitis classically starts in one eye and spreads to the other eye within 2–3 days of onset. Bacterial conjunctivitis will likely be bilateral and may be associated with sinusitis or nasolacrimal duct obstruction. Staphylococcal marginal blepharoconjunctivitis or infection secondary to lacrimal apparatus stasis can be unilateral or asymmetric in appearance.

Herpes-related conjunctivitis is often unilateral, though bilateral disease can be seen and is more common in atopic or immunocompromised patients. These patients may also have experienced previous episodes of redness, irritation, and light sensitivity.

Systemic diseases may need to be ruled out. Viral etiologies are presumed in the presence of preauricular lymphadenopathy and the absence of other more severe signs of illness. Patients at risk or with suggestive histories should be asked if they have known sexually transmitted diseases. Other important factors would be previous trauma, surgery, long-term topical medication use, topical steroid use, and history of radiation to the face.

A focused physical examination can confirm a diagnosis or lead the astute physician to make a less likely diagnosis. Morphology focuses on the type of conjunctival

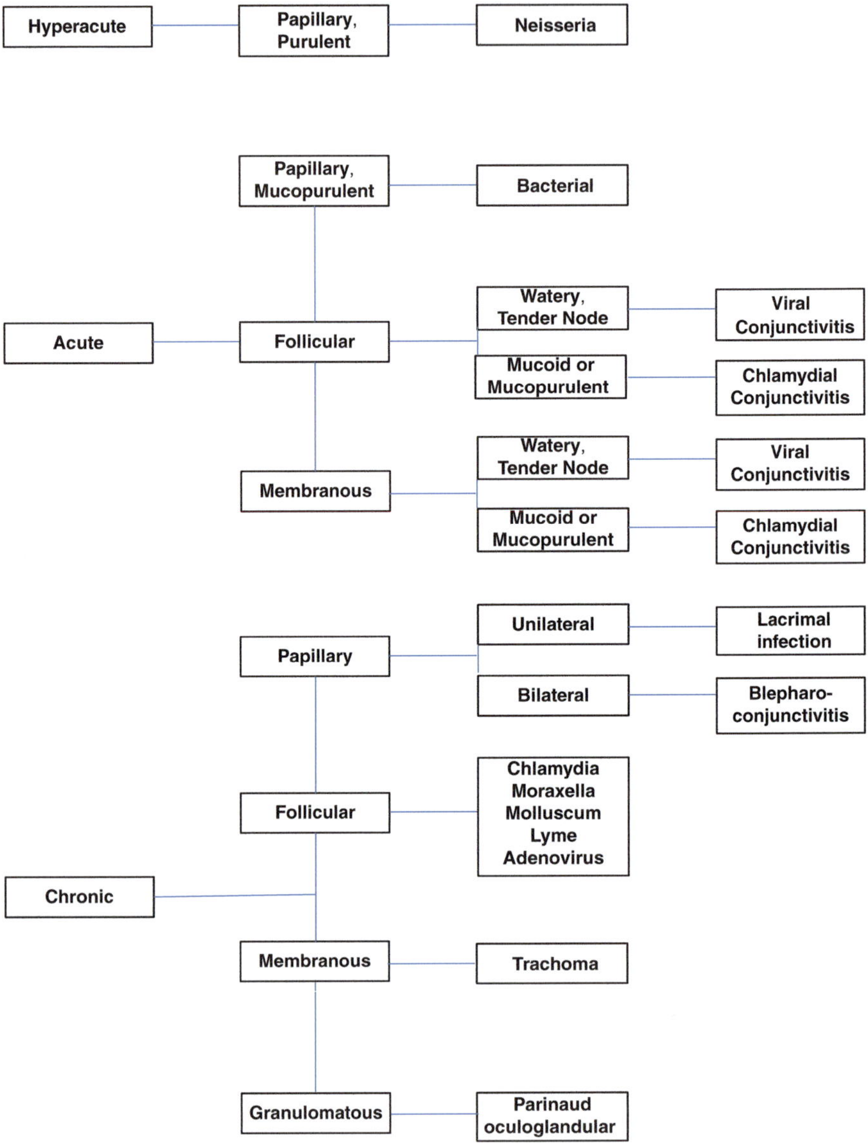

Fig. 4.1 Most likely cause of conjunctivitis based on rapidity of onset and morphological features (Adapted from Figures 42.1 and 42.2 in Lindquist [1])

reaction: papillary versus follicular. There may be a mixed response, but often one type will predominate. Classically papillary conjunctivitis is bacterial or allergic in origin. Follicles suggest a viral or chlamydial etiology. Other factors to look for are the presence of membranous or granulomatous disease.

Enumeration and Presentation of Common Pathogens

Understanding which organisms not only are the most common causes of conjunctivitis but also are most pathogenic is important in order to provide appropriate therapy. Knowing the risk factors associated with various microbes also assists in diagnosis.

Viral Conjunctivitis

Adenovirus

Adenoviral conjunctivitis (Fig. 4.2) is the most common cause of infectious conjunctivitis [20, 21] and is seen most often in the summer [22]. The virus has over 60 serotypes and seven subgroups; of the seven subgroups, group D is the most frequent source of adenoviral keratoconjunctivitis. There are four main ocular manifestations of adenoviral conjunctivitis, of which acute follicular conjunctivitis is the most benign [5]. Another frequent manifestation is epidemic keratoconjunctivitis (EKC). EKC is more aggressive and can be associated with pseudomembranes and symblepharon, as well as with corneal subepithelial infiltrates (SEIs). Pharyngoconjunctival fever (PCF) is characterized by fever, pharyngitis, follicular reaction, and preauricular adenopathy. Chronic conjunctivitis can wax and wane for months to years after the initial bout but eventually has spontaneous resolution. It can present with a mixed papillary and follicular reaction as well as with SEIs [23, 24].

Patients complain of bilateral symptoms, and classically the second eye becomes involved 2–3 days after the first. People in healthcare settings, day-cares, and other situations where there is close contact are at higher risk. The disease is biphasic and an inflammatory phase follows the initial infective phase at about 7–10 days after initial inoculation. Patients remain infected for up to 2–3 weeks after initial symptoms.

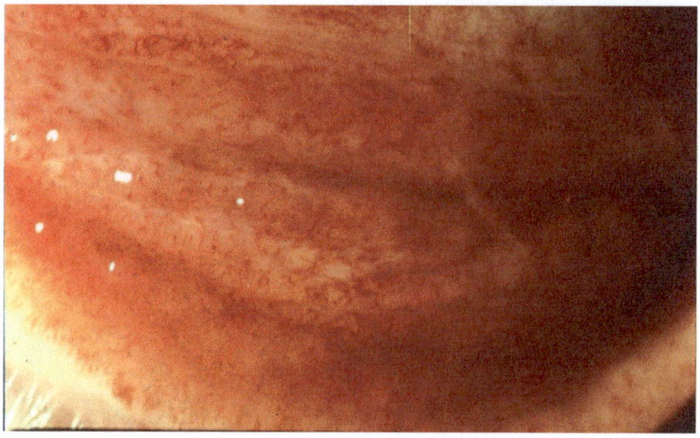

Fig. 4.2 Classic follicular response with a watery discharge, suggestive of adenoviral conjunctivitis

Herpes

Herpetic disease rarely presents as a simple follicular conjunctivitis without eyelid or corneal involvement. Nevertheless, almost 5 % of isolated follicular conjunctivitis cases that were thought to be adenovirus (due to the absence of clinical herpes) were found to be culture positive for herpes simplex virus (HSV) [25]. HSV conjunctivitis is typically unilateral and has a watery discharge. Vesicular eyelid lesions or a keratouveitis may be present [5, 26].

Primary varicella zoster virus rarely causes conjunctivitis. Infection after latency that manifests as herpes zoster ophthalmicus (HZO) can present as a conjunctivitis, scleritis, or keratouveitis and will typically be associated with the classic, dermatomal shingles rash. Involvement of the nasociliary branch of the trigeminal nerve (CN V), Hutchinson's sign, has a high correlation with ocular involvement and should be followed closely [5].

When herpetic infection is suspected, a dilated eye exam should be performed, especially if associated with a decrease in vision or worsening of symptoms, to ensure that there is no chorioretinal spread.

Atypical Viral Pathogens

Many viruses can cause conjunctivitis with a range of clinical appearances from a mild follicular reaction to significant membrane development with associated keratitis; Epstein–Barr virus [27], cytomegalovirus [28], paramyxovirus [5], or togavirus [29] may be involved. Molluscum contagiosum, secondary to poxvirus, is often associated with lid margin lesions that are raised, umbilicated, and flesh colored, as depicted in Fig. 4.3. Surgical removal [30] and other treatment options such as topical cidofovir [31] have been tried with some success for molluscum lesions.

Interest in flavivirus infection has increased since the 2015 outbreak of Zika virus in Latin America. The viruses that cause dengue, yellow fever, Japanese encephalitis, and West Nile disease are also flaviviruses. Zika virus can present with a maculopapular skin rash, fever, arthralgias, and conjunctivitis; these signs and symptoms are similar to those of dengue and chikungunya [32]. Treatment is typically supportive and conservative management is recommended for all of the abovementioned viral pathogens. Travelers to endemic areas are recommended to take proper precautions to avoid mosquito bites, as treatment is mainly preventative [33].

Bacterial Conjunctivitis

Bacterial infection is the second most common cause of conjunctivitis overall and is the source of most cases in children; it presents more frequently in winter [34]. Spread is typically through oculodigital contact or fomites [34, 35], but infection

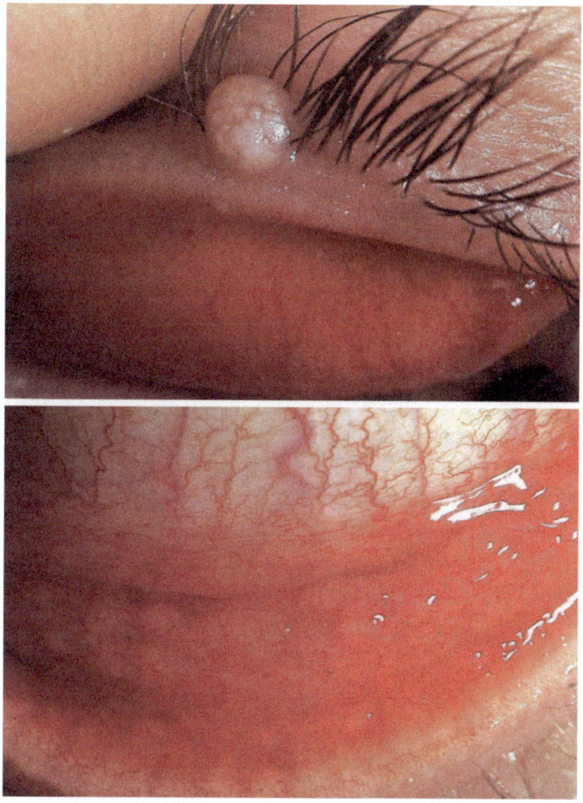

Fig. 4.3 *Upper image*: dome-shaped, waxy lesion suggestive of molluscum contagiosum, secondary to the poxvirus. *Lower image*: follicular conjunctivitis secondary to molluscum

can result from abnormal proliferation of native flora, trauma, and oculogenital or transvaginal spread as in neonatal conjunctivitis [26, 36]. Moreover, certain virulent pathogens can invade intact conjunctival and corneal epithelial surfaces, leading to deeper spread and even to perforation of the globe [17].

Staphylococcus

Staphylococcal species are the most common pathogens of adult bacterial conjunctivitis [36]. Acute bacterial conjunctivitis secondary to *Staphylococcus aureus* presents as a mucoid or mucopurulent, papillary conjunctivitis that affects the bulbar more than the palpebral conjunctiva. Typically, there is an associated matting and sticky closure of the eyelashes. It can become a chronic conjunctivitis if there is an associated blepharitis. Other normal eyelid flora includes *Staphylococcus epidermidis*, which can also become a chronic blepharoconjunctivitis [37].

Streptococcus

Although any streptococcal species can cause conjunctivitis, the second most common cause of bacterial disease is *Streptococcus pneumoniae*. It occurs more commonly in temperate climates during the winter and is observed more frequently in children [38]. Acute disease is associated with a mucopurulent discharge and a papillary reaction, as seen in other bacterial conjunctivitises.

Haemophilus

Haemophilus influenzae is the most common cause of bacterial conjunctivitis in young children [38, 39]. There is an encapsulated and a nonencapsulated form [17]. The encapsulated form often presents with mucoid or mucopurulent conjunctivitis that is highly contagious and requires treatment for resolution and prevention of recurrence [3, 17]. The nonencapsulated form is prevalent in more temperate environments and is seen in the springtime. It is often associated with upper respiratory tract infections and *H. influenza*-associated otitis media [38]; this form is self-limiting and often resolves within 1–2 weeks of onset [3, 17].

Moraxella

Moraxella catarrhalis can cause a chronic conjunctivitis and is often associated with an angular blepharitis [17].

Neisseria

Neisseria gonorrhoeae causes a hyperacute, profuse, and purulent conjunctivitis accompanied by severe chemosis, eyelid swelling, and keratitis [40]. The incubation period is typically 3 days to 3 weeks, and the urethral symptoms often precede the ocular findings by several weeks [40]. Still, cases without any urethral discharge and longer incubation periods have been reported [41]. If inadequately treated, gonococcal conjunctivitis can progress rapidly and may lead to corneal perforation within 24 h. Aggressive systemic therapy with antibiotics can reduce the risk of vision loss associated with perforation and other significant sequelae. The Centers for Disease Control recommend that patients being treated for gonococcal conjunctivitis be hospitalized and given high-dose parenteral antibiotics for 5 days [42]. Recently, there has been an increased incidence of gonococcal conjunctivitis, as well as increased levels of resistance to penicillin [40, 43]. Thus, cases that have rapid progression, that are refractory to treatment, or where there is a high suspicion for a sexually transmitted disease should have cultures and sensitivities performed in order to rule out more virulent or resistant pathogens.

Chlamydia

Chlamydia trachomatis is the primary species that causes conjunctivitis. Serovars A-C are associated with trachoma, the leading cause of preventable blindness worldwide [44]. The disease spreads via direct contact but also can be transmitted via fomites and flies; low socioeconomic status is a significant risk factor [18, 44, 45]. Trachoma manifests as a follicular conjunctivitis with mucoid discharge and hyperemia. In the later stages of the disease, classic findings include Herbert's pits along the limbus and Arlt's line along the superior tarsus. The inflammatory phase is followed by cicatricial changes; the stages of the disease are listed in Table 4.4 [44, 46].

Serovars D-K cause inclusion conjunctivitis, a sexually transmitted disease that is seen more commonly in industrialized nations [47]. It presents as a follicular reaction in adults about 1–2 weeks after inoculation, which occurs via direct contact with genital secretions and can be seen in up to 2 % of patients with urogenital *Chlamydia* infection [48]. Though less virulent, similar to gonorrheal conjunctivitis, it must be treated as a systemic disease requiring oral treatment with doxycycline or azithromycin [49]. Neonatal disease is discussed separately below.

Additionally, serovars L1–3 lead to lymphogranuloma venereum. In patients with high-risk sexual activity and a chronic follicular conjunctivitis, this rare entity should remain on the differential. *Chlamydia psittaci*, in patients who handle pigeons and certain other birds, may also present with a rare follicular conjunctivitis [50].

Atypical Bacterial Pathogens

Any number of bacteria can cause conjunctival inflammation, typically manifesting as a papillary conjunctivitis with a granulomatous component. One example is *Bartonella henselae*, which causes cat-scratch disease [51]. Cat-scratch disease can present with a nodular conjunctivitis and local lymphadenopathy and is a leading cause of Parinaud's oculoglandular syndrome. There may be history of a cat scratch, though this is not necessary [52, 53]. The list of possible pathogens

Table 4.4 Stages of trachoma [44, 46]

Stage
TF: Follicular inflammation – five or more follicles (0.5 mm) in upper tarsus
TI: Intense inflammation – significant tarsal thickening that obscures > ½ of the deep vessels
TS: Trachomatous scarring – tarsal scarring
TT: Trachomatous trichiasis – one or more eyelashes rubbing on surface
CO: corneal opacity – opacification over the pupil

Table 4.5 More frequent causes of Parinaud's oculoglandular syndrome

Cat-scratch *B. henselae*
Tularemia
Sporotrichosis
Tuberculosis
Syphilis
Coccidioidomycosis

Adapted from Gruzensky [54], which contains the complete differential

causing oculoglandular conjunctivitis is extensive [54], but *Francisella tularensis* [54], *Mycobacterium tuberculosis* [55], and *Treponema pallidum* [56] are high in the etiological differential diagnosis. Any of these organisms can cause granulomatous inflammation. If risk factors are present and the clinical picture is not that of a typical form of conjunctivitis, conjunctival scrapings should include acid fast and gram stains as well as cultures on Löwenstein–Jensen medium and chocolate agar. Giemsa stain and Sabouraud agar can be added if there is suspicion for a fungal etiology. Table 4.5 lists the most likely cause of Parinaud's oculoglandular syndrome.

Neonatal Conjunctivitis (Ophthalmia Neonatorum)

Ophthalmia neonatorum is a sight-threatening disease that manifests within the first 3–4 weeks of life and requires urgent treatment. Time to incubation and onset of disease are important factors in determining the cause of disease. Most often, neonatal conjunctivitis presents as a hyperacute papillary reaction; a follicular response is atypical before 6–8-week postpartum due to an inability to mount an immune response until that age [57].

Noninfectious conjunctivitis, or chemical conjunctivitis, often presents within the first 24–48 h of birth [58] and is generally secondary to the use of silver nitrate solution for prophylaxis against ophthalmia neonatorum. Chemical conjunctivitis is much less common in current neonatal practice, as the less toxic erythromycin ointment or povidone iodide eye drops have replaced silver nitrate solution for prophylaxis against ocular infections.

Conjunctivitis in the neonate can be secondary to infection with bacterial, viral, or rarely fungal organisms. Gonococcal conjunctivitis usually presents within 2–5 days after birth and will manifest with copious thick, purulent discharge [59] Urgent treatment is required in order to prevent scarring and corneal perforation. Other less common causes of bacterial neonatal conjunctivitis include *Haemophilus* spp., *Streptococcus pneumoniae*, and *Staphylococcus aureus* [60, 61]. Neonatal inclusion conjunctivitis is caused by *C. trachomatis* and is the most common cause of infectious neonatal conjunctivitis in the industrialized world [62]. It typically presents between 5 and 14 days after rupture of membranes. While membranes and conjunctival scarring can cause long-term sequelae, the disease is typically

Table 4.6 Neonatal conjunctivitis: diagnosis and treatment

Time to onset (postpartum)	Likely pathogen	Treatment
24–48 h	Chemical	Artificial tears and lubrication
2–5 days	*Neisseria gonorrhoeae*	Ceftriaxone 125 mg IM ×1 [60] OR Cefotaxime 25 mg/kg IM or IV BID-TID × 7 days [65] OR Penicillin G 100,000 U/kg/day IV divided QID × 7 days [58, 66] PLUS saline irrigation
5–14 days	*Chlamydia*	Erythromycin 12.5 mg/kg/day PO or IV divided QID × 14 days OR Azithromycin 20 mg/kg PO daily × 3 days PLUS erythromycin 0.5 % ointment QID [49]
>5 days	Fungal (*Candida*)	Natamycin 5 % drops Q1 hour × 14 days [6]
1–2 weeks	Herpes simplex	Acyclovir 30 mg/kg/day × 10 days OR Vidarabine 30 mg/kg/day × 10 days PLUS topical drops or ointment (trifluorothymidine 1 % Q2 hour OR ganciclovir ointment 5×/day) [59, 66, 67]

self-limiting. Systemic treatment is required because chlamydial pneumonitis is often associated with this condition [58, 63].

Herpes-related neonatal conjunctivitis typically presents 6–14 days after birth and is associated with eyelid swelling and a watery discharge. In addition to a vesicular skin rash, the cornea may be involved. Similar to chlamydial conjunctivitis, herpetic conjunctivitis needs to be treated systemically due to the mortality rate associated with disease dissemination [64].

Though infrequent, conjunctivitis due to infection by *Candida* spp. has been reported and typically will present five or more days after birth [6, 57]. Table 4.6 describes time to onset for neonatal conjunctivitis, as well as treatment options [65–67].

Diagnostic and Treatment Algorithm

Guidelines for treatment of conjunctivitis vary based on the characteristics of a given patient population (adults, neonates, the presence or absence of specific risk factors). Nevertheless, certain pathogens are seen at such a high frequency that an algorithm based on onset of disease can be used for most clinic situations (Fig. 4.1).

Meta-analysis of clinical features that would help accurately identify the type of infectious conjunctivitis shows that complete redness of the conjunctiva including tarsus, purulent discharge, and matting of both eyes in the morning increases the likelihood of a bacterial source [68]. Matting of the eyelids is the most important of these three factors [69]. Classically, preauricular lymphadenopathy is associated with viral conjunctivitis; however, this has not been shown to be diagnostically accurate [68].

Conjunctival cultures are not performed routinely but are indicated in cases of recurrent or recalcitrant disease, high suspicion for gonococcal or chlamydial infection, or in cases of neonatal conjunctivitis. Frequently used smears and culture media are listed in Tables 4.7 and 4.8, as it is imperative to culture on media that is most likely to grow the suspected organism.

In-office rapid antigen testing for adenoviral conjunctivitis can be instituted in the primary care setting; this may lead to a reduction in inappropriate therapy and visits [8]. This testing could also be useful in the ophthalmologist's office, as it is relatively inexpensive and provides the patient with the reassurance needed to continue with conservative management when indicated [21]. The mainstay of treatment for adenoviral conjunctivitis is conservative management with cool compresses and artificial tears. Strict hand-washing and limiting the spread of the disease by using separate hand towels, pillowcases, and refraining from going to regularly scheduled crowded places like day-care and work are important factors to discuss with the patient.

Herpes-related conjunctivitis typically has additional clinical features with possible involvement of the eyelids, cornea, and sclera. If the clinical picture remains unclear, shave biopsy of eyelid lesions, viral culture of the fornix, or impression cytology of corneal epithelial lesions can be performed. Herpes-associated conjunctivitis often resolves on its own. If there is corneal involvement or if symptomatic

Table 4.7 Frequently used smears and their corresponding organisms

Stain	Organisms seen
Gram stain	Bacteria (gram positive vs. gram negative), fungi, *Acanthamoeba*
Giemsa stain	Bacteria, fungi, *Chlamydia*, *Acanthamoeba*
Acid fast	*Mycobacterium*, *Nocardia*
Calcofluor white	Fungi

Table 4.8 Frequently used culture media and the common isolates grown on them

Culture media	Common isolates	Comment
Blood agar	Aerobic and facultative anaerobic bacteria	Incubate at 35°
Chocolate agar	Primarily anaerobic bacteria and facultative anaerobic, but may also grow aerobic	Incubate at 35°
Sabouraud agar	Primarily fungi, but may also grow filamentous bacteria, i.e., *Nocardia* spp.	Incubate at room temperature
Thioglycollate broth	Aerobic, anaerobic, and facultative anaerobic bacteria	Incubate at 35°
Lowenstein–Jensen medium	*Mycobacterium* and *Nocardia* spp.	Incubate at 35°
Thayer–Martin agar	*Neisseria* spp.	Incubate at 35°

Table 4.9 Common bacterial pathogens and their treatment in adults

Pathogen	Type of conjunctivitis	Treatment
Neisseria	Hyperacute	Ceftriaxone 1 g IM PLUS saline lavage [42]
Gram-positive bacteria (*S. aureus* or *S. pneumoniae*)	Acute	Vancomycin Cefazolin Fluoroquinolones (4th generation)
Gram-negative (*H. influenza*)	Acute	Tobramycin Gentamicin Ceftazidime Fluoroquinolones

Table 4.10 Management options for acute conjunctivitis

Artificial tears during day and ointment at night for adults and school-aged children
Artificial tear ointment in infants and toddlers
Strict hand-washing
Cool compresses
Avoid direct contact with others for 1–2 weeks
Antibiotic eye drops for bacterial conjunctivitis 2–4×/day
Steroid eye drops if associated subepithelial corneal infiltrates with VA < 20/40
Steroid eye drops for membranous conjunctivitis
Membrane peeling
Symblepharon ring +/– amniotic membrane to prevent aggressive membranes from forming a symblepharon
Rapid antigen testing or cultures to verify etiology or when conjunctivitis persists > 4 weeks

relief is needed, a 10-day course of antivirals should be used. Conjunctivitis secondary to atypical viruses is treated conservatively. Common causes of bacterial conjunctivitis and useful topical medications are listed in Table 4.9.

For many cases of viral or bacterial conjunctivitis, follow-up can be scheduled for 7–14 days after initial symptoms or first clinic visit based on the extent of disease. Typically, if patients are asymptomatic and have no visual complaints, they do not require a repeat ophthalmic examination. The authors leave follow-up for simple conjunctivitis up to the patient. In cases where there are pseudomembranes, risk for symblepharon formation, and visually significant subepithelial infiltrates, visits should be scheduled more frequently and compliance stressed. Membranes should be peeled every 3–5 days, if not more frequently, and sequelae of aggressive disease monitored closely. Therapy should be tailored based on etiology. Common treatment options are listed in Table 4.10.

Conjunctival infection that arises as a complication of surgical or nonsurgical trauma rarely remains limited to the conjunctiva. If there is significant pain, decrease in vision, or conjunctival injection that does not blanch with a drop of phenylephrine, a full dilated eye examination should be performed so that conjunctival epithelial defects, lacerations, foreign bodies, uveitis, or any posterior segment involvement can be identified.

Neonatal conjunctivitis requires rapid, accurate diagnosis and treatment. The time of onset, mother's medical history, and cultures are key factors to determine the underlying cause. Table 4.6 lists the most likely causes of neonatal conjunctivitis based on onset of disease and describes available treatments.

Additional Treatment Options

Steroids are rarely required when treating conjunctivitis and may prolong the disease course by increasing viral shedding. They may also exacerbate the disease if the conjunctivitis is accompanied by herpetic epithelial keratitis or a fungal infection.

Still, judicious use is indicated in cases that are associated with a strong inflammatory component, such as pseudomembranes or corneal subepithelial infiltrates causing vision less than 20/40 on the Snellen chart. For patients with recurrent, aggressive membranes, especially those who cannot be seen for frequent visits, symblepharon rings may be an option (Fig. 4.4), as well as amniotic membrane on a ring or sutured to the conjunctiva and positioned in the fornix.

Prognosis

Most cases of conjunctivitis, whether viral or bacterial, are self-limiting and resolve without any visually significant sequelae [26]. Infection with an aggressive viral strain or resistant bacteria may lead to symblepharon formation and post-infectious

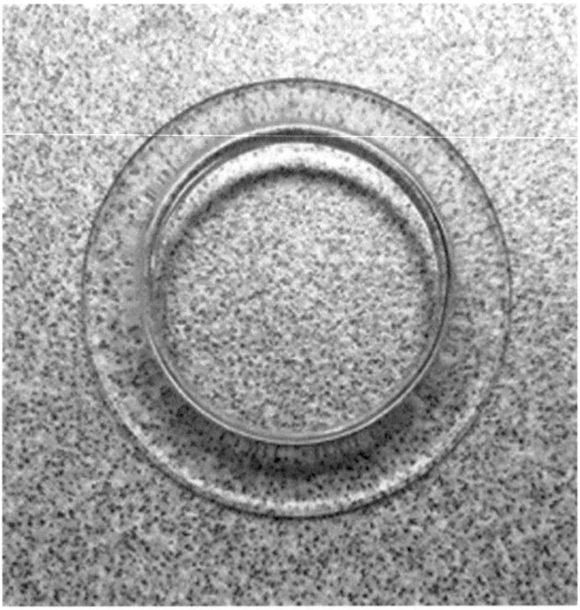

Fig. 4.4 Plastic ring placed within the fornices to prevent further cicatrization and symblepharon formation. Amniotic membrane attached to the ring (ProKera) or sutured in place to cover the fornices can be used for additional treatment

cicatrization. If treated appropriately and aggressively early in the disease course with judicious use of steroids or physical removal, permanent damage may be avoided. When dealing with virulent pathogens like *N. gonorrhoeae* or potentially chronic, progressive conditions like chlamydial conjunctivitis, early diagnosis and aggressive treatment that includes systemic therapy can limit damage to the ocular surface and prevent visual compromise. Ultimately, preventing spread of disease is critical and remains the mainstay of treatment, as most conjunctivitis is secondary to direct inoculation via hand–eye touch or fomites.

References

1. Lindquist T. Conjunctivitis: an overview and classification. In: Krachmer JH, Mannis MJ, Holland EJ, editors. Cornea. China: Mosby; 2011. p. 509–20.
2. Faraj HG, Hoang-Xuan T. Chronic cicatrizing conjunctivitis. Curr Opin Ophthalmol. 2001;12:250–7.
3. Duke-Elder S. System of ophthalmology. St. Louis: Mosby; 1965. p. 159–61.
4. Landers J, Kleinschmidt A, Wu J, Burt B, Ewald D, Henderson T. Prevalence of cicatricial trachoma in an indigenous population of Central Australia: the Central Australian Trachomatous Trichiasis Study (CATTS). Clin Experiment Ophthalmol. 2005;33:142–6.
5. Alvarenga L, Scaarpi M, Mannis M. Viral conjunctivitis. In: Krachmer JH, Mannis MJ, Holland EJ, editors. Cornea. China: Mosby; 2011. p. 535–44.
6. Arffa RC, Grayson M. Grayson's diseases of the cornea. 4th ed. St. Louis: Mosby; 1997. p. 125–56.
7. Kaufman HE. Adenovirus advances: new diagnostic and therapeutic options. Curr Opin Ophthalmol. 2011;22:290–3.
8. Udeh BL, Schneider JE, Ohsfeldt RL. Cost effectiveness of a point-of-care test for adenoviral conjunctivitis. Am J Med Sci. 2008;336:254–64.
9. Smith AF, Waycaster C. Estimate of the direct and indirect annual cost of bacterial conjunctivitis in the United States. BMC Ophthalmol. 2009;9:13.
10. Gilger BC. Immunology of the ocular surface. Vet Clin North Am Small Anim Pract. 2008;38:223–31, v.
11. Dawson CR. How does the external eye resist infection. Invest Ophthalmol. 1976;15:971–4.
12. Selinger DS, Selinger RC, Reed WP. Resistance to infection of the external eye: the role of tears. Surv Ophthalmol. 1979;24:33–8.
13. Williams RC, Gibbons RJ. Inhibition of bacterial adherence by secretory immunoglobulin A: a mechanism of antigen disposal. Science. 1972;177:697–9.
14. Stuchell RN, Farris RL, Mandel ID. Basal and reflex human tear analysis. II. Chemical analysis: lactoferrin and lysozyme. Ophthalmology. 1981;88:858–61.
15. Ford LC, DeLange RJ, Petty RW. Identification of a nonlysozymal bactericidal factor (beta lysin) in human tears and aqueous humor. Am J Ophthalmol. 1976;81:30–3.
16. Chandler JW, Gillette TE. Immunologic defense mechanisms of the ocular surface. Ophthalmology. 1983;90:585–91.
17. Soukiasian SaB J. Bacterial conjunctivitis. In: Krachmer JH, Mannis MJ, Holland EJ, editors. Cornea. China: Mosby; 2011. p. 521–34.
18. Schemann JF, Sacko D, Malvy D, Momo G, Traore L, Bore O, et al. Risk factors for trachoma in Mali. Int J Epidemiol. 2002;31:194–201.
19. Givner LB, Rennels MB, Woodward CL, Huang SW. Chlamydia trachomatis infection in infant delivered by cesarean section. Pediatrics. 1981;68:420–1.
20. Woodland RM, Darougar S, Thaker U, Cornell L, Siddique M, Wania J, et al. Causes of conjunctivitis and keratoconjunctivitis in Karachi, Pakistan. Trans R Soc Trop Med Hyg. 1992;86:317–20.

21. Jhanji V, Chan TC, Li EY, Agarwal K, Vajpayee RB. Adenoviral keratoconjunctivitis. Surv Ophthalmol. 2015;60:435–43.
22. Ariga T, Shimada Y, Shiratori K, Ohgami K, Yamazaki S, Tagawa Y, et al. Five new genome types of adenovirus type 37 caused epidemic keratoconjunctivitis in Sapporo, Japan, for more than 10 years. J Clin Microbiol. 2005;43:726–32.
23. Darougar S, Grey RH, Thaker U, McSwiggan DA. Clinical and epidemiological features of adenovirus keratoconjunctivitis in London. Br J Ophthalmol. 1983;67:1–7.
24. Pettit TH, Holland GN. Chronic keratoconjunctivitis associated with ocular adenovirus infection. Am J Ophthalmol. 1979;88:748–51.
25. Uchio E, Takeuchi S, Itoh N, Matsuura N, Ohno S, Aoki K. Clinical and epidemiological features of acute follicular conjunctivitis with special reference to that caused by herpes simplex virus type 1. Br J Ophthalmol. 2000;84:968–72.
26. Azari AA, Barney NP. Conjunctivitis: a systematic review of diagnosis and treatment. JAMA. 2013;310:1721–9.
27. Slobod KS, Sandlund JT, Spiegel PH, Haik B, Hurwitz JL, Conley ME, et al. Molecular evidence of ocular Epstein-Barr virus infection. Clin Infect Dis. 2000;31:184–8.
28. Brown HH, Glasgow BJ, Holland GN, Foos RY. Cytomegalovirus infection of the conjunctiva in AIDS. Am J Ophthalmol. 1988;106:102–4.
29. Hara J, Fujimoto F, Ishibashi T, Seguchi T, Nishimura K. Ocular manifestations of the 1976 rubella epidemic in Japan. Am J Ophthalmol. 1979;87:642–5.
30. Wheaton AF, Timothy NH, Dossett JH, Manders EK. The surgical treatment of Molluscum contagiosum in a pediatric AIDS patient. Ann Plast Surg. 2000;44:651–5.
31. Zabawski Jr EJ, Cockerell CJ. Topical and intralesional cidofovir: a review of pharmacology and therapeutic effects. J Am Acad Dermatol. 1998;39:741–5.
32. Musso D, Nilles EJ, Cao-Lormeau VM. Rapid spread of emerging Zika virus in the Pacific area. Clin Microbiol Infect. 2014;20:O595–6.
33. Summers DJ, Acosta RW, Acosta AM. Zika virus in an American recreational traveler. J Travel Med. 2015;22:338–40.
34. Hovding G. Acute bacterial conjunctivitis. Acta Ophthalmol. 2008;86:5–17.
35. Sattar SA, Dimock KD, Ansari SA, Springthorpe VS. Spread of acute hemorrhagic conjunctivitis due to enterovirus-70: effect of air temperature and relative humidity on virus survival on fomites. J Med Virol. 1988;25:289–96.
36. Mannis MJ. Bacterial conjunctivitis. In: Tasman W, Jaeger E, editors. Duane's clinical ophthalmology, vol. 4. Philadelphia: JB Lippincott; 1990. p. 1–8.
37. Valenton MJ, Okumoto M. Toxin-producing strains of Staphylococcus epidermidis (albus). Isolates from patients with staphylococcic blepharoconjunctivitis. Arch Ophthalmol. 1973;89: 186–9.
38. Gigliotti F, Williams WT, Hayden FG, Hendley JO, Benjamin J, Dickens M, et al. Etiology of acute conjunctivitis in children. J Pediatr. 1981;98:531–6.
39. Brook I. Anaerobic and aerobic bacterial flora of acute conjunctivitis in children. Arch Ophthalmol. 1980;98:833–5.
40. Kestelyn P, Bogaerts J, Stevens AM, Piot P, Meheus A. Treatment of adult gonococcal keratoconjunctivitis with oral norfloxacin. Am J Ophthalmol. 1989;108:516–23.
41. Lee JS, Choi HY, Lee JE, Lee SH, Oum BS. Gonococcal keratoconjunctivitis in adults. Eye (Lond). 2002;16:646–9.
42. Control CfD. Antibiotic-resistant strains of Neisseria gonorrhoeae. Policy guidelines for detection, management, and control. MMWR. 1987:244.
43. Rothenberg R, Voigt R. Epidemiologic aspects of control of penicillinase-producing Neisseria gonorrhoeae. Sex Transm Dis. 1988;15:211–6.
44. Wright HR, Turner A, Taylor HR. Trachoma. Lancet. 2008;371:1945–54.
45. Lietman T, Porco T, Dawson C, Blower S. Global elimination of trachoma: how frequently should we administer mass chemotherapy? Nat Med. 1999;5:572–6.

46. Bowman RJ, Jatta B, Cham B, Bailey RL, Faal H, Myatt M, et al. Natural history of trachomatous scarring in The Gambia: results of a 12-year longitudinal follow-up. Ophthalmology. 2001;108:2219–24.
47. Prevention CfDCa. Recommendations for the prevention and management of Chlamydia trachomatis infections. MMWR. 1993:RR-12.
48. Stenberg K, Mardh PA. Genital infection with Chlamydia trachomatis in patients with chlamydial conjunctivitis: unexplained results. Sex Transm Dis. 1991;18:1–4.
49. Hammerschlag MR. Chlamydial infections. J Pediatr. 1989;114:727–34.
50. Singal N, Rootman D. Chlamydial infections. In: Krachmer JH, Mannis MJ, Holland EJ, editors. Cornea. China: Mosby; 2011. p. 545–52.
51. Carithers HA. Cat-scratch disease. An overview based on a study of 1,200 patients. Am J Dis Child. 1985;139:1124–33.
52. Tobin EH, McDaniel H. Oculoglandular syndrome. Cat-scratch disease without the cat scratch. Postgrad Med. 1992;91:207–8, 10.
53. Ridder GJ, Boedeker CC, Technau-Ihling K, Sander A. Cat-scratch disease: otolaryngologic manifestations and management. Otolaryngol Head Neck Surg. 2005;132:353–8.
54. Gruzensky W. Parinaud's oculoglandular syndrome. In: Krachmer JH, Mannis MJ, Holland EJ, editors. Cornea. China: Mosby; 2011. p. 559–66.
55. Archer D, Bird A. Primary tuberculosis of the conjunctiva. Br J Ophthalmol. 1967;51: 679–84.
56. Spektor FE, Eagle Jr RC, Nichols CW. Granulomatous conjunctivitis secondary to Treponema pallidum. Ophthalmology. 1981;88:863–5.
57. Lindquist T. Ophthalmia neonatorum. In: Krachmer JH, Mannis MJ, Holland EJ, editors. Cornea. China: Mosby; 2011. p. 553–8.
58. Grosskreutz C, Smith LB. Neonatal conjunctivitis. Int Ophthalmol Clin. 1992;32:71–9.
59. Overall Jr JC, Glasgow LA. Virus infections of the fetus and newborn infant. J Pediatr. 1970;77:315–33.
60. Laga M, Plummer FA, Nzanze H, Namaara W, Brunham RC, Ndinya-Achola JO, et al. Epidemiology of ophthalmia neonatorum in Kenya. Lancet. 1986;2:1145–9.
61. Chandler JW, Rapoza PA. Ophthalmia neonatorum. Int Ophthalmol Clin. 1990;30:36–8.
62. Rours IG, Hammerschlag MR, Ott A, De Faber TJ, Verbrugh HA, de Groot R, et al. Chlamydia trachomatis as a cause of neonatal conjunctivitis in Dutch infants. Pediatrics. 2008;121: e321–6.
63. McCormack WM, Evrard JR, Laughlin CF, Rosner B, Alpert S, Crockett VA, et al. Sexually transmitted conditions among women college students. Am J Obstet Gynecol. 1981;139:130–3.
64. Gutierrez KM, Falkovitz Halpern MS, Maldonado Y, Arvin AM. The epidemiology of neonatal herpes simplex virus infections in California from 1985 to 1995. J Infect Dis. 1999;180:199–202.
65. Lepage P, Bogaerts J, Kestelyn P, Meheus A. Single-dose cefotaxime intramuscularly cures gonococcal ophthalmia neonatorum. Br J Ophthalmol. 1988;72:518–20.
66. de Toledo AR, Chandler JW. Conjunctivitis of the newborn. Infect Dis Clin North Am. 1992;6:807–13.
67. Whitley RJ. Herpes simplex virus infections of women and their offspring: implications for a developed society. Proc Natl Acad Sci U S A. 1994;91:2441–7.
68. Narayana S, McGee S. Bedside diagnosis of the 'red eye': a systematic review. Am J Med. 2015;128:1220–4.e1.
69. Rietveld RP, ter Riet G, Bindels PJ, Sloos JH, van Weert HC. Predicting bacterial cause in infectious conjunctivitis: cohort study on informativeness of combinations of signs and symptoms. BMJ. 2004;329:206–10.

Chapter 5
Corneal Infection and Ulceration

Seth M. Pantanelli and Tayyeba K. Ali

Introduction

Microbial keratitis is a common, sight-threatening infection of the cornea that results in a reactive inflammatory response. Infection may be caused by bacteria, viruses, fungi, or parasites. Normal lid function, tear film constituents, and the corneal epithelium all act as effective barriers against these organisms. However, a defect in any one of these defenses (e.g., lid function) can cascade and cause failure of the others (e.g., dry eye, integrity of the corneal epithelium). Likewise, external insults (e.g., trauma) can directly injure the corneal epithelium and create a passage by which organisms may enter the deeper cornea. As the organisms invade and proliferate, they cause release of inflammatory cytokines and matrix metalloproteinases, which in turn lead to proteolytic stromal degradation, tissue necrosis, and corneal thinning or ulceration.

Clinically, the diagnosis of microbial keratitis is not always straightforward. It must be differentiated from autoimmune causes of corneal ulceration like rheumatoid arthritis-associated peripheral ulcerative keratitis or neurotrophic ulceration secondary to previous herpes zoster ophthalmicus (HZO). Moreover, microbial

The authors of this article have no financial disclosures.

S.M. Pantanelli, MD, MS (✉)
Cornea and External Diseases, Department of Ophthalmology, Penn State College of Medicine, Penn State Health-Milton S. Hershey Medical Center,
500 University Drive, HU19, Hershey, PA 17033, USA
e-mail: spantanelli@hmc.psu.edu

T.K. Ali, MD
Department of Ophthalmology, University of Arkansas for Medical Sciences,
Little Rock, AR, USA

Jones Eye Institute, University of Arkansas for Medical Sciences,
Little Rock, AR 72205, USA
e-mail: tkali@uams.edu

N.V. Laver, C.S. Specht (eds.), *The Infected Eye*,
DOI 10.1007/978-3-319-42840-6_5

keratitis can coexist with one of these other causes for the ulcer. Generally speaking, a high index of suspicion for infection must be maintained. When there is doubt as to the cause of ulceration, empiric cultures and treatment with broad-spectrum antibiotics are the mainstay of initial therapy.

The short-term goal of the clinician should be to clear the infection and prevent corneal perforation, endophthalmitis, or loss of the eye. To achieve this, the astute clinician will usually treat empirically and conservatively with broad-spectrum antibiotics to start. Tapering or modifying the medications is guided by culture results, response to therapy, or a clear decompensation in the clinical picture as represented by corneal perforation, extension of the infection to or beyond the limbus, or endophthalmitis. When devastating complications occur, surgical therapy is then indicated. On the other hand, most infections can be halted and the inflammatory response quelled. With patience, effort may then slowly be shifted toward vision restoration.

Epidemiology of Corneal Infection

The incidence of microbial keratitis is not accurately known. It was estimated that, in 1992, there were approximately 30,000 cases per year in the United States [1, 2]. Although there are not any more recent estimates, the incidence within the United States, and other industrialized nations, is likely to increase over time with the increasing prevalence of contact lens use – one of the most common risk factors for microbial keratitis. Estimating its incidence has become more challenging with the availability of commercialized fourth-generation fluoroquinolones (e.g., Vigamox (moxifloxacin)). Having easy access to these effective topical medications has led to the widespread adoption of empiric treatment by those that lack resources to perform corneal scraping and cultures; thus, fewer patients are making their way to tertiary care centers where estimates of incidence might be more easily ascertained.

Of the 40 million people affected by blindness worldwide, approximately half are due to either cataract or trachoma [3]. In contrast, infectious keratitis is thought to be responsible for 5 % of the world's unilateral blindness. As a result, its importance is often overlooked and underappreciated. Worldwide, there are still 1.5–2.0 million new cornea infections (not including viral) each year [4]. The developing world bears the majority of this burden – in the United States, the incidence of microbial keratitis is estimated to be 11.0 per 100,000, while in Madurai, India, it is 113.0 per 100,000 [5]. Examined another way, there are approximately 1500 new cases of microbial keratitis per year in Great Britain but possibly as many as 840,000 per year in India [6]. In China, 85 % of corneal blindness is due to microbial keratitis [7, 8].

Most cases of microbial keratitis can be treated medically. However, complications including corneal perforation or endophthalmitis are reasons for surgery. The risk of endophthalmitis in the setting of microbial keratitis is thought to be approximately 0.5 % [9]. Risk factors for progression to endophthalmitis include a

Table 5.1 Host defenses

Host defenses
Orbital rim
Eyelids
Eyebrows/eyelashes
Blink reflex
Bell's phenomenon
Tear film
Lysozyme
Beta-lysine
Lactoferrin
Immunoglobulins IgA/IgG
Complement
Conjunctiva-associated lymphoid tissue (CALT)
Corneal epithelium

fungal etiology, use of topical steroids, or infectious keratitis developing adjacent to a surgical wound. Similarly, between 0.5 and 1.0% of microbial keratitis cases in the United States require a surgical intervention. These might include corneal gluing, corneal transplant, pars plana vitrectomy for endophthalmitis, or evisceration/enucleation. The need for surgical interventions in developing countries is likely just as great or greater, but the lack of an eye banking infrastructure may limit the number of people that receive those services.

Host Defenses (Table 5.1)

The human eye has so many defense mechanisms in place that it is a wonder any organism can evade them all and cause infection. The orbital rim and eyelids serve as a physical barrier against penetration by large blunt objects. Likewise, the eyebrows and eyelashes prevent small particles from trickling into the eye. The blink reflex has two important functions – first, it is a rapid and involuntary activation of the physical lid barrier; secondly, it rinses tears over the eye and washes away foreign matter or microorganisms. Similarly, the Bell's phenomenon, or upward and outward movement of the eye that occurs with lid closure, protects the cornea from direct trauma.

The tear film, which is continually renewed and replaced, not only dilutes toxins but also contains natural antimicrobial proteins [10]. The aqueous layer contains lysozyme, the most abundant tear film protein, and beta-lysine, which are both especially effective in lysing the cell walls of bacteria. Lactoferrin binds iron used in microbial metabolism. Immunoglobulins IgA and IgG prevent bacterial adherence by neutralizing critical surface receptors. They also promote phagocytosis and complement mediated cell lysis. The lipid and mucin layers of the tear film are also important, as they help to stabilize both the inner and outer surfaces of the aqueous layer; a deficiency in either of these decreases the tear breakup time and creates an

Table 5.2 Risk factors

Risk factors	
Intrinsic	Extrinsic
Abnormal/absent blink reflex	Tropical/humid climate
Abnormal/absent Bell's response	Trauma
Parkinson's disease	Agricultural habitat
Elderly	Exposure to contaminated water
Intubated/unconscious	Contact lens use
Abnormal tear film	Previous ocular surgery
Mucin layer	Topical steroids
Vitamin A deficiency	Contaminated topical medications
Aqueous layer	Topical anesthetic abuse
Rheumatoid arthritis	
Sjögren's syndrome	
Lipid layer	
Rosacea	
Meibomian gland dysfunction	
Chronic cicatrizing conjunctivitis	
Neurotrophic keratopathy	

opportunity for microorganisms to gain access to the corneal epithelium [11]. Finally, the conjunctiva-associated lymphoid tissue (CALT) contains B lymphocytes, which, when bound by an antigen, trigger an inflammatory cascade via release of cytokines [12].

The corneal epithelium is the defense mechanism of last resort. It forms a barrier by adhering to adjacent epithelial cells via desmosomes and tight junctions and to the basement membrane via hemidesmosomes. There are only a few pathogenic organisms known to have the ability to penetrate intact epithelium, namely, *Neisseria*, *Haemophilus influenzae*, *Listeria*, *Corynebacterium*, and *Shigella* spp. Other organisms require a prior insult that disrupts the normal epithelial architecture and exposes the underlying corneal stroma.

Risk Factors (Table 5.2)

Intrinsic

Isolated problems with the host defenses listed above contribute to the existence of ocular surface disease. A decreased or absent blink reflex or Bell's response, as seen in patients with Parkinson's disease, the elderly, or the unconscious, compromises the lid as an effective barrier to trauma. It also prevents the redistribution of all three layers of the tear film and puts the epithelium at risk for exposure and erosion. Vitamin A deficiency might result in a deficient mucin layer, Sjögren's syndrome or rheumatoid arthritis might result in a deficient aqueous layer, and rosacea might result in meibomian gland dysfunction and an abnormal lipid layer. Obliteration of the meibomian glands from a chronic cicatrizing conjunctivitis like Stevens-Johnson syndrome or ocular cicatricial pemphigoid might also result in a deficient lipid layer. Ocular infection with herpes simplex virus (HSV) or reactivation of the varicella zoster virus (VZV) along the ophthalmic division of the trigeminal nerve (V1) leads to a neurotrophic cornea. This in turn is thought to disrupt normal reflex tearing, which results in dry eye and sterile neurotrophic corneal ulcers. Even uncontrolled, long-standing diabetes can cause a "peripheral neuropathy" of the cornea. All of the above "first hits" lead to punctate epithelial erosions and epithelial defects, which are chronically at risk for superinfection.

Extrinsic

Local climate contributes to the frequency of microbial keratitis. Increasing temperature, from either proximity to the equator or change in season, is directly proportional to the number of infections seen within a region. Tropical climate also seems to correlate strongly with the proportion of infections with a fungal etiology. In South India, the incidence of fungal keratitis is higher between June and September than the rest of the year [13]. In Hong Kong, the fungal/bacterial ratio is 1:17 but ranges between 1:5 (Singapore) and 1:2 (South India) in more tropical climates [14]. While the temperature and humidity are both strongly correlated with the frequency of infection, humidity itself does not appear to be an independent risk factor for a particular type of infection (e.g., fungal) [15].

The industrialization, or lack thereof, of a person's habitat also contributes to his or her risk for microbial keratitis and the profile of organisms he or she is most vulnerable to. People living in rural habitats may have occupations centered on agriculture; trauma, especially with vegetable matter, is strongly correlated with developing microbial keratitis, in particular fungal keratitis [16, 17]. Exposure to contaminated water may also increase the risk of microbial keratitis. For example, it has been suggested that changes to the water disinfection practices in Chicago, Illinois, enforced between 2002 and 2004 are responsible for the ongoing outbreak of Acanthamoeba keratitis in that metropolitan area [18, 19].

Contact lens use is the strongest risk factor for microbial keratitis in developed countries. The overall incidence of microbial keratitis in the United States is 11 per 100,000, but the incidence among contact lens wearers is between 2- and 20-fold higher, depending on the lens type and pattern of use [20]. Rigid gas permeable lenses appear to increase the risk the least of all lens types (12 per 100,000), low Dk lenses increase the risk moderately (19–22 per 100,000), and silicone hydrogel lenses increase the risk the most (55–119 per 100,000). Overnight use of any contact lens dramatically increases the risk over daily use (195–254 per 100,000), and there is a strong correlation with the duration of continuous overnight wear. As the number of contact lens users in the United States increases, the proportion of microbial keratitis cases associated with contact lenses has also increased and is most recently reported to be as high as 44 % [21]. Orthokeratology lenses have also been implicated in microbial keratitis, and the incidence with these lenses is similar to that of other overnight wear lenses [22]. One multipurpose disinfecting solution, ReNu with MoistureLoc (Bausch & Lomb, Rochester, NY), was implicated in *Fusarium* outbreaks in Singapore and the United States between 2004 and 2006 before being subsequently removed from the global market in May of 2006 [23].

Trauma is a significant risk factor for infection; as such, it is unsurprising that a history of ocular surgery also puts patients at risk [24]. The pathogenesis for infection in these eyes likely depends on whether it occurs in the immediate postoperative period, subacutely, or chronically. When the infection occurs early, it may be a direct result of an epithelial defect of which an invading microorganism subsequently takes advantage. This temporal relationship between the creation of an epithelial defect and acutely documented infection has been well studied in patients receiving LASIK or surface ablations, where 36–72 % of all infections occur within the first 7 days [25, 26]. On the other hand, when the infection occurs late, the surgery itself is less likely to be the inciting factor. Instead, a history of ocular surgery may simply identify an eye that was at high risk for ocular surface disease. For instance, eyes with a history of cornea transplant are at increased risk for late infection, but it is more likely the ocular surface disease secondary to graft failure or the chronic use of topical steroids that puts the eye at risk for late infection, not the surgery itself [27, 28].

Contamination of topical medications was a documented cause of microbial keratitis in the 1980s [29], but guidelines for the preparation of sterile solutions have since been adopted by commercial manufacturers. On the other hand, compounded medications for ophthalmic use (e.g., autologous serum tears and fortified antibiotics) continue to play an important role in many subspecialty practices. Appropriate precautions and patient counseling are still warranted when prescribing these medications.

Presentation

The symptoms of microbial keratitis that bring a patient to the attention of a physician include eye redness, photophobia, vision loss, and pain. However, the rapidity of symptom onset is highly variable and dependent upon the infecting organism and preexisting corneal disease. *Pseudomonas aeruginosa* infection has a characteristically rapid onset that drives the patient to seek medical care within 24–48 h. In contrast, organisms like nontuberculous *Mycobacterium*, *Nocardia*, or *Fusarium* might have a more indolent course, and patients may not present for 5 days or more from symptom onset. If there is a preexisting eye condition, such as a sterile neurotrophic corneal ulcer that gets subsequently superinfected, presentation might be further delayed, as the patient might only seek care when a dramatic change in vision or seemingly incidental increase of redness is noticed. Likewise, presentation to an ophthalmologist might be delayed if the patient is seen first by another healthcare provider and is treated with suboptimal antibiotics (e.g., sulfacetamide) or topical steroids.

History and Clinical Examination

A carefully obtained history helps to differentiate microbial keratitis from noninfectious (autoimmune/inflammatory) keratitis, elucidate risk factors so that they may be altered, and counsel the patient appropriately on prognosis. The timing of symptom onset (redness, photophobia, blurry vision, and pain) and duration should be well understood. A detailed medical history should include a list of systemic diseases, with special attention to the presence of any autoimmune or immune-compromising conditions. Even a history of poorly controlled diabetes can be important, as it can clue the physician in to the possibility of a neurotrophic cornea. Ocular history should focus on any previous surgery, current topical medications, and whether the patient has had a previous episode of herpes simplex virus keratitis or herpes zoster ophthalmicus. A history of ptosis repair associated with an infectious ulcer inferiorly may suggest exposure as the risk factor most responsible for the infection. Likewise, a recent history of LASIK might increase suspicion for an atypical organism like *Mycobacterium.*

A search for risk factors predisposing to infection is important, since risk factor modification will help to clear the current infection and decrease the patient's risk for future infections. The patient should be questioned for occupational hazards (e.g., agricultural work), a recent history of trauma, and exposure to freshwater, swimming pools, hot tubs, or contact lens use. If there is a history of trauma, knowing whether the object contained vegetable matter (e.g., tree branch) will help to gauge the patient's risk for fungal keratitis. If the patient is a contact lens user, the physician should document the type of contact lens and precise cleaning solution used. Contact lens hygiene can be assessed by asking the patient how often the lenses are designed to be replaced, how often the patient actually replaces them, and whether they sleep in the contact lenses. Knowing the answers to these questions establishes the foundation for a conversation on contact lens hygiene, so that questionable habits can be identified and corrected later if the patient wishes to use them again.

The purpose of the clinical examination is to evaluate for any predisposing factors not already disclosed in the history, document the severity of the disease, and narrow the differential diagnosis so that appropriate workup and treatment can be instituted. The exam starts with documentation of visual acuity, which should correlate with the anterior segment findings. Next, corneal sensation should be ascertained, before the instillation of a topical anesthetic. Intraocular pressure is then tested. Examination is best begun with the lights on and without the ophthalmic microscope. The patients face should be examined grossly, at first, for rash (e.g., as in HZO), facial droop, and both the quality and frequency of blink function (e.g., decreased in elderly or patients with Parkinson's disease). The level of conjunctival hyperemia is also usually best ascertained without the microscope. Slit-lamp biomicroscopy can then be used to look at the puncta for evidence of chronic inflammation and stenosis, lashes for trichiasis or collarettes suggestive of blepharitis, and meibomian glands for inspissation or dysfunction. The lid margin should be inspected for keratinization. Both the superior and inferior fornices should be inspected for the presence of follicles, papillae, membrane formation, cicatrization, ulceration, or foreign bodies. The bulbar conjunctiva and sclera are then similarly assessed for injection, ulceration, and ischemia. Limbal ischemia or neovascularization should be noted; the latter is especially important as it is suggestive of either a long-standing preexisting condition or chronicity of the active process under question.

Attention is then turned toward the cornea. The location of any infiltrate is carefully documented and usually referred to as central, paracentral, mid-peripheral, or peripheral. The widest and shortest dimensions of the infiltrate are measured and recorded, as is the presence or absence of an overlying epithelial defect. The infiltrate can be further characterized as discrete, feathery, multicentric with satellite lesions, suppurative, necrotic, or crystalline. Any areas of corneal thinning should be noted. If the cornea is perforated, an attempt should be made to estimate the size of the perforation and assess whether it is actively leaking or has been sealed by prolapsed iris tissue. Finally, the endothelium is inspected for the presence of plaques or keratic precipitates.

The remainder of the slit-lamp exam focuses on evaluation for intraocular inflammation and spread of infection. The anterior chamber is assessed for cell, flare, and the presence of fibrin or a hypopyon. The eye is dilated unless a contraindication exists, and vitritis, retinitis, or choroiditis ruled out. If the view is poor through the corneal infiltrate, a B-scan ultrasound can help to rule out endophthalmitis.

Enumeration and Presentation of Pathogens

It is helpful to know which organisms are the most infectious isolates within a region. Knowing the risk factors that put patients at risk for specific organisms is also helpful. However, there is considerable overlap in the history and clinical presentation among patients infected with bacteria, fungus, parasites, and even viral isolates. It cannot be overemphasized that speculative treatment for suspected organisms is likely to result in a high proportion of incorrectly diagnosed and managed ulcers. In one study, cornea specialists were only able to differentiate between bacterial and fungal ulcers 66 % of the time [30]. As such, a more universally accepted strategy is to provisionally start all patients on broad-spectrum antimicrobials that cover the majority of isolates found in a region and simultaneously perform microbiologic workup (e.g., cultures, stains, confocal microscopy) that might allow for tailoring of treatment later. With that being said, an attempt will be made to identify characteristic features and treatment recommendations for a few causal organisms.

Staphylococcus spp.

Staphylococci are gram-positive cocci and are part of the normal human skin flora. The two species most relevant to cornea infections include *Staphylococcus aureus* and *Staphylococcus epidermidis*. Both are facultative anaerobes; however, *S. aureus* is coagulase positive and *S. epidermidis* is coagulase negative. The leading risk factor for *Staphylococcus* keratitis is ocular surface disease, but whether the surface disease itself is caused by *Staphylococcus* colonization or some other cause requires careful consideration [31]. For instance, severe blepharitis from *S. aureus* can cause meibomian gland dysfunction, dry eye, and ocular surface disease, which in turn can put the patient at risk for *Staphylococcus* marginal keratitis and subsequent abscess or ulcer formation. Alternatively, the ocular surface disease might be caused by HSV-associated neurotrophic keratopathy, which subsequently leads to epithelial breakdown and opportunistic corneal infection by *Staphylococcus* spp. Thus, understanding the relationship between the ocular surface disease and the microbial keratitis is an important step in identifying and eliminating risk factors for recurrent infections.

Staphylococcus marginal keratitis is the most common presentation for *Staphylococcus*-associated keratitis. The clinical picture is characterized by small, round, peripheral, sterile corneal infiltrates that usually lack an overlying epithelial defect. This presentation is not due to a primary *Staphylococcus* infection of the cornea. It is a type III hypersensitivity reaction to exotoxin secreted by the bacteria that leads to immune complex deposition, activation of complement, neutrophil recruitment, and infiltrate formation. As such, treatment is geared toward management of the inflammatory response and elimination of the exotoxin. Judicious use of topical steroids, warm compresses, and lid scrubs usually lead to symptom resolution over days to weeks.

When true *S. aureus* infection occurs, it produces a rapidly progressive stromal infiltrate, anterior chamber reaction, endothelial plaque, and hypopyon. Methicillin-resistant *Staphylococcus aureus* (MRSA) keratitis used to be confined to the hospital setting, but an increasing number of community acquired isolates are being seen. One study from Taiwan found that the hospital-acquired MRSA isolates were also more likely to be resistant to trimethoprim/sulfamethoxazole [31]. Fortunately, all strains of *S. aureus* remain sensitive to topical fortified vancomycin [32].

Coagulase-negative staphylococcus is the most commonly isolated organism cultured from the ocular surface. In fact, it is more often considered a contaminant of cultures than the cause of infectious keratitis. However, this assumption is an oversimplification, since *S. epidermidis* can cause corneal ulceration, especially in the injured cornea or in the elderly. Moreover, not all coagulase-negative staphylococcus is *S. epidermidis*; other pathogenic organisms (e.g., *S. hominis*, *S. lugdunensis*, and *S. simulans*) are identifiable with further speciation [33]. This group of organisms is most susceptible to vancomycin or gentamicin and has variable susceptibility to the fluoroquinolones [33].

Streptococcus pneumoniae

S. pneumoniae is a gram-positive, alpha-hemolytic, facultative anaerobe. Its associated keratitis most often occurs after corneal trauma or surgery [34]. It is characterized by rapid onset, suppuration, and vigorous anterior chamber reaction with endothelial fibrin plaque and hypopyon. As with other gram-positive organisms, topical fortified vancomycin or cefuroxime is extremely effective and considered first line. Gentamicin has also been found effective. Although the role for topical corticosteroids remains controversial for microbial keratitis in general, this may be a particular situation in which complementary treatment with antibiotics is beneficial [34].

Pseudomonas aeruginosa

Pseudomonas spp. are gram-negative, aerobic, bacillus bacteria. They also have the ability to grow in oxygen deficient or depleted environments; as such, they might also be considered facultative anaerobes. They are the most common causative organism for microbial keratitis in contact lens wearers (specifically *P. aeruginosa*), and may account for greater than 60 % of the culture isolates in this group [21]. This pattern holds true in studies across the globe, including those from the United States, Hong Kong, and the Netherlands [21, 35–37]. The pathogenesis for this association is not precisely understood but is certainly driven by the ability of *P. aeruginosa* to form biofilms on contact lenses. In one study in rabbits, corneas exposed to extended wear contact lenses had a *P. aeruginosa* bacterial load between three and eight times that of control eyes [38]. Additionally, the contact lens acts as a barrier between the cornea and the lids, allowing for adherence of the organism to the corneal surface without risk of being mechanically washed away with lid blink.

P. aeruginosa tends to produce a rapidly progressive corneal infiltrate. It also creates proteolytic enzymes (e.g., collagenase) that can rapidly destroy tissue and lead to corneal perforations. The infiltrate is usually singular, round or oval in shape, white in color, and suppurative in nature (Fig. 5.1). It can be associated with a significant anterior chamber response and sterile hypopyon. *Pseudomonas* spp. are susceptible to topical tobramycin, gentamicin, and ceftazidime. They are also susceptible to the fluoroquinolones; however, the temptation to use ciprofloxacin because of cost must be weighed against the possibility of resistance [39, 40]. Fourth-generation fluoroquinolones like moxifloxacin and gatifloxacin are still extremely effective.

Nocardia spp.

Nocardia spp. are weakly gram-positive, variably acid-fast, aerobic bacilli. On culture media, they are seen to form pseudohyphae. They are a relatively rare cause of microbial keratitis, accounting for between 0.3 and 8.3 % of

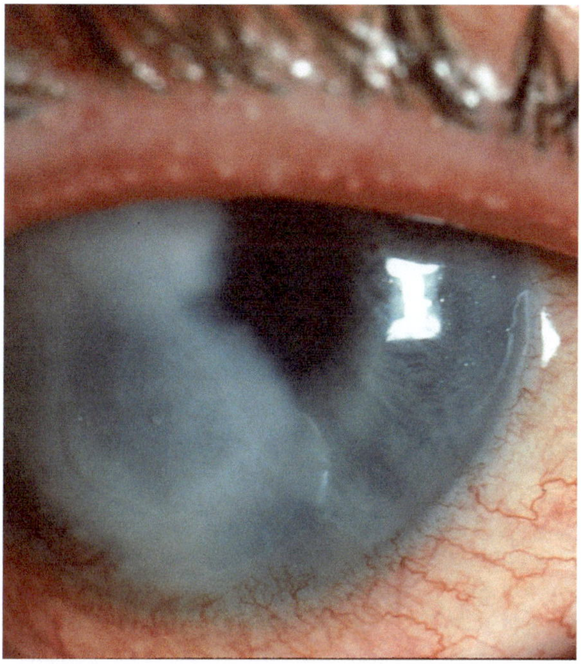

Fig. 5.1 Pseudomonas corneal ulcer. Note the suppurative nature of the infiltrates

culture-positive isolates [41, 42]. It is most often reported after minor trauma but has also previously been associated with ocular surgery like photorefractive keratectomy (PRK) [43]. Many species within this genus, including *N. transvalensis*, *N. asteroides*, *N. arthritidis*, and *N. farcinica*, have been implicated in causing keratitis. *Nocardia* characteristically produces an ulcer with an indolent course. If a patient presents early, they may complain of pain out of proportion to objective findings, and visual acuity is generally good. This may prompt the clinician to diagnose the patient with noninfectious keratitis and start topical steroids. Even if infection is suspected, the patient might be started on fortified vancomycin and tobramycin, a combination that is ineffective against *Nocardia* spp. As the infection progresses, a ring-shaped, subepithelial or anterior stromal infiltrate develops. The ring has a characteristic brushfire border and consists of yellow-white pinhead-sized infiltrates and satellite lesions (Fig. 5.2). An epithelial defect, anterior chamber reaction, and hypopyon may or may not be present. These findings might be confused with fungal keratitis or another atypical bacterial infection like nontubercular mycobacterium. Once the correct diagnosis is made, therapy can be switched to topical amikacin. Patients must be followed closely for possible resistance and switched to topical compounded trimethoprim +/− sulfamethoxazole if indicated [44]. Visual acuity after treatment of *Nocardia* keratitis is generally better than with other causes of bacterial keratitis [45].

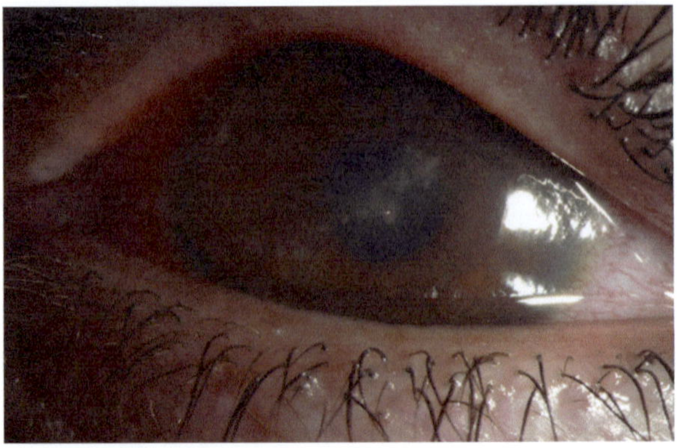

Fig. 5.2 Nocardia corneal ulcer. Note the brushfire borders, wreathlike configuration, and relative lack of suppurative infiltrate

Neisseria spp.

N. gonorrhoeae and *N. meningitidis* are obligate intracellular gram-negative cocci. *N. gonorrhoeae* is often thought of in association with neonatal conjunctivitis [46] but can also occur in adults [47]. If left untreated, it can quickly progress to cause corneal ulceration and perforation. Discharge is characteristically hyperpurulent. Treatment is with systemic ceftriaxone. If the patient is a neonate, it is important to also treat the mother and any sexual partners to prevent transmission to other adults or future children.

Nontuberculous Mycobacteria

Nontuberculous mycobacteria (NTM) are a group of aerobic, acid-fast mycobacteria that are ubiquitously found in soil and water. *M. fortuitum* and *M. chelonae* are the two species most often implicated in cornea infections. Ascertaining the incidence of NTM is difficult, but it seems that they are increasing in frequency [48]. This can likely be attributed to the association of NTM infection with cornea surgery and the increase in popularity of keratorefractive surgery (e.g., LASIK and PRK) over the past three decades. In fact, LASIK is the predisposing factor in nearly half of reported NTM cases [48]. History of trauma or a foreign body is another risk factor that is commonly elicited. In stark contrast to *Pseudomonas aeruginosa* keratitis, which causes rapid stromal infiltration and a flagrant inflammatory response, NTM infections are indolent and presentation is delayed. The average time from exposure to presentation is 5.6 weeks [48]. The infiltrate is nonsuppurative and may have indiscriminate borders or satellite lesions (Fig. 5.3). These features mimic those of fungal keratitis. NTM also has poor growth characteristics on standard culture media. All of these attributes result in a frequent delay in diagnosis.

Diagnosis of NTM requires a high index of suspicion, which usually comes about when the infiltrate does not respond to conventional antibiotic therapy.

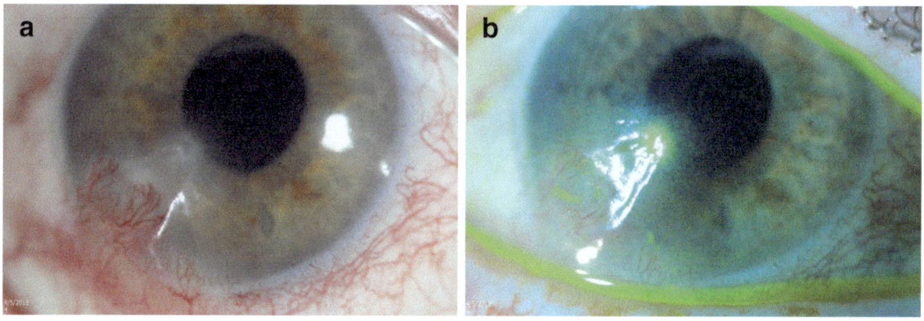

Fig. 5.3 Nontubercular mycobacterial corneal ulcer without (**a**) and with (**b**) fluorescein stain

Ziehl-Neelsen acid-fast stain and Löwenstein-Jensen culture medium are best for isolating the organism. Once confirmed, treatment can be narrowed to include drugs such as amikacin and clarithromycin. Topical fourth-generation fluoroquinolones seem to have anti-NTM activity as well but should probably not be used as monotherapy given conflicting reports on susceptibility [49, 50]. Generally speaking, treatment with two topical antibiotics is preferred, and therapy is usually tapered over 1–3 months, as recrudescence of infection can occur.

Fungal Keratitis

Fungi causing keratitis may be categorized as yeast, filamentous septated, or filamentous nonseptated. *Aspergillus* spp. are filamentous septated fungi and are the most common cause of fungal keratitis worldwide [42, 51]. Other more common causes include *Candida* spp. (yeast) and *Fusarium* spp. (filamentous septated). A large number of other species (e.g., *Paecilomyces* spp., *Alternaria* spp., *Curvularia* spp., and *Acremonium* spp.) have also been reported in the literature in smaller numbers. Fungal infections are more common in tropical and rural climates; as such, even though they are a relatively uncommon occurrence in comparison to bacterial keratitis worldwide, they make up as much as a third of microbial keratitis cases in Southern India [52]. There is also a geographic predilection for certain fungi; for instance, *Fusarium* spp. are more common in the southern United States.

Fungal keratitis has a more indolent course compared to other forms of microbial keratitis, especially that caused by *Pseudomonas* spp. Instead of presenting within 24–48 h of symptom onset, patients may first experience slight foreign body sensation with increasing pain over 4–5 days. The clinical appearance at presentation is similar in many ways to bacterial keratitis: an epithelial defect is usually but not necessarily present, the infiltrate is typically suppurative, and there may be an anterior chamber reaction with hypopyon. On the other hand, fungal keratitis is more likely to have feathery margins, satellite lesions, and macroscopic gray or

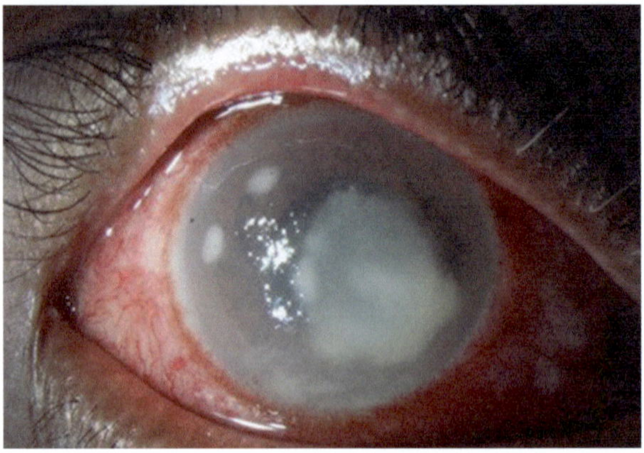

Fig. 5.4 *Fusarium* corneal ulcer. Typically characterized by suppurative infiltrate with soft or feathery borders and satellite lesions

brown pigmentation (Fig. 5.4). With this being said, there is no definitive way to distinguish between bacterial and fungal keratitis clinically. Microbiologic workup is absolutely required and obviates speculative treatment and mismanagement.

Once the diagnosis is made, treatment may be narrowed to cover the infecting organism. In the United States, topical natamycin 5 % is commercially available and remains the first choice for the treatment of filamentous fungi (e.g., *Fusarium* spp.). If the infection does not respond, or in the case of a yeast infection, Amphotericin B (compounded in the United States) may be substituted. Topical voriconazole can also be compounded; though expensive, its spectrum of activity and improved toxicity profile makes it an attractive choice as another first-line agent [53]. The role for the addition of an oral imidazole (e.g., ketoconazole, fluconazole, or voriconazole) is controversial in the treatment of keratitis but is likely beneficial if the infiltrate approaches the limbus or in the case of fungal sclerokeratitis. There are no guidelines on the duration of treatment for fungal keratitis; this is decided on a case by case basis, though most agree that the treatment time required to clear the infection and prevent recurrence is longer than that of bacterial keratitis.

Acanthamoeba

Acanthamoeba spp. are protozoa universally found in soil and freshwater that live by preying on other microorganisms. They exist in two forms – an active trophozoite form and an inactive cyst form. Infection likely occurs while the organism is a trophozoite. However, when challenged with antimicrobial medication, it can encyst rapidly and remain viable and dormant for weeks, months, or even years. It is best known for its role in acanthamoeba keratitis (AK) but can rarely manifest in other ways systemically (e.g., granulomatous amoebic encephalitis).

It is important to keep in mind that AK is a rare infection, making up approximately 0–2.4 % of culture-proven microbial keratitis isolates [7, 13, 17]. With that being said, contact lens wear is the largest risk factor for AK. It is interesting to note that while 400–800 per 10,000 contact lens storage cases are contaminated with *Acanthamoeba*, the incidence of AK among contact lens wearers is thought to be only 0.01–1.49 per 10,000 [54]. Other risk factors include a history of exposure to contaminated water, such as natural streams, lakes, or hot tubs. If the patient presents early, he or she may complain of foreign body sensation or photophobia, visual acuity will be variable, and examination might reveal nothing more than an epitheliopathy, often described as granular or cystic appearing. Alternatively, epithelial pseudodendrites might misleadingly suggest a diagnosis of herpes simplex keratitis (Fig. 5.5). If the diagnosis is not considered at this point, the disease process continues, and the patient is likely to return complaining of increasing, excruciating pain out of proportion to physical exam findings. An anterior stromal infiltrate and radial perineuritis are classic findings in the middle stages of the

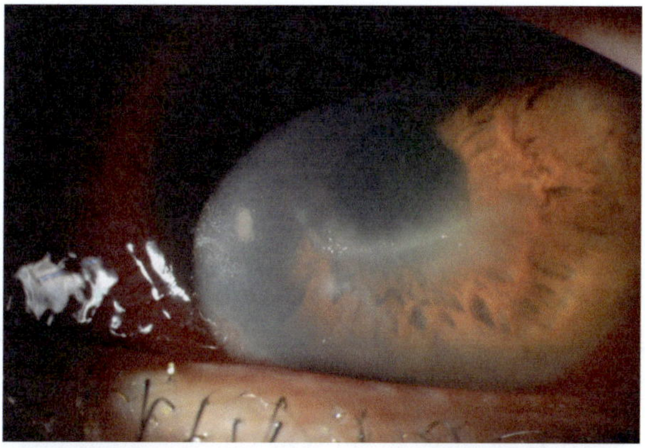

Fig. 5.5 Acanthamoeba keratitis with dendritiform appearance. These manifestations of early acanthamoeba infection cause frequent confusion with herpes simplex keratitis

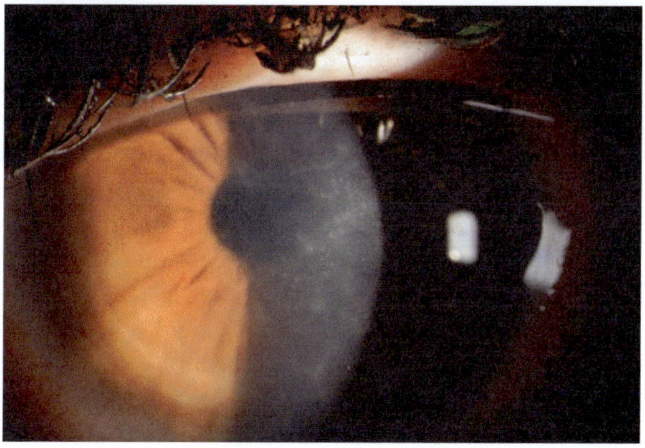

Fig. 5.6 Acanthamoeba-associated perineuritis

disease (Fig. 5.6). If untreated, a "ring infiltrate" develops in late-stage AK. Although the ring infiltrate often clues the physician in to the diagnosis, beginning treatment at this late stage comes with a more guarded prognosis and risk for complications requiring surgical management. As such, maintaining a high index of suspicion when evaluating any keratitis helps to minimize the missed opportunities for early treatment.

Diagnosis of AK starts with a high index of suspicion, as the protozoa are unlikely to grow on standard culture media or broth. Since *Acanthamoeba* spp. characteristically feed on other microorganisms, they are best cultured on a non-nutrient agar with E. coli overlay. Corneal smears or biopsies incorporating corneal epithelium and stroma are extremely helpful and are more sensitive than cultures. Gram or calcofluor-white stains can be useful. Lastly, confocal microscopy has an emerging and increasingly important role in the diagnosis of AK. The cysts are round and between 15 and 35 μm in size; since no other cell or structure native to the cornea fits this description, identification of such structures on confocal imaging, in the context of a supportive clinical history, has a sensitivity and specificity of 90 and 77 %, respectively [55]. However, the reliability of a confocal microscopy study is highly dependent upon both the operator's familiarity with using the confocal microscope and the clinician's experience interpreting the images.

There are no universally accepted guidelines for the medical treatment of AK. However, most agree that therapy should include a biguanide, either polyhexamethylene 0.02 % or chlorhexidine 0.02 % [56]. There are several studies that also support the addition of a diamidine (propamidine 0.1 % or hexamidine 0.1 %) [57, 58]. Diamidines have anti-trophozoite activity and retard the transformation to cyst form, while the biguanides have both anti-trophozoite and cysticidal activity. Monotherapy or dual therapy is applied topically every hour around the clock for the first 48 h and then during the day only for an additional 1–3 days. This intense early therapy is indicated to kill acanthamoebae while they are most susceptible, in the trophozoite form, and before they have a chance to encyst. Therapy is then tapered slowly over 4–6 weeks down to four times daily dosing and then tailored appropriately on a case-by-case basis. Six months of therapy is not uncommon and is occasionally indicated for even a year or longer. Corneal toxicity associated with use of the above medications is common. A short drug holiday, which results in improvement in the case of toxicity and worsening in the case of recalcitrant disease, helps to differentiate the two.

Surgical management of AK is centered upon therapeutic penetrating keratoplasty, but its role in the acute setting is controversial. Since it is nearly impossible to determine clear margins in the operating room, and cure rate with medical therapy is high, cornea transplantation should probably be reserved for those patients that develop eye-threatening complications of disease (e.g., corneal perforation or impending infection of the limbus or sclera). On the other hand, penetrating keratoplasty does have a role as a sight-restoring procedure once the infection has subsided. This is generally done no less than 3 months after the cessation of topical anti-amoebic agents, with documented absence of recurrent disease.

Diagnostic and Therapeutic Algorithm

The algorithm used to manage a patient with suspected microbial keratitis is dependent upon the environment in which a physician practices. For the majority of ophthalmologists practicing in the United States, culture media are not readily available at all times. Furthermore, prescribing topical fortified antibiotics requires ready access to a compounding pharmacy. For these reasons, small peripheral corneal ulcers that are not vision threatening on presentation are often empirically treated with commercially available fluoroquinolones like Vigamox (moxifloxacin) or Zymar (gatifloxacin). This is especially true when the patient has a history of contact lens use and the suspected organism is *Pseudomonas* spp. There is good evidence to support the position that this practice is as efficacious as therapy with fortified antibiotics [59, 60]. At the same time, careful attention should be paid to situations in which empiric coverage is inappropriate and likely to only delay proper treatment. When the patient gives a history of trauma, is hospitalized or ventilator dependent and immunocompromised, or has a central or severe corneal ulcer, a culture-guided approach is preferred, and the patient may be better served at an academic or tertiary care center.

A culture-guided algorithm is depicted in Fig. 5.7. When cultures are obtained, the scrapings must be plated on media that support growth of the most commonly encountered organisms. Common culture media are listed in Table 5.3 and include blood agar, chocolate agar, Sabouraud agar, and thioglycolate broth. These are the media on which initial cultures are usually plated. It is only when there is a risk factor for an atypical infection or the clinical picture worsens and cultures are inconclusive that ancillary plates are typically used. A standard stain such as the gram stain is also often obtained simultaneously (Table 5.4). Once cultures have been

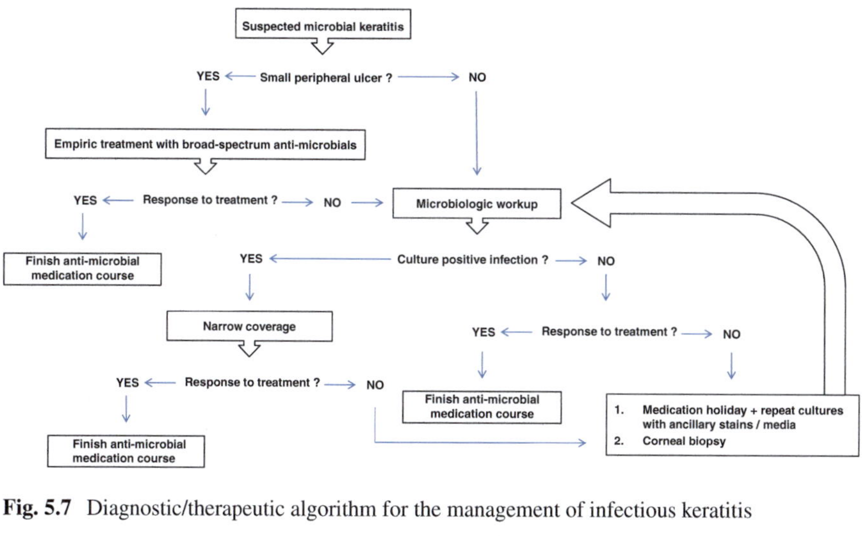

Fig. 5.7 Diagnostic/therapeutic algorithm for the management of infectious keratitis

Table 5.3 Common culture media

Culture media	Common isolates	Comment
Blood agar	Aerobic and facultative anaerobic bacteria	Incubate at 35°
Chocolate agar	Primarily anaerobic bacteria and facultative anaerobic, but may also grow aerobic	Incubate at 35°
Sabouraud agar	Primarily fungi, but may also grow filamentous bacteria e.g., *Nocardia* spp.	Incubate at room temperature
Thioglycolate broth	Aerobic, anaerobic, and facultative anaerobic bacteria	Incubate at 35°
Löwenstein-Jensen medium	*Mycobacterium* and *Nocardia* spp.	Incubate at 35°
Thayer-Martin agar	*Neisseria* spp.	Incubate at 35°
Non-nutrient agar with *E. coli* overlay	*Acanthamoeba* spp.	Incubate at room temperature

Table 5.4 Stains

Stain	Organism seen
Gram stain	Bacteria (gram-positive vs. gram-negative), fungi, acanthamoebae
Giemsa stain	Bacteria, fungi, chlamydia, acanthamoebae
Acid fast	Mycobacteria, nocardia
Calcofluor white	Fungi, acanthamoebae

obtained, the patient may be started on empiric broad-spectrum topical fortified antibiotics. Vancomycin 25 mg/ml is usually combined with either tobramycin 14 mg/ml or ceftazidime 50 mg/ml.

After the initial evaluation, the patient is seen within 24–48 h, depending on the severity of the ulcer. The goal of the follow-up visit is to assess for interval change, alter medical therapy in concert with microbiologic culture results, and rule out eye-threatening complications requiring surgical management. Unfortunately, the yield from corneal cultures is only 50 % [61]. If, however, culture results are positive, topical medical therapy is narrowed to cover the infecting organism and limit the effects of toxicity from unnecessary medications (Table 5.5). If culture results are negative, but there is significant improvement in the clinical picture, empiric therapy may be continued and tapered over 1–3 weeks. If culture results are negative and the clinical picture has worsened, the clinician must make a choice between (1) instituting a medication holiday for 24 h to allow the infecting organism to grow uninhibited before repeating cultures or (2) performing a corneal biopsy, which is subsequently emulsified and plated on culture media for higher yield [62]. If and when repeat cultures are taken, ancillary culture media are added at the physician's discretion (e.g., Löwenstein-Jensen medium, or non-nutrient agar with E. coli overlay) to further explore the possibility of an atypical bacterial or parasitic infection.

The role for topical corticosteroids in the setting of microbial keratitis is controversial. There is no literature to suggest that adding corticosteroids alters the clinical

Table 5.5 Common infecting organisms and preferred antimicrobial agents

Organism	Preferred antimicrobial
Gram-positive cocci (e.g., *Staphylococcus aureus*)	Vancomycin Cefazolin Fluoroquinolones (4th generation)
Gram-negative bacilli (e.g., *Pseudomonas aeruginosa*)	Tobramycin Gentamucin Ceftazidime Fluoroquinolones
Gram-negative cocci (e.g., *Neisseria gonorrhoeae*)	Ceftriaxone Ceftazidime Fluoroquinolones
Nontuberculous mycobacteria (e.g., *Mycobacteria chelonae*)	Amikacin Clarithromycin Azithromycin
Nocardia	Amikacin Trimethoprim/sulfamethoxazol
Candida	Amphotericin

course [63]. Nevertheless, some clinicians choose to use topical corticosteroid therapy judiciously with the belief that its use decreases inflammation and scarring. Opponents argue that its use may rekindle a clearing infection, promote corneal melt through inhibition of collagen synthesis, and promote persistent epithelial defects through inhibition of epithelial cell migration. If corticosteroids are to be started, institution of therapy is usually delayed until 48–72 h after antibiotic therapy is begun. It is especially helpful if culture results are known, but steroids might also be considered so long as the infection has shown steady and consistent improvement over 2–3 days with empiric antibiotic therapy.

Other Therapeutic Management Options

Surgical Management of Complications

Surgical interventions for the management of active microbial keratitis are generally considered an option of last resort, when the alternative is an impending vision or eye-threatening complication. For instance, cytokine and matrix metalloproteinase release at the site of active infection leads to proteolytic stromal degradation and necrosis, and, in severe cases, descemetocele or perforation. Whether the perforation is impending or realized, application of cyanoacrylate tissue adhesive is a reasonable option. The glue may be used to seal perforations or cover descemetoceles up to 2–3 mm in size. It is especially helpful when the ulcer is bacterial, being appropriately treated with antibiotics, and simply requires a tectonic reinforcement where active necrosis is occurring. The minimum amount of glue needed is applied, followed by a therapeutic bandage contact lens. Successful cyanoacrylate gluing avoids an emergent therapeutic keratoplasty, allowing the infection to finish clearing and the eye to quiet. The glue and contact lens generally remains in place until it either spontaneously dislodges or the patient undergoes another surgical intervention. Glue may be less helpful in the setting of fungal, atypical mycobacterial, or parasitic infections that are more indolent or associated with smoldering necrosis.

Therapeutic penetrating keratoplasty is an option of last resort and is reserved for cases in which there is either a perforation that cannot be closed with tissue adhesive or limbal involvement of the infection with risk for developing infectious scleritis. In either case, it is important to counsel the patient preoperatively on the goals of surgery in this setting: namely to reestablish a formed globe to avoid endophthalmitis and to avoid progression of the infection to the sclera, which carries a much poorer prognosis. The patient must also understand that the risk of bleeding, suprachoroidal hemorrhage, subsequent permanent vision loss, or loss of the eye is higher than with penetrating keratoplasty in a quiet eye. Furthermore, the patient should be counseled on the increased risk of graft rejection and failure in this setting, and the possible need for a second optical penetrating keratoplasty 3–6 months after the inflammatory response is controlled.

Management of Persistent Epithelial Defects

Microbial keratitis almost universally results in an epithelial defect. Treatment often entails use of fortified antibiotics that are toxic to the corneal epithelium. As the infection clears, a scar usually forms; Bowman's membrane is destroyed and replaced by an irregular network of collagen and fibrous scar tissue. Lastly, in the case of concurrent corticosteroid treatment, collagen synthesis and epithelial cell migration may be inhibited. All of the above factors contribute to the development of a nonhealing epithelial defect. This sequela requires careful consideration so that reinfection, prolonged pain, progressive thinning, and perforation do not occur.

Table 5.6 Management options for persistent epithelial defects

Management options for persistent epithelial defects
Frequent lubrication with preservative-free artificial tears
Discontinue topical medications containing benzalkonium chloride
Decrease or discontinue topical corticosteroids
Punctal occlusion
Debridement
Therapeutic soft contact lens
Amniotic membrane transplant
Autologous serum tears
Pressure patch
Tarsorrhaphy
Scleral contact lens (e.g., PROSE)

The management of persistent epithelial defects is challenging but can be approached in a stepwise fashion (Table 5.6). The most conservative, cheapest, and convenient interventions might be tried first. Judiciously decreasing toxic topical antibiotic (potentially containing benzalkonium chloride) and corticosteroid drops, along with frequent lubrication with preservative-free artificial tears and ointments, is a logical first step. If, after this, the patient returns with a persistent epithelial defect, a therapeutic soft contact lens might be considered [64]. The contact lens acts as a mechanical barrier between the corneal epithelium and the lids and allows the epithelial cells to migrate without being sloughed. Similarly, an amniotic membrane can be placed over the defect. The amniotic membrane not only provides the mechanical barrier of a contact lens but also may act as a scaffold for migrating corneal epithelial cells. Other options include pressure patching, temporary or permanent tarsorrhaphy, or the administration of autologous serum tears. Regardless of the intervention used, an antibiotic should remain part of the treatment regimen to prevent reinfection in this unstable situation.

Prognosis

The prognosis of microbial keratitis is highly variable and dependent upon patient access to appropriate resources, time to presentation, causative organism, and compliance with the treatment regimen. Outcomes are more favorable in developed countries with accessible ophthalmologists and tertiary care centers. In one study from the Netherlands, 67 % of contact lens-associated keratitis cases had best-corrected visual acuities better than 20/100 [35]. Conversely, a study from East Africa showed that 66 % of patients with microbial keratitis had BCVA outcomes worse than 20/200 [65]. Low BCVA at the time of presentation, previous care by another provider with subsequent referral, and topical corticosteroid use before diagnosis are all predictors of poor final BCVA and need for surgical intervention. Rarely, microbial keratitis progresses to endophthalmitis. These high-risk eyes have particularly poor outcomes, with upward of 60 % requiring evisceration/enucleation [66]. Whether the infecting organism is bacterial, fungal, or parasitic is a less important prognostic indicator; this fact undermines the importance of timely referral to eye care providers well versed in the proper diagnosis and management of microbial keratitis.

References

1. Pepose JS, Wilhelmus KR. Divergent approaches to the management of corneal ulcers. Am J Ophthalmol. 1992;114:630–2.
2. Erie JC, Nevitt MP, Hodge DO, Ballard DJ. Incidence of ulcerative keratitis in a defined population from 1950 through 1988. Arch Ophthalmol. 1993;111:1665–71.
3. Thylefors B. Present challenges in the global prevention of blindness. Aust N Z J Ophthalmol. 1992;20:89–94.

4. Whitcher JP, Srinivasan M, Upadhyay MP. Corneal blindness: a global perspective. Bull World Health Organ. 2001;79:214–21.
5. Gonzales CA, Srinivasan M, Whitcher JP, Smolin G. Incidence of corneal ulceration in Madurai district, South India. Ophthalmic Epidemiol. 1996;3:159–66.
6. Dart JK. Disease and risks associated with contact lenses. Br J Ophthalmol. 1993;77:49–53.
7. Cao J, Yang Y, Yang W, Wu R, Xiao X, Yuan J, et al. Prevalence of infectious keratitis in Central China. BMC Ophthalmol. 2014;14:43.
8. Song X, Xie L, Tan X, Wang Z, Yang Y, Yuan Y, et al. A multi-center, cross-sectional study on the burden of infectious keratitis in China. PLoS One. 2014;9, e113843.
9. Henry CR, Flynn Jr HW, Miller D, Forster RK, Alfonso EC. Infectious keratitis progressing to endophthalmitis: a 15-year study of microbiology, associated factors, and clinical outcomes. Ophthalmology. 2012;119:2443–9.
10. Selinger DS, Selinger RC, Reed WP. Resistance to infection of the external eye: the role of tears. Surv Ophthalmol. 1979;24:33–8.
11. Sommer A. Effects of vitamin A deficiency on the ocular surface. Ophthalmology. 1983;90:592–600.
12. Knop N, Knop E. Conjunctiva-associated lymphoid tissue in the human eye. Invest Ophthalmol Visual Sci. 2000;41:1270–9.
13. Bharathi MJ, Ramakrishnan R, Meenakshi R, Padmavathy S, Shivakumar C, Srinivasan M. Microbial keratitis in South India: influence of risk factors, climate, and geographical variation. Ophthalmic Epidemiol. 2007;14:61–9.
14. Houang E, Lam D, Fan D, Seal D. Microbial keratitis in Hong Kong: relationship to climate, environment and contact-lens disinfection. Trans R Soc Trop Med Hyg. 2001;95:361–7.
15. Stapleton F, Keay LJ, Sanfilippo PG, Katiyar S, Edwards KP, Naduvilath T. Relationship between climate, disease severity, and causative organism for contact lens-associated microbial keratitis in Australia. Am J Ophthalmol. 2007;144:690–8.
16. Bharathi MJ, Ramakrishnan R, Vasu S, Meenakshi R, Palaniappan R. Epidiomiological characteristics and laboratory diagnosis of fungal keratitis. A three-year study. Indian J Ophthalmol. 2003;51:315–21.
17. Gopinathan U, Sharma S, Garg P, Rao GN. Review of epidemiological features, microbiological diagnosis and treatment outcome of microbial keratitis: experience of over a decade. Indian J Ophthalmol. 2009;57:273–9.
18. Joslin CE, Tu EY, McMahon TT, Passaro DJ, Stayner LT, Sugar J. Epidemiological characteristics of a Chicago-area Acanthamoeba keratitis outbreak. Am J Ophthalmol. 2006;142:212–7.
19. Joslin CE, Tu EY, Shoff ME, Anderson RJ, Davis FG. Shifting distribution of Chicago-area Acanthamoeba keratitis cases. Arch Ophthalmol. 2010;128:137–9.
20. Stapleton F, Keay L, Edwards K, Naduvilath T, Dart JK, Brian G, et al. The incidence of contact lens-related microbial keratitis in Australia. Ophthalmology. 2008;115:1655–62.
21. Yildiz EH, Airiani S, Hammersmith KM, Rapuano CJ, Laibson PR, Virdi AS, et al. Trends in contact lens-related corneal ulcers at a tertiary referral center. Cornea. 2012;31:1097–102.
22. Bullimore MA, Sinnott LT, Jones-Jordan LA. The risk of microbial keratitis with overnight corneal reshaping lenses. Optom Vis Sci. 2013;90:937–44.
23. Ma SK, So K, Chung PH, Tsang HF, Chuang SK. A multi-country outbreak of fungal keratitis associated with a brand of contact lens solution: the Hong Kong experience. Int J Infect Dis. 2009;13:443–8.
24. Green M, Apel A, Stapleton F. Risk factors and causative organisms in microbial keratitis. Cornea. 2008;27:22–7.
25. de Rojas V, Llovet F, Martinez M, Cobo-Soriano R, Ortega-Usobiaga J, Beltran J, et al. Infectious keratitis in 18,651 laser surface ablation procedures. J Cataract Refract Surg. 2011;37:1822–31.
26. Ortega-Usobiaga J, Llovet-Osuna F, Djodeyre MR, Llovet-Rausell A, Beltran J, Baviera J. Incidence of corneal infections after laser in situ keratomileusis and surface ablation when moxifloxacin and tobramycin are used as postoperative treatment. J Cataract Refract Surg. 2015;41:1210–6.

27. Das S, Constantinou M, Ong T, Taylor HR. Microbial keratitis following corneal transplantation. Clin Experiment Ophthalmol. 2007;35:427–31.
28. Nielsen SE, Nielsen E, Julian HO, Lindegaard J, Hojgaard K, Ivarsen A, et al. Incidence and clinical characteristics of fungal keratitis in a Danish population from 2000 to 2013. Acta Ophthalmol. 2015;93:54–8.
29. Schein OD, Wasson PJ, Boruchoff SA, Kenyon KR. Microbial keratitis associated with contaminated ocular medications. Am J Ophthalmol. 1988;105:361–5.
30. Dalmon C, Porco TC, Lietman TM, Prajna NV, Prajna L, Das MR, et al. The clinical differentiation of bacterial and fungal keratitis: a photographic survey. Invest Ophthalmol Vis Sci. 2012;53:1787–91.
31. Hsiao CH, Ong SJ, Chuang CC, Ma DH, Huang YC. A comparison of clinical features between community-associated and healthcare-associated methicillin-resistant Staphylococcus aureus keratitis. J Ophthalmol. 2015;2015:923941.
32. Chang VS, Dhaliwal DK, Raju L, Kowalski RP. Antibiotic resistance in the treatment of Staphylococcus aureus keratitis: a 20-year review. Cornea. 2015;34:698–703.
33. Manikandan P, Bhaskar M, Revathy R, John RK, Narendran K, Narendran V. Speciation of coagulase negative staphylococcus causing bacterial keratitis. Indian J Ophthalmol. 2005;53:59–60.
34. Charteris DG, Batterbury M, Armstrong M, Tullo AB. Suppurative keratitis caused by Streptococcus pneumoniae after cataract surgery. Br J Ophthalmol. 1994;78:847–9.
35. Hoddenbach JG, Boekhoorn SS, Wubbels R, Vreugdenhil W, Van Rooij J, Geerards AJ. Clinical presentation and morbidity of contact lens-associated microbial keratitis: a retrospective study. Graefes Arch Clin Exp Ophthalmol. 2014;252:299–306.
36. Ng AL, To KK, Choi CC, Yuen LH, Yim SM, Chan KS, et al. Predisposing factors, microbial characteristics, and clinical outcome of microbial keratitis in a tertiary centre in Hong Kong: a 10-year experience. J Ophthalmol. 2015;2015:769436.
37. Ni N, Nam EM, Hammersmith KM, Nagra PK, Azari AA, Leiby BE, et al. Seasonal, geographic, and antimicrobial resistance patterns in microbial keratitis: 4-year experience in eastern Pennsylvania. Cornea. 2015;34:296–302.
38. Klotz SA, Misra RP, Butrus SI. Contact lens wear enhances adherence of Pseudomonas aeruginosa and binding of lectins to the cornea. Cornea. 1990;9:266–70.
39. Chaudhry NA, Flynn Jr HW, Murray TG, Tabandeh H, Mello Jr MO, Miller D. Emerging ciprofloxacin-resistant Pseudomonas aeruginosa. Am J Ophthalmol. 1999;128:509–10.
40. Garg P, Sharma S, Rao GN. Ciprofloxacin-resistant Pseudomonas keratitis. Ophthalmology. 1999;106:1319–23.
41. Lalitha P. Nocardia keratitis. Curr Opin Ophthalmol. 2009;20:318–23.
42. Upadhyay MP, Karmacharya PC, Koirala S, Tuladhar NR, Bryan LE, Smolin G, et al. Epidemiologic characteristics, predisposing factors, and etiologic diagnosis of corneal ulceration in Nepal. Am J Ophthalmol. 1991;111:92–9.
43. Faramarzi A, Feizi S, Javadi MA, Rezaei Kanavi M, Yazdizadeh F, Moein HR. Bilateral nocardia keratitis after photorefractive keratectomy. J Ophthalmic Vis Res. 2012;7:162–6.
44. Pandya VB, Petsoglou C. Nocardia transvalensis resistant to amikacin: an unusual cause of microbial keratitis. Cornea. 2008;27:1082–5.
45. Lalitha P, Srinivasan M, Rajaraman R, Ravindran M, Mascarenhas J, Priya JL, et al. Nocardia keratitis: clinical course and effect of corticosteroids. Am J Ophthalmol. 2012;154:934–9, e1.
46. Glasgow LA, Overall JC. Infections of the newborn. In: Vaughan VC, Behrman RE, Nelson WE, editors. Nelson textbook of pediatrics. Philadelphia: WB Saunders; 1983. p. 399–406.
47. Lee JS, Choi HY, Lee JE, Lee SH, Oum BS. Gonococcal keratoconjunctivitis in adults. Eye (Lond). 2002;16:646–9.
48. Kheir WJ, Sheheitli H, Abdul Fattah M, Hamam RN. Nontuberculous mycobacterial ocular infections: a systematic review of the literature. Biomed Res Int. 2015;2015:164989.
49. Abshire R, Cockrum P, Crider J, Schlech B. Topical antibacterial therapy for mycobacterial keratitis: potential for surgical prophylaxis and treatment. Clin Ther. 2004;26:191–6.

50. Girgis DO, Karp CL, Miller D. Ocular infections caused by non-tuberculous mycobacteria: update on epidemiology and management. Clin Experiment Ophthalmol. 2012;40:467–75.
51. Foster CS. Fungal keratitis. Infect Dis Clin North Am. 1992;6:851–7.
52. Lalitha P, Prajna NV, Manoharan G, Srinivasan M, Mascarenhas J, Das M, et al. Trends in bacterial and fungal keratitis in South India, 2002–2012. Br J Ophthalmol. 2015;99:192–4.
53. Tuli SS. Fungal keratitis. Clin Ophthalmol. 2011;5:275–9.
54. Lorenzo-Morales J, Khan NA, Walochnik J. An update on Acanthamoeba keratitis: diagnosis, pathogenesis and treatment. Parasite. 2015;22:10.
55. Tu EY, Joslin CE, Sugar J, Booton GC, Shoff ME, Fuerst PA. The relative value of confocal microscopy and superficial corneal scrapings in the diagnosis of Acanthamoeba keratitis. Cornea. 2008;27:764–72.
56. Lim N, Goh D, Bunce C, Xing W, Fraenkel G, Poole TR, et al. Comparison of polyhexamethylene biguanide and chlorhexidine as monotherapy agents in the treatment of Acanthamoeba keratitis. Am J Ophthalmol. 2008;145(1):130–5.
57. Duguid IG, Dart JK, Morlet N, Allan BD, Matheson M, Ficker L, et al. Outcome of acanthamoeba keratitis treated with polyhexamethyl biguanide and propamidine. Ophthalmology. 1997;104:1587–92.
58. Seal D, Hay J, Kirkness C, Morrell A, Booth A, Tullo A, et al. Successful medical therapy of Acanthamoeba keratitis with topical chlorhexidine and propamidine. Eye (Lond). 1996;10: 413–21.
59. Constantinou M, Daniell M, Snibson GR, Vu HT, Taylor HR. Clinical efficacy of moxifloxacin in the treatment of bacterial keratitis: a randomized clinical trial. Ophthalmology. 2007;114:1622–9.
60. Shah VM, Tandon R, Satpathy G, Nayak N, Chawla B, Agarwal T, et al. Randomized clinical study for comparative evaluation of fourth-generation fluoroquinolones with the combination of fortified antibiotics in the treatment of bacterial corneal ulcers. Cornea. 2010;29:751–7.
61. Alexandrakis G, Alfonso EC, Miller D. Shifting trends in bacterial keratitis in south Florida and emerging resistance to fluoroquinolones. Ophthalmology. 2000;107:1497–502.
62. Alexandrakis G, Haimovici R, Miller D, Alfonso EC. Corneal biopsy in the management of progressive microbial keratitis. Am J Ophthalmol. 2000;129:571–6.
63. Srinivasan M, Mascarenhas J, Rajaraman R, Ravindran M, Lalitha P, Glidden DV, et al. Corticosteroids for bacterial keratitis: the Steroids for Corneal Ulcers Trial (SCUT). Arch Ophthalmol. 2012;130:143–50.
64. Lois N, Cohen EJ, Rapuano CJ, Laibson PR. Contact lens use after contact lens-associated infectious ulcers. CLAO J. 1997;23:192–5.
65. Burton MJ, Pithuwa J, Okello E, Afwamba I, Onyango JJ, Oates F, et al. Microbial keratitis in East Africa: why are the outcomes so poor? Ophthalmic Epidemiol. 2011;18:158–63.
66. O'Neill EC, Yeoh J, Fabinyi DC, Cassidy D, Vajpayee RB, Allen P, et al. Risk factors, microbial profiles and prognosis of microbial keratitis-associated endophthalmitis in high-risk eyes. Graefes Arch Clin Exp Ophthalmol. 2014;252:1457–62.

Chapter 6
Intraocular Infection

Andre J. Witkin

Introduction

Intraocular infections are uncommon but potentially devastating to vision and to the eye. There is a broad range of pathogens that can cause infection in the eye. Intraocular infections can be grouped into two categories: *exogenous*, those caused by introduction of pathogens through penetration of the eye wall, or *endogenous*, those caused by introduction of the pathogen through the bloodstream to the eye [1]. Exogenous infections can be introduced via surgery, intraocular injection of medication, or trauma, and pathogens are typically either bacterial or fungal in nature [2–6]. Endogenous infections are caused by introduction of a systemic infection to the eye via the ophthalmic (usually choroidal) circulation, and therefore pathogens can be much more varied and include bacteria, fungi, viruses, protozoa, and other parasites. This chapter categorizes and describes different types of intraocular infections and their treatments.

Exogenous Endophthalmitis

Exogenous endophthalmitis is one of the most dreaded complications of intraocular surgery, intravitreal injection, or penetrating ocular trauma. It is most often classified based on the mechanism of introduction, as different organisms are associated with different mechanisms of introduction into the eye. Postoperative endophthalmitis usually presents after recent intraocular surgery, but it can also have a delayed presentation or can be associated with distant surgery (e.g., bleb-associated

A.J. Witkin, MD
Retina Service, Tufts Medical Center-New England Eye Center, Tufts University School of Medicine, 800 Washington Street, Box 450, Boston, MA 02111, USA
e-mail: awitkin@tuftsmedicalcenter.org

N.V. Laver, C.S. Specht (eds.), *The Infected Eye*,
DOI 10.1007/978-3-319-42840-6_6

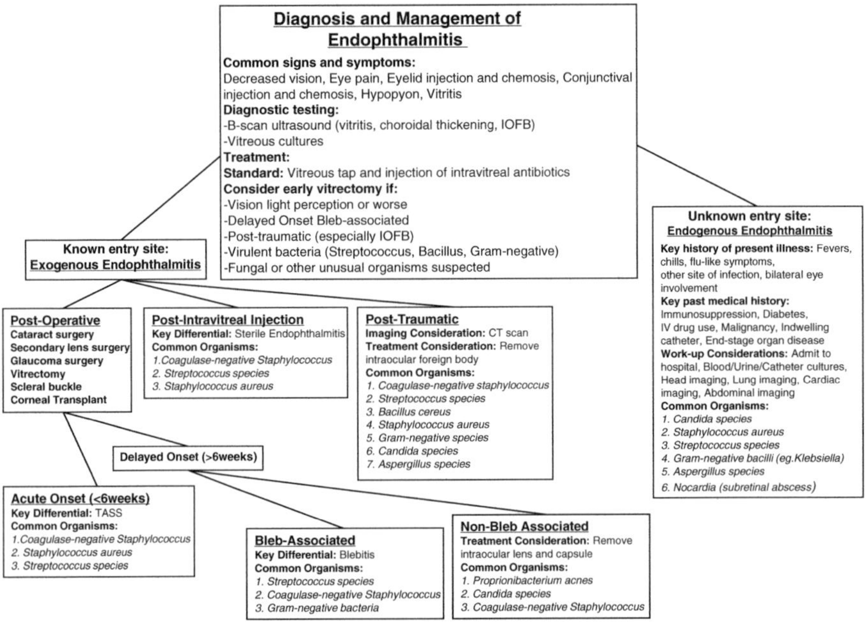

Fig. 6.1 Diagnosis and management of endophthalmitis. *IOFB* intraocular foreign body, *TASS* toxic anterior segment syndrome

endophthalmitis). Post-injection endophthalmitis has become more common with the advent of intravitreal injections for treatment of a variety of ocular diseases. Posttraumatic endophthalmitis is rare but can be associated with a greater variety of bacteria as well as fungi. Distinguishing features of these various types of exogenous endophthalmitis are discussed in more detail below, but many of the presenting features and management decisions are similar. For a summary of diagnosis and management of endophthalmitis, see Fig. 6.1.

Presentation

Patients with exogenous endophthalmitis most commonly present with blurred vision after a known introductory event, whether it be surgery, intraocular injection, or trauma [1–7]. Other symptoms include ocular pain, conjunctival or eyelid redness and/or swelling, ocular irritation, and/or photophobia. Onset may be acute (<6 weeks) or delayed (>6 weeks) after the inciting event [8]. Signs of infection on ophthalmic examination may include decreased visual acuity, relative afferent papillary defect, increased or decreased intraocular pressure, conjunctival and/or eyelid injection and chemosis, anterior chamber inflammation, hypopyon, vitritis on examination and B-scan ultrasound, and choroidal thickening (Figs. 6.2, 6.3, and 6.4). If the retina is visible in the eyes with endophthalmitis, retinal hemorrhages, nerve fiber layer infarcts, retinitis, perivasculitis, and subretinal exudation may also be seen [9]. More virulent organisms are associated with a more guarded prognosis [10] and should be suspected if there is an early presentation (<3 days after inciting

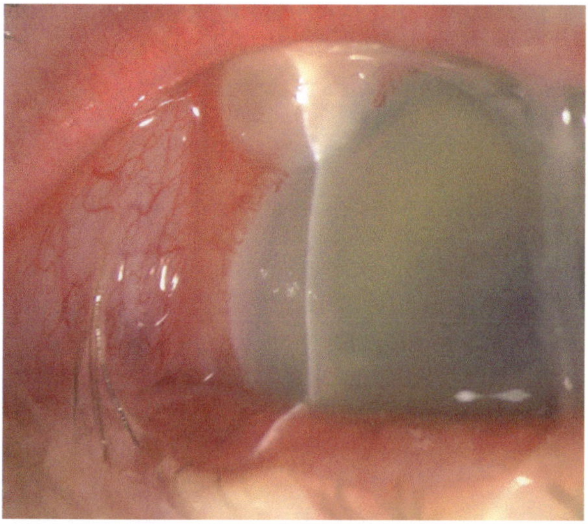

Fig. 6.2 Bleb-associated endophthalmitis. Cultures grew out *Streptococcus pneumoniae*. Purulent material is visible within the bleb. There is severe ecchymosis and chemosis of the conjunctiva. The cornea is edematous, and there is a severe anterior chamber reaction

event), trauma as the inciting event, severe eye pain, very poor visual acuity on presentation (light perception or no light perception), low intraocular pressure, conjunctival and/or eyelid chemosis, and/or dense intraocular inflammation.

Diagnostic Testing

B-scan ultrasound is often useful to detect presence and amount of vitritis. Choroidal thickening on B-scan is a poor prognostic sign. Intraocular foreign bodies may be visualized using B-scan, although radiographic imaging is often warranted in post-traumatic cases suspected of having intraocular foreign material.

A vitreous or aqueous tap is often performed at the time of intravitreal antibiotic injection. This procedure is not only helpful in allowing more space for intravitreal fluid to be injected, but the specimen may also be sent for stain and culture [1, 3, 7, 11]. Vitreous cultures may have higher yield after pars plana vitrectomy (PPV) cases with difficult-to-culture organisms, such as in fungal endophthalmitis; however, the Endophthalmitis Vitrectomy Study (EVS) showed no difference in culture positivity between the tap and PPV groups [12].

In acute postoperative endophthalmitis, vitreous cultures may be negative in up to 30 % of cases [1, 13]; aqueous cultures are more often negative than vitreous cultures. In fact, in one study, 50 % of eyes that had negative aqueous cultures had positive vitreous cultures [14]. Vitreous cultures in delayed-onset postoperative endophthalmitis are often negative. In post-injection endophthalmitis, the percentage of negative vitreous cultures is higher than in postoperative endophthalmitis (50 % vs. 75 % culture-positive rates) [15]. This may be due to an increased percentage of sterile or noninfectious endophthalmitis cases included in these numbers.

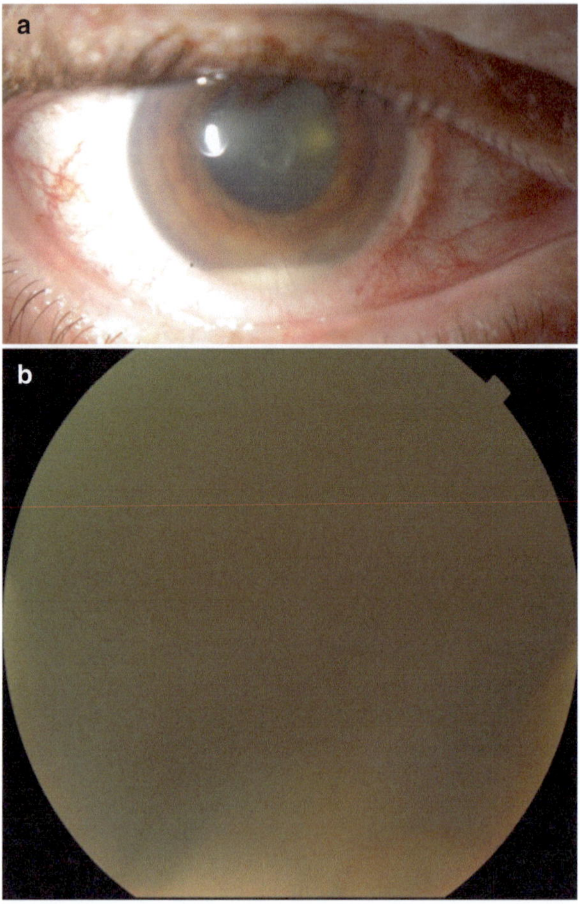

Fig. 6.3 Endogenous bacterial endophthalmitis. (**a**) There is mild corneal edema, moderate anterior chamber fibrin and white cells, and a 3 mm hypopyon. (**b**) Dense vitritis is evident (Fig. 6.2b). Cultures of the vitreous were negative, but a wrist abscess was present and grew methicillin-resistant *Staphylococcus aureus* (MRSA). The patient also had uncontrolled diabetes mellitus

Treatment

Because it is rare, much of our understanding of the treatment of endophthalmitis has come from retrospective case series. One of the largest and well-known prospective studies of endophthalmitis was the Endophthalmitis Vitrectomy Study (EVS), which was a large multicenter prospective interventional randomized controlled trial funded by the National Institute of Health, which compared intravitreal antibiotic injection alone to pars plana vitrectomy with intravitreal antibiotic injection for treatment of lens surgery-related postoperative endophthalmitis [7]. Although the study was only specific to acute post-cataract surgery endophthalmitis, many discoveries by the EVS have been used to generally guide treatment for

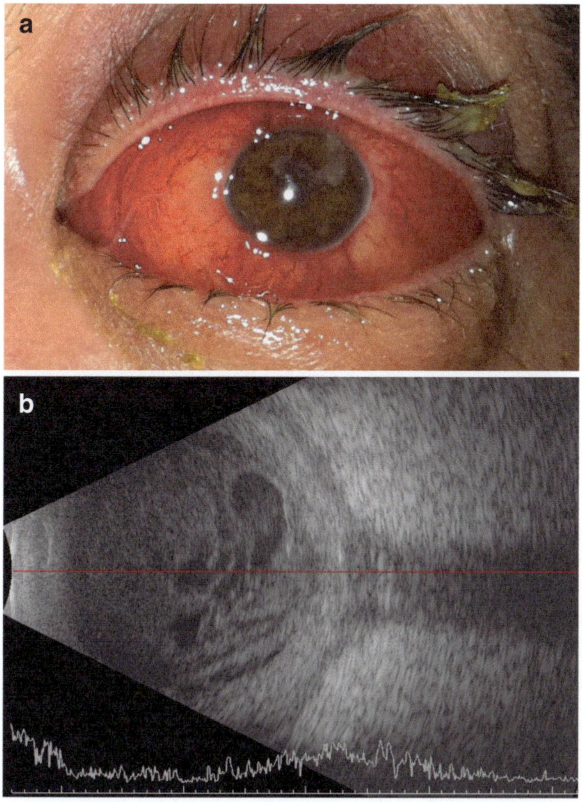

Fig. 6.4 Endogenous bacterial endophthalmitis. Infection was due to *Escherichia coli* from a liver abscess. (**a**) There is severe eyelid and conjunctival erythema and chemosis, dense microcystic corneal edema, neovascularization of the iris, severe anterior chamber inflammation, and no view to the posterior pole. (**b**) A B-scan ultrasound showed dense vitritis and severe choroidal and scleral thickening with a "T-sign" (Fig. 6.3b)

endophthalmitis. In general, the clearest evidence for prophylaxis to prevent endophthalmitis has been with the use of povidone iodine [16, 17].

Patients with suspected endophthalmitis should be treated acutely with intravitreal injections of antibacterial antibiotics with broad gram-positive and gram-negative coverage [1, 3, 7, 11]. Most studies have recommended use of vancomycin (1 mg/0.1 ml) in addition to a broad-spectrum cephalosporin, usually ceftazidime (2.25 mg/0.1 ml). This combination of medications has been shown to cover nearly 100% of organisms in culture-positive bacterial endophthalmitis [18, 19]. If the patient is allergic to penicillins, amikacin (0.4 mg/0.1 ml), which also has excellent gram-negative coverage, may be substituted for ceftazidime. Addition of intravitreal clindamycin (450 ug/0.1 ml) may be considered for penicillin-resistant strains of

Table 6.1 Doses of common intravitreal antibiotics

Antibacterial	
Vancomycin	1 mg/0.1 ml
Ceftazidime	2.25 mg/0.1 ml
Amikacin	400 μg/0.1 ml
Clindamycin	450 μg/0.1 ml
Antifungal	
Amphotericin B	5–10 μg/0.1 ml
Voriconazole	50–100 μg/0.1 ml
Antiviral	
Foscarnet	2.4 mg/0.1 ml
Ganciclovir	2 mg/0.1 ml

bacteria [11]. Antibiotic doses are summarized in Table 6.1. If the post-injection or postoperative course does not improve after 2–3 days, a repeat intravitreal injection may be given, and the possibility of a resistant or fungal infection, or a masquerade syndrome, should also be considered.

A short course of systemic antibiotics may also be considered in the case of a particularly severe infection or associated with trauma, either a third- or fourth-generation oral fluoroquinolone, such as moxifloxacin, which have excellent intraocular penetration, or intravenous antibiotics with broad coverage for suspected organisms [11, 20, 21]. It is unclear if systemic antibiotics play an additional role in routine treatment for exogenous endophthalmitis. Notably, the EVS showed that intravenous antibiotics did not provide significant visual benefits, and the cost and risk of hospital stay outweighed the small theoretical benefit of intravenous antibiotics in most cases [7].

Topical antibiotics are typically used during the initial treatment period. Either fortified antibiotics such as vancomycin and ceftazidime or tobramycin may be used or fourth-generation fluoroquinolones such as moxifloxacin or gatifloxacin may be used. Topical administration of antibiotics should be frequent in cases of post-traumatic, bleb-associated, or postoperative endophthalmitis, particularly in cases where there appears to be active infection at the wound or entry site into the eye [11, 22].

Fungal endophthalmitis is treated similarly to bacterial endophthalmitis, with antibiotics that target the most common species of intraocular infection (*Candida*, *Aspergillus*, and *Fusarium*, followed by other species) [23, 24]. Intravitreal amphotericin B (5–10 μg/0.1 ml) combined with systemic antifungal medication is often used to treat exogenous fungal endophthalmitis [11, 23]. Intravenous antifungal medication, such as amphotericin B, may be considered, although oral antifungal medications such as fluconazole or voriconazole also have good intraocular penetration and have lower toxicity profiles. Instead of intravitreal amphotericin B, which has been shown to have retinal toxicity at higher concentrations, intravitreal voriconazole (50–100 ug/0.1 ml) may be used to successfully treat fungal endophthalmitis; voriconazole may be particularly helpful in cases of drug-resistant fungal infections [24, 25].

If the patient is suspected to have a particularly virulent organism, or if the vision is extremely poor on presentation (light perception or no light perception), urgent pars plana vitrectomy (PPV) with anterior chamber and vitreous washout and intravitreal antibiotic injection should be considered. The role of vitrectomy in endophthalmitis is similar to the role of incision and drainage of infection in other regions of the body. Vitrectomy can decrease the pathogen load and remove toxins and inflammatory material from the eye, remove the vitreous scaffolding, and may help clear the media more quickly [7, 26, 27].

Notably, the EVS showed that visual outcomes were better in acute postoperative endophthalmitis patients with LP or NLP vision treated with PPV with intravitreal antibiotics versus intravitreal antibiotic injection alone; this benefit was not seen in the eyes with better than LP vision [7]. PPV is likely helpful in cases of infection with particularly toxigenic or pathogenic organisms, such as *Streptococcus* species or gram-negative bacteria [27]. However, PPV performed during the acute infectious phase is often limited due to difficulty with visualization and can be associated with higher risk of retinal detachment during the postoperative period than vitrectomy for other conditions [11].

Intravitreal steroids (dexamethasone 0.4 mg/0.1 cc) have been used by some physicians to treat acute endophthalmitis. The rationale has been to decrease the amount of inflammatory damage to the retina; however, the utility of intravitreal steroids in the setting of endophthalmitis has been debated [28, 29]. If there is a possibility of fungal endophthalmitis, intraocular corticosteroids should probably be avoided. Otherwise, intravitreal corticosteroids may be considered at the treating physician's discretion.

Prognosis

Visual prognosis is highly dependent on the virulence of the organism. Coagulase-negative *Staphylococcus* species and culture-negative endophthalmitis tend to have better visual prognoses [30]. In acute postoperative endophthalmitis, where coagulase-negative *Staphylococcus* is the predominant organism, the EVS showed that patients regained visual acuities of 20/40 or better 50 % of the time, while only 15 % had outcomes of 20/200 or worse [7]. Delayed-onset postoperative endophthalmitis after cataract surgery is also associated with less virulent organisms, and it tends to have better visual prognosis [8]. Delayed-onset bleb-associated endophthalmitis, on the other hand, is associated with much worse visual prognoses due to the higher virulence of organisms, with *Streptococcus* species being the most prevalent organism. Up to 1/3 of patients had final visual outcomes of NLP in one study [5, 27]. In posttraumatic endophthalmitis, visual acuity outcomes are also highly dependent on organism, but in general visual prognosis is guarded. The presence of an intraocular foreign body in endophthalmitis portends a worse prognosis, with 50 % of patients achieving visual outcomes of hand motions or worse [31]. Post-injection endophthalmitis visual outcomes also tend to be worse than outcomes after acute postoperative endophthalmitis due to the higher prevalence of *Streptococcus* species in the post-injection eyes [32].

Specific Considerations in Exogenous Endophthalmitis

Acute Postoperative Endophthalmitis

Acute postoperative endophthalmitis presents less than 6 weeks after eye surgery, by definition [8]. The most common causative surgery is cataract surgery, but other eye surgeries can also cause endophthalmitis, including penetrating keratoplasty, trabeculectomy, glaucoma drainage device implantation, pars plana vitrectomy, and scleral buckle [1].

Acute postoperative endophthalmitis can often be distinguished from a noninfectious inflammatory syndrome called toxic anterior segment syndrome (TASS), which may also occur acutely after intraocular surgery [33]. TASS is thought to be related to instillation of inflammatory agents (such as residues, preservatives, denatured medications, etc.) into the eye during surgery [16, 33]. TASS usually presents in the hyperacute phase after surgery, often in the 12–48 h period. The distinguishing features of TASS are diffuse limbus-to-limbus corneal edema, severe anterior chamber reaction but minimal vitritis, and minimal ocular pain on presentation. However, it can be difficult to distinguish TASS from endophthalmitis in some cases, and these patients often must be presumed to have bacterial endophthalmitis.

Preoperative risk factors for acute postoperative endophthalmitis include blepharitis, immunosuppression (including diabetes mellitus), and older age [1, 34]. Intra- and postoperative risk factors include intraoperative complications, particularly posterior capsular rupture with vitreous loss, inexperienced surgeons, and postoperative wound leak [35]. Injection of prophylactic intracameral antibiotics, use of acrylic intraocular lenses (versus silicon), and use of scleral tunnel (versus clear corneal incision) have been shown to be protective against endophthalmitis in some studies, although these associations have been debated [1, 36].

Acute postoperative endophthalmitis is nearly always caused by a bacterial infection, although acute postoperative fungal endophthalmitis is a prevalent complication in developing countries [1]. Vitreous cultures may be negative in up to 30 % of cases [1, 13]. Of culture-positive cases, the most common organisms found are gram-positive cocci. Of these, coagulase-negative *Staphylococcus* is most common, followed by *Staphylococcus aureus* and then *Streptococcus* species [7, 13, 14, 18].

Chronic Postoperative Endophthalmitis

Delayed-onset or chronic postoperative endophthalmitis presents later than 6 weeks after surgery [8]. Diagnosis may sometimes be further delayed, because of the insidious onset of these cases. Delayed-onset postoperative endophthalmitis is relatively uncommon, accounting for less than 8 % of all postoperative endophthalmitis cases in one study [37]. Patients often present with remitting and relapsing intraocular inflammation, many times without a frank hypopyon. Patients often do not have pain or redness on presentation. The characteristic finding of chronic postoperative endophthalmitis is a white plaque within the lens capsule, which is a nidus of the infection [8].

Vitreous or aqueous cultures in these cases are often negative. Of culture-positive cases, the most common causative organism is *Propionibacterium acnes*, followed by coagulase-negative *Staphylococcus* species. Fungal infections may also be a cause of delayed-onset endophthalmitis, accounting for up to 25 % of these cases [1, 8].

Treatment of chronic bacterial endophthalmitis can sometimes be challenging. Although simple injection with antibacterial antibiotics may be curative in some cases, often the infection is not completely eradicated with intravitreal injection alone. Pars plana vitrectomy with partial capsulectomy and intravitreal antibiotic injection can increase the rate of cure; however, some patients will still go on to harbor persistent infection. The definitive procedure in these patients is pars plana vitrectomy with complete removal of the intraocular implant and lens capsule with injection of intravitreal antibiotics, but this procedure should be reserved for recurrent cases, as the patients will typically later need an additional operation to insert a secondary intraocular lens implant [38].

Bleb-Associated Endophthalmitis

Trabeculectomy is associated with a particular subset of exogenous endophthalmitis, referred to as *bleb-associated endophthalmitis*. Onset can be acute or delayed, often many months or years after the initial surgery [22]. Acute-onset bleb-associated endophthalmitis is similar to other forms of acute postoperative endophthalmitis, as described above, but delayed-onset bleb-associated endophthalmitis can be associated with more virulent bacteria with more guarded visual prognosis (Fig. 6.2). *Streptococcus* species and gram-negative bacteria such as *Haemophilus influenzae* are the most common organisms causing delayed-onset bleb-associated endophthalmitis [5, 27].

Bleb-associated endophthalmitis must be distinguished from blebitis, which may often be treated with topical antibacterial antibiotics alone [22]. Both bleb-associated endophthalmitis and blebitis often present with a purulent filtering bleb and anterior ocular inflammation, but blebitis presents with little vitritis and no hypopyon. Despite proper treatment, blebitis may still develop into bleb-associated endophthalmitis; therefore these patients must be monitored closely.

Risk factors for bleb-associated intraocular infections include a history of previous blebitis, late-onset bleb leak, younger age, antimetabolite use during surgery, inferior blebs, thin avascular blebs, myopia, and blepharitis. Fornix-based trabeculectomy surgery may be associated with less risk than limbus-based surgery, but this has been debated [1, 39].

Because of the association of delayed-onset bleb-associated endophthalmitis with more virulent organisms, more aggressive management of this disease, including urgent PPV, should be considered [27]. During the operation, the surgeon may consider injecting antibiotic subconjunctivally around the bleb in addition to intravitreally, to help with clearance of the inciting bleb infection.

Post-injection Endophthalmitis

Intravitreal injections, the most common of which are anti-vascular endothelial growth factor (anti-VEGF) medication injections, are routinely given for the treatment of a variety of retinal conditions including diabetic macular edema, age-related macular degeneration, and macular edema secondary to retinal vein occlusion. Although the risk of endophthalmitis with this treatment is low (0.02–0.32 %) [15], because intravitreal injections are becoming more and more common, the incidence of post-injection endophthalmitis has risen dramatically in the past 10 years. Incidence of endophthalmitis may be higher with injection of intravitreal triamcinolone acetonide than with other intravitreal medications, although this may be related to higher incidence of sterile endophthalmitis with triamcinolone [40].

Sterile or noninfectious endophthalmitis can occur after intravitreal injection and has been reported after injection of aflibercept, bevacizumab, ranibizumab, and triamcinolone [1]. It may be related to an immune response to the medication itself, or in the case of triamcinolone, it may be related to migration of small medication particles into the anterior chamber of the eye [41]. Usually, sterile endophthalmitis presents with minimal pain, less inflammation, and more acute presentation than bacterial endophthalmitis, but distinction between noninfectious and infectious endophthalmitis can be difficult, and it is often prudent to treat these cases as infectious.

Risk factors for post-injection endophthalmitis may include older age, diabetes mellitus, blepharitis, subconjunctival anesthesia, patient moving/squeezing during the injection, use of prophylactic antibiotic eye drops, and use of a conjunctival mold, although it is challenging to find definitive risk factors given the low incidence of the disease and lack of prospective studies [4, 42]. The use of compounded medications for intravitreal injection has also been a recent topic of debate, as there have been several outbreaks of bacterial and fungal endophthalmitis related to contaminated batches of compounded bevacizumab and triamcinolone [43, 44]. However, with proper sterile compounding techniques, the dreaded occurrence of a batch-related endophthalmitis outbreak can be avoided.

Similar to postoperative endophthalmitis, organisms associated with post-injection endophthalmitis are nearly always gram-positive cocci [4, 42]. Coagulase-negative *Staphylococcus* species are most common, followed by *Streptococcus* species and then *Staphylococcus aureus* [4, 42]. However, infection with *Streptococcus* species is up to three times more common in post-injection endophthalmitis versus postoperative endophthalmitis, suggesting there may be increased incidence of contamination of the injection site with oral flora in these cases [32].

Posttraumatic Endophthalmitis

Posttraumatic bacterial endophthalmitis is a rare type of exogenous endophthalmitis but can be associated with the most virulent and varied organisms. Endophthalmitis occurrence after open globe trauma ranges from 2 to 12 % [1, 11, 45, 46]; percentages may be as high as 50 % with intraocular foreign body [11], although this percentage is highly variable depending on geographic region and mechanism of injury [45, 47]. Risk factors include presence of an intraocular foreign body, injury with dirty or plant material, traumatic lens rupture, corneal wound, retinal break/detachment, long hospital stay, rural location, and delayed wound closure [11].

In addition to the typical presenting signs of endophthalmitis, posttraumatic endophthalmitis may be associated with retained foreign bodies that are either partially embedded in the cornea or sclera, or intraocular foreign bodies (IOFB), or, if there is a perforating injury, there can be intraorbital or intracranial foreign bodies. Additional orbital and/or brain imaging is warranted via ultrasound, plain radiography, or CT scan to evaluate for the presence and location of a foreign body if suspected, as it may help determine surgical approach for removal of the foreign body [11, 48, 49]. Of note, some metallic foreign bodies, particularly 100 % copper ones, can cause sterile inflammation including hypopyon and vitritis, which may be difficult to differentiate from infectious endophthalmitis [11].

Most (80–90 %) of culture-positive cases of posttraumatic endophthalmitis are caused by bacteria, but the incidence of fungal endophthalmitis is higher than with other mechanisms of exogenous endophthalmitis [50]. Gram-positive cocci are the most common bacterial isolates, followed by gram-positive bacilli (e.g., *Bacillus cereus*) and then gram-negative organisms [50, 51]. Among gram-positive cocci, coagulase-negative *Staphylococcus* species and *Streptococcus* species are the predominant groups. The gram-positive *Bacillus cereus* is particularly devastating to the eye and is a common causative organism of endophthalmitis after trauma. *B. cereus* is often associated with a hyperacute presentation and fulminant bacterial endophthalmitis, and infection with this organism has extremely guarded visual prognosis [11, 52]. *Enterobacter* and *Pseudomonas*es are the most common gram-negative pathogens in a traumatic setting and also portend a poor visual prognosis [1, 11, 53].

Candida species are the most prevalent fungal infections after trauma, but infection with *Aspergillus* and *Fusarium* species is also common [23, 50]. Clinical features suggestive of fungal infection include delayed onset of infection, usually between 1 and 5 weeks after injury, or unresponsiveness to standard antibacterial antibiotics. Clinical signs suggestive of fungal endophthalmitis include minimal pain and minimal conjunctival redness or chemosis on presentation, slowly progressive intraocular inflammation, and the presence of inflammatory infiltrates in the vitreous or anterior chamber that resemble “fluff balls,” “snowballs,” or a “string of pearls” [1, 11]. Infections with yeast (e.g., *Candida*) are more indolent than infections with molds (e.g., *Aspergillus*) and portend better visual prognoses [23].

Endogenous Endophthalmitis

Endogenous endophthalmitis is an uncommon form of endophthalmitis, accounting for about 5 to 10% of all endophthalmitis cases [1]. It is due to hematogenous spread of infection to the eye and is nearly always caused by bacterial or fungal infection (Figs. 6.3 and 6.4). There is a high prevalence of systemic comorbid illnesses and factors in patients who present with endogenous endophthalmitis, including uncontrolled diabetes mellitus, malignancies, intravenous drug use, organ abscess, immunosuppressive therapy, indwelling catheter, end-stage renal or liver disease, and endocarditis [1, 24, 54, 55]. However, some patients have no predisposing factors, and rarely no source of infection is found [55].

Unlike in exogenous endophthalmitis, fungal infection is more prevalent than bacterial infection in many series of endogenous endophthalmitis [54, 56, 57]. The most common type of fungal infection is by *Candida* species, followed by *Aspergillus* (Fig. 6.5) [24, 58]. Mold species such as *Aspergillus* are more commonly associated with systemic immunosuppression and organ transplantation, and signs of endophthalmitis manifest rapidly [59]. Endogenous *Candida* endophthalmitis is often more indolent and presentation can be delayed; misdiagnosis in these cases is common [60]. *Candida* may start as choroidal lesions with minimal vitreous involvement, and these early candidal infections may resolve with systemic antifungal medications alone [61].

Endogenous bacterial endophthalmitis is usually due to gram-positive bacteria such as *Staphylococcus* (usually *S. aureus*) and *Streptococcus* species (e.g., *S. pneumoniae*, *Group B Streptococcus*, *Enterococcus*) in the Western world [2, 57]. However, in Asian countries, gram-negative species, particularly *Klebsiella* species, are the most common cause of endogenous bacterial endophthalmitis, and prevalence of gram-negative infections is also increasing in Western countries [3, 54, 56].

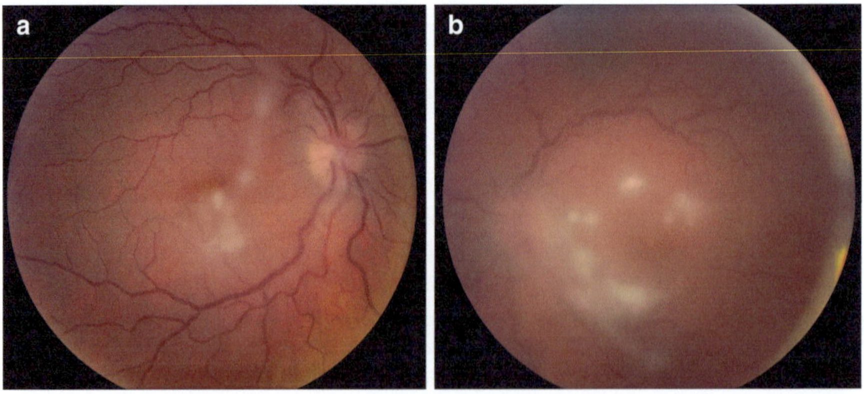

Fig. 6.5 Endogenous fungal endophthalmitis. Infection was due to *Candida albicans*, introduced into the bloodstream via intravenous heroin abuse. (**a**, **b**) There was moderate vitritis in the right eye and severe vitritis in the left eye, with multifocal fluffy vitreous balls of inflammation. In the right eye, the vitritis appeared to emanate from a fluffy chorioretinal lesion in the posterior pole, just inferior to the macula

In these cases, liver abscess is typically the source of infection. In a series from a major Taiwanese hospital, nearly 2/3 of all endogenous endophthalmitis patients had liver abscesses, and most of these patients had *Klebsiella* endophthalmitis [56].

Nocardia endophthalmitis is typically seen in patients with underlying immunosuppression, although it may also occur in otherwise healthy individuals [9, 62]. It is commonly associated with pulmonary infection, although ocular symptoms are often the presenting complaints [63].

Presentation

The presenting ocular symptoms and signs are similar to exogenous endophthalmitis, as discussed above. Symptoms can vary from patient to patient, with some having more indolent presentation if less pathogenic organisms are involved or more acute presentations if highly virulent pathogens are the culprit. However, since the pathogenesis involves the hematogenous spread of infection to the eye from another source, often there may also be systemic signs and symptoms, with fever and flu-like symptoms being most common and occurring in approximately 1/3 of patients. In fact, nearly 75 % of patients have some form of preceding or accompanying sign of systemic infection [3, 54]. In addition, because of the hematogenous spread of the infection, bilateral involvement can occur in up to 1/3 of cases [1, 3, 54]. Diagnosis of endogenous endophthalmitis may be difficult, as there is often no inciting illness noted by history. Up to 25 % of cases were misdiagnosed or had a delayed diagnosis in one study [3].

Also, because endogenous infections spread from the choroid, intraocular infections may only involve the choroid or subretinal space without causing fulminant endophthalmitis (Fig. 6.6) [9, 58, 63]. Subretinal abscess is an uncommon manifestation of

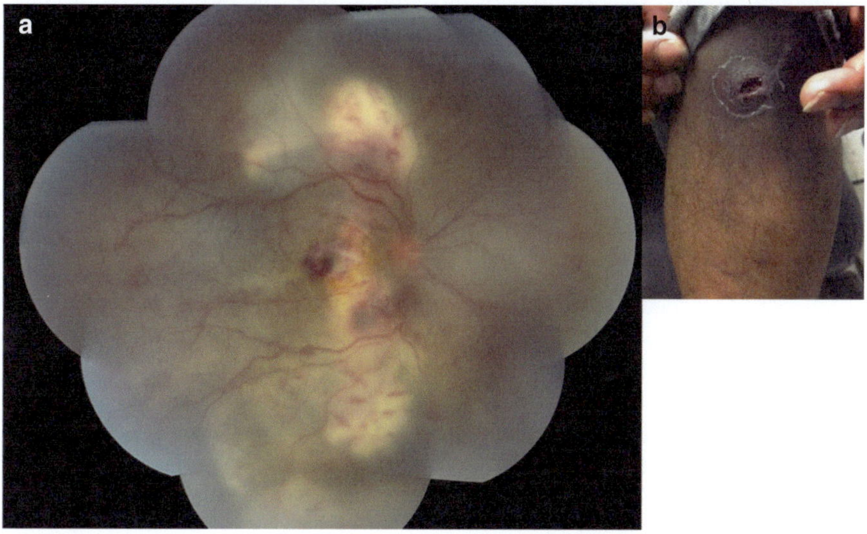

Fig. 6.6 Subretinal abscess. Infection was to methicillin-sensitive *Staphylococcus aureus* introduced into the bloodstream via a skin abscess. (**a**) Examination revealed moderate vitritis and a large multilobular subretinal white mass with overlying exudative retinal detachment, as well as multiple white-centered intraretinal hemorrhages. (**b**) An open skin wound

endogenous endophthalmitis. Subretinal abscesses usually appear in the posterior fundus as yellow-white circumscribed lesions, often with hemorrhages in the overlying retina, and mild to moderate vitreous inflammation. Subretinal pseudohypopyon and more extensive exudative detachment may occur in advanced cases [9]. *Nocardia* is the organism most commonly associated with these lesions, although other organisms may also cause subretinal abscess [9].

Diagnostic Testing

Diagnosis of the causative organism in endogenous endophthalmitis is often aided by vitreous biopsy, as blood cultures are negative in many of these cases. Blood cultures may only be positive 33–50 % of the time [3, 64], while vitreous biopsy may be positive in up to 87 % of patients [64]. In cases of fungal endophthalmitis or subretinal abscess, PPV with vitreous or subretinal fine needle biopsy may be particularly helpful to obtain adequate specimen for culture [9, 59]. Diagnosis of *Nocardia* can be particularly challenging, and a PPV with subretinal biopsy is often necessary to obtain an adequate sample for culture [63].

Additional systemic testing may be tailored to symptoms and suspected organisms. Management should be done in conjunction with an infectious disease expert. Blood and serological testing is often helpful to detect systemic disease. There may be a leukocytosis, with increased neutrophil count. Erythrocyte sedimentation rate and C-reactive protein, which are nonspecific tests of inflammation, are often elevated, particularly in cases of endocarditis. Other niduses of infection are common and can be found in a variety of extraocular tissues. Indwelling intravenous catheters may be removed and cultured. If there are signs of a urinary tract infection, urine cultures may be sent. Lung, liver, endocardium, and soft tissue were most commonly reported sites of primary infection in one study [2]. Therefore, lung, abdominal, and cardiac imaging, with radiography or echography or both, is important in many cases of endogenous endophthalmitis. To detect infection of the aortic valve, transesophageal ultrasound may be more sensitive than transthoracic ultrasound. In cases of gram-negative bacterial endogenous endophthalmitis, particularly in *Klebsiella* species infections, a liver abscess is often the primary infection site; therefore diagnostic imaging of the abdomen is often advisable in these cases [54]. Head and orbital imaging may be helpful in some cases.

Treatment

Treatment of endogenous endophthalmitis typically includes hospitalization and systemic intravenous antibacterial and/or antifungal medications, in addition to intravitreal antibiotic injections. Intravitreal medications and doses are identical to those used in exogenous endophthalmitis, as discussed above. Often it is prudent to inject antifungal medications in addition to antibacterial medications intravitreally if the causative organism is not known. Systemic medications are important in treatment of endogenous endophthalmitis, as there is typically an occult or manifest systemic infection in these cases [3].

In fungal endophthalmitis, instead of intravenous amphotericin B or other intravenous antifungal agents, oral fluconazole or voriconazole may be used in some cases as an adjunctive therapy, as the ocular penetration is relatively good [59, 65]. Intravitreal amikacin and oral trimethoprim/sulfamethoxazole should be considered for treatment of intraocular *Nocardia* [63].

The role of therapeutic PPV is unclear in endogenous endophthalmitis, but as in cases of exogenous endophthalmitis, PPV should be considered in cases where more virulent organisms are suspected. In one large series of endogenous endophthalmitis, visual outcomes were better in patients who underwent PPV than in those who did not [3]. PPV may also be used to aid in obtaining a specimen for diagnosis.

Prognosis

Visual prognosis in these cases is guarded, due to the virulence of organisms typical of endogenous endophthalmitis. In one study, visual results were worse prior to 2001, when visual acuities of better than 20/200 were seen in only 1/3 of patients, while after 2001, up to 41 % of patients were able to obtain 20/200 or better vision [2, 3]. Up to 20 % of eyes needed enucleation or evisceration in the same study [3]. Of cases of endogenous fungal endophthalmitis, molds such as *Aspergillus* species portend the worst visual prognosis (up to 25 % enucleation rate), while yeasts such as *Candida* species are associated with the best visual prognoses [1, 59].

Atypical Bacteria

Tuberculosis

Tuberculosis (TB) is a disease caused by infection with *Mycobacterium tuberculosis*. It is a systemic disease that can have "protean manifestations" and mainly involves the lung [66]. Although most commonly found in the lung, the disease may manifest anywhere in the body; extrapulmonary sites may include the gastrointestinal tract, genitourinary tract, skin, central nervous system, and eye. In some cases, the organism can disseminate from the lungs by hematogenous spread to various organs resulting from seeding of tissues with small nodules of infection; this is termed miliary tuberculosis [66].

There is an annual incidence of approximately nine million cases per year, and TB is the cause of three million deaths yearly worldwide [66]. The disease is uncommon in the USA but is becoming increasingly more common in underdeveloped regions of the world. In the USA, immigrants and racial and ethnic minorities are most affected, with the most common groups being Asian immigrants. Most of the new cases of TB in the USA are due to reactivation of latent TB in HIV-infected individuals [67].

Presentation

Mycobacterium tuberculosis (TB) is an acid-fast bacillus that spreads via airborne droplets, which can remain suspended in the air for a few hours. Over 90 % of people infected with TB never develop symptoms, 5 % develop the disease in the first

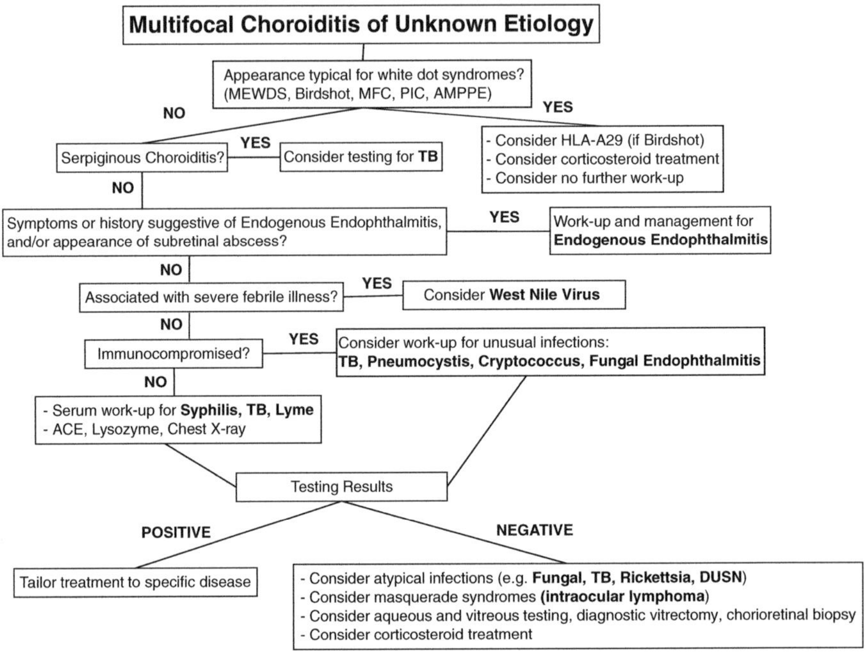

Fig. 6.7 Multifocal choroiditis of unknown etiology. *MEWDS* multiple evanescent white dot syndrome, *AMPPE* acute multifocal placoid posterior epitheliopathy, *PIC* punctate inner choroidopathy, *MFC* multifocal choroiditis, *TB* tuberculosis, *DUSN* diffuse unilateral subacute neuroretinitis

few years after infection, and the remaining 5 % develop symptoms later because of a weakened immune system. In this last group of patients, termed latent TB, most patients remain asymptomatic, but a few surviving dormant bacilli occasionally reactivate and can cause a wide variety of symptoms. There is no radiographic evidence of pulmonary involvement in latent TB [68].

TB is considered to be a "great masquerader," along with Lyme disease and syphilis, and can manifest in the eye as inflammation in a large variety of ocular structures. The most common ocular manifestations are posterior uveitis and panuveitis, and intraocular manifestations often also include choroidal granulomas (Figs. 6.7 and 6.8). Other presentations include subretinal abscess, serpiginous-like choroiditis, intermediate uveitis, and retinal vasculitis and/or vascular occlusion (Eales' disease) [68]. Anterior segment manifestations are less common, and appearance can include anterior uveitis, phlyctenulosis, episcleritis and scleritis, and peripheral ulcerative keratitis [67]. Of the anterior segment presentations, granulomatous anterior uveitis is most common and may be associated with anterior segment granulomas or nodules [66].

Choroidal granulomas are the most common manifestation of ocular TB and usually are found in conjunction with systemic TB infection, either pulmonary or extrapulmonary. They can be unifocal or multifocal, are white or yellow in color, and can

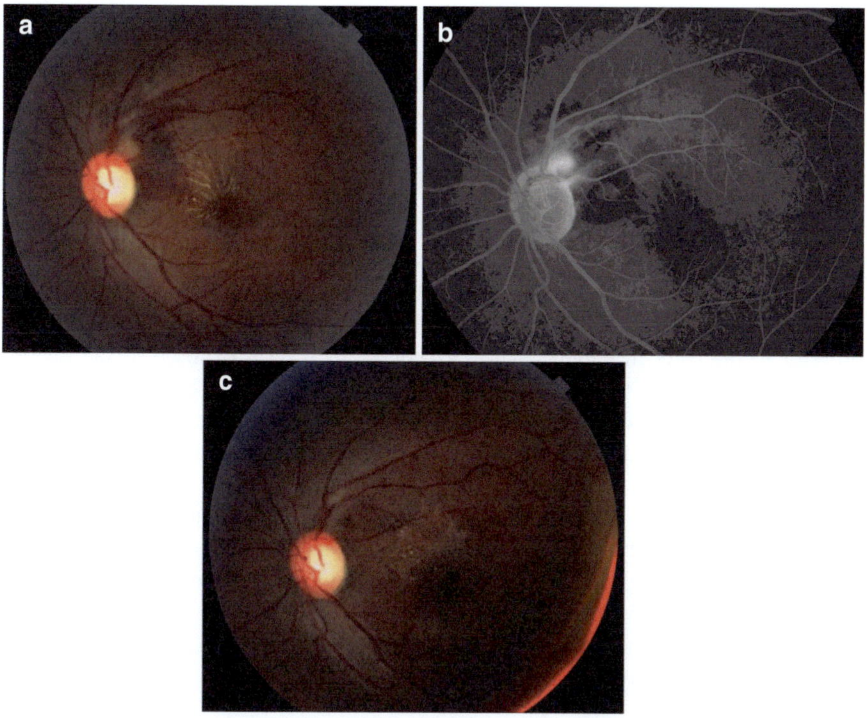

Fig. 6.8 Tuberculosis neuroretinitis. CT scan of the chest and positive interferon-gamma immunoassay confirmed presumed intraocular tuberculosis. (**a**) Granulomatous peripapillary chorioretinal lesion with surrounding subretinal hemorrhage and an associated partial macular star. (**b**) Fluorescein angiography showed early hyperfluorescence and late leakage from the granuloma and associated mild retinal vascular staining and leakage. (**c**) Visual acuity gradually returned to normal and retinal findings improved after 4 months of treatment

have overlying hemorrhage, exudate, or subretinal fluid [66]. Small granulomas are termed tubercles, and larger ones are termed tuberculomas [66]. If they enlarge further, a subretinal abscess may form.

Eales' disease is caused by periphlebitis, secondary retinal non-perfusion, and often leads to subsequent retinal neovascularization with vitreous hemorrhage or tractional retinal detachment. The precise mechanism is unknown but is thought to be due to hypersensitivity to an antigen of *Mycobacterium tuberculosis* [69].

Serpiginous-like choroiditis is a more recently recognized manifestation of TB. Like Eales' disease, serpiginous-like choroiditis may be related to hypersensitivity to a mycobacterial antigen and results in multifocal plaque-like choroiditis that may or may not be contiguous in the posterior pole. Distinguishing features from noninfectious serpiginous choroiditis may include associated vitritis, unilateral presentation, and sparing of the peripapillary region, but the two entities may be difficult to distinguish from each other, and testing for TB and subsequent response to TB treatment is often necessary to make the distinction.

Diagnostic Testing

Diagnosis of TB may be difficult due to the paucity and difficulty of obtaining organisms for culture or staining. To aid in diagnosis, tuberculin skin testing (TST) has long been used to assess for prior exposure to *Mycobacterium tuberculosis*. In this test, a small amount of mycobacterial antigen, or purified protein derivative (PPD), is injected subcutaneously. A positive TST appears as a raised reddish skin reaction at the site of injection.

One of the disadvantages of the TST is that the skin reaction is delayed, and the test must be read between 48–72 h after administration, which may delay diagnosis and requires patients to return to the clinic for reading. Additionally, results may be difficult to interpret in patients who have previously been exposed to the bacille Calmette–Guerin (BCG) vaccine, as this vaccine can produce false-positive skin testing results. More recently, T-cell interferon-gamma release assays have been developed, which have the advantage of permitting same-day results from a single blood serum sample and increased specificity for *Mycobacterium tuberculosis* which avoids false-positive results due to previous BCG vaccination [70].

If organisms can be obtained, and a patient has ocular manifestations of TB, the patient is said to have *confirmed* ocular TB. If no organism specimen is obtained but the patient has ocular manifestations along with positive testing for TB which may include tuberculin skin testing, positive interferon-gamma serum testing, a lesion on chest radiography consistent with TB, or extrapulmonary imaging consistent with TB, then the patient is said to have *presumed* ocular TB [68]. The disadvantage of relying on a positive TST or interferon-gamma serum assay is that these tests cannot distinguish between latent and active tuberculosis infection [67]. In these cases, mycobacterium DNA may sometimes be obtained by sampling of the ocular fluid, which may then be sent for PCR assay. However, the yield of ocular fluid biopsy and PCR testing is low in TB; therefore routine ocular fluid sampling is not warranted in most cases of presumed ocular TB [66, 67].

Treatment

The management of ocular tuberculosis is complex, even more so in the era of multidrug-resistant TB. Management should be done in conjunction with an infectious disease expert. Treatment of ocular TB is the same as treatment for pulmonary or extrapulmonary TB [71]. In general, the Centers for Disease Control (CDC) recommends use of the four common anti-TB drugs (isoniazid, rifampicin, pyrazinamide, and ethambutol) for an initial 2-month period followed by a choice of different options over the next 4–7 months for treatment of tuberculosis. Usually, pyrazinamide and ethambutol are stopped, and isoniazid and rifampin are continued to complete a 9–12-month treatment course, although recommendations vary [66].

Corticosteroids may be used in conjunction with the anti-TB therapy but should not be used alone when treating ocular TB. If a patient has inflammatory uveitis unrelated to TB, but also has latent TB (a positive TST or interferon-gamma assay), corticosteroids or immunomodulators may be given but only in conjunction with isoniazid or rifampin monotherapy for a full treatment course for latent TB [66].

Syphilis

Syphilis, infection by the spirochete *Treponema pallidum*, is another rare but important cause of intraocular infection and secondary uveitis. It is spread by sexual contact, transplacentally to the fetus, or rarely by blood transfusion [68]. There are three clinical stages of syphilis. In primary syphilis, a painless chancre is often observed at the site of inoculation, which disappears spontaneously over 4–6 weeks. Secondary syphilis may then follow, presenting with fever, malaise, and mucocutaneous lesions. This is the most infectious stage of syphilis, and ocular involvement occurs in up to 10 % of cases. Tertiary syphilis occurs later, months or years after primary infection, and is characterized by gummas, which are soft, tumor-like nodules of inflammation. Latent syphilis may also occur, which implies seropositivity but no symptoms of active disease. Neurosyphilis can occur at any stage and is classified as early or late [68].

Rates of syphilis in the developed world, including the USA, have been increasing over the past two decades, probably due to an increase in unprotected sex in the era of antiretroviral therapy for the human immunodeficiency virus (HIV) [72]. In the USA, the rate of primary and secondary syphilis in 2013 was more than double that in 2000. Young men account for the majority of cases in the USA, and men having sex with men represents the highest risk group [73]. Tertiary syphilis is the most common presentation of the disease, representing over 2/3 of cases in the USA in 2012 [74]. In the current era, coinfection with HIV is common, occurring in approximately 1/2 of newly diagnosed syphilis cases [74]. Therefore, if a new diagnosis of syphilis is made, additional testing for HIV infection is crucial.

Presentation

Like tuberculosis, ocular syphilis is a "great masquerader," as it can present with inflammation in any part of the eye and can have a large variety of appearances. Syphilitic uveitis usually presents with granulomatous inflammation and can present as nonspecific anterior, intermediate, or posterior uveitis or as panuveitis, episcleritis/scleritis, or keratitis. Posterior manifestations are most common and include vitreous inflammation, chorioretinitis, retinal vasculitis, serous retinal detachment, and, rarely, necrotizing retinitis. Optic nerve manifestations include inflammatory disk edema, neuroretinitis, pallor, or optic nerve nodules (gummas). Because of the variety of presentations, testing for syphilis infection should be considered for many cases of chronic uveitis.

There are distinctive appearances of retinal infection that can assist in rapid diagnosis of syphilitic uveitis. The first is the presence of superficial retinal precipitates in panuveitis [75]. The precipitates are small and creamy and can migrate over the infected regions of retina. Retinitis caused by syphilis has a mildly opacified appearance, which is often distinct from the typical chalky white appearance of necrotizing retinitis seen with viral infections (Figs. 6.9 and 6.10). One of the other features of syphilitic retinitis is that it leaves behind minimal disruption of the retinal pigment epithelium when it heals [75].

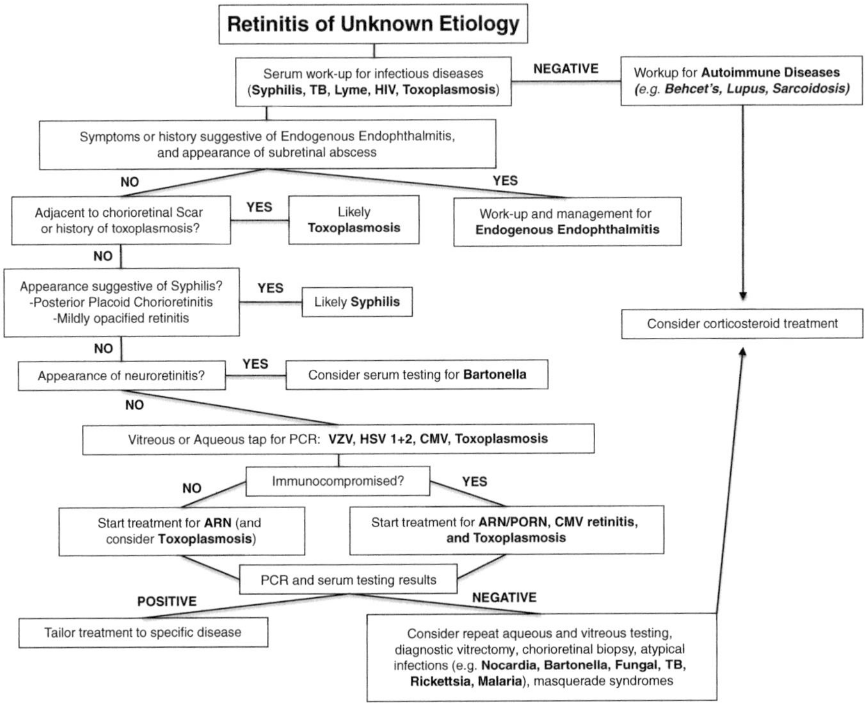

Fig. 6.9 Retinitis of unknown etiology. *TB* tuberculosis, *HIV* human immunodeficiency virus, *PCR* polymerase chain reaction, *HSV* herpes simplex virus, *VZV* varicella zoster virus, *CMV* cytomegalovirus, *ARN* acute retinal necrosis, *PORN* progressive outer retinal necrosis

Another distinctive pattern is that of acute syphilitic posterior placoid chorioretinitis [76, 77]. This appears as a discrete nummular area of outer retinal and inner choroidal inflammation in the posterior pole (Fig. 6.11). The lesion is gray-white or pale yellow, with evidence of central fading and a coarsely stippled hyperpigmentation pattern [77].

Congenital or latent syphilis can produce ophthalmic abnormalities such as optic neuropathies or pseudoretinitis pigmentosa but may not have active evidence of clinical disease and should be considered in patients with an appearance of unexplained optic neuropathy or retinal pigmentary changes with visual loss [74].

Diagnostic Testing

Clinical appearance can be further defined with multimodal retinal imaging, including fluorescein angiography (FA), indocyanine green angiography (ICGA), fundus autofluorescence, and optical coherence tomography [74]. In particular, posterior placoid chorioretinitis has the characteristic appearance of early and late hypofluorescence on ICGA, stippled hyperautofluorescence, and small amounts of subretinal fluid on OCT [76, 78].

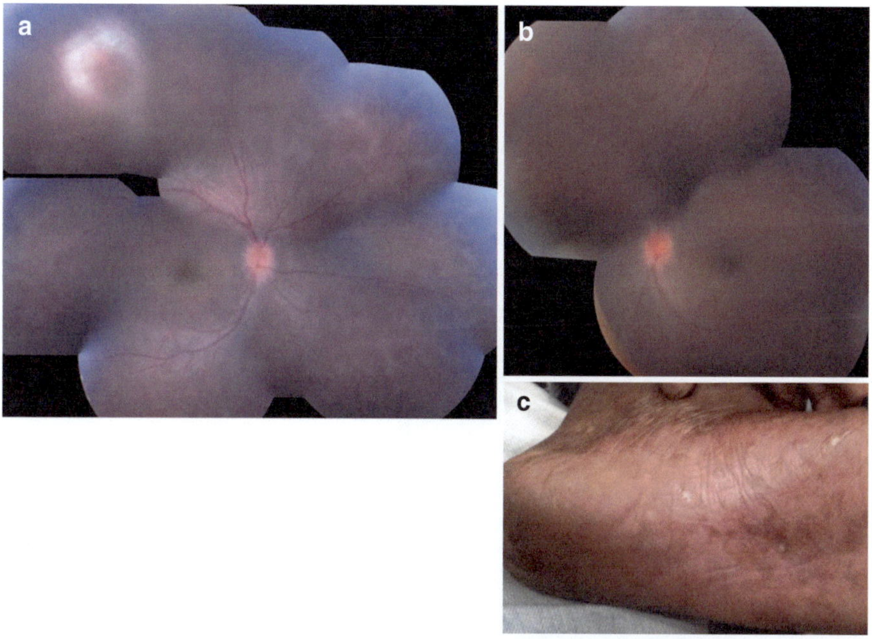

Fig. 6.10 Syphilitic retinitis. Diagnosis confirmed with serologic testing. (**a**, **b**) Vitritis and diffuse retinal vascular sheathing in both eyes. In the right eye, there was a patch of peripheral nummular and grayish-colored retinitis. The optic disks were mildly elevated and edematous. (**c**) Further review of systems revealed a maculopapular rash on the soles of both feet

Serologic testing is the standard for diagnosis of syphilitic uveitis. Seronegativity is rare but can occasionally occur, most commonly in HIV-positive patients. Commonly, two categories of tests may be ordered: treponemal and nontreponemal tests. The CDC currently recommends enzyme immunoassays and chemoluminescent immunoassays as the primary screening tests for syphilis to detect antibodies to treponemal antigens, followed by reflex testing of positive specimens with a nontreponemal test: the rapid plasma reagin (RPR) or the Venereal Disease Research Laboratory test (VDRL) [74].

The reason for this sequence of testing is that some patients will be positive by treponemal-specific tests but negative by RPR/VDRL. Because sensitivity of the treponemal-specific tests is higher than RPR/VDRL and specificity is lower, discordant results are expected. Specimens positive by treponemal-specific tests and negative on RPR/VDRL are submitted for a confirmatory *Treponema pallidum* particle agglutination test (TP-PA), and if that test is positive, a diagnosis of syphilis is confirmed [74]. Once a diagnosis of syphilis is made, the nontreponemal tests (RPR or VDRL) are useful to monitor response to treatment.

Patients with a new diagnosis of syphilitic uveitis should also have examination of the cerebrospinal fluid. Patients who have a prior diagnosis of syphilis as well as

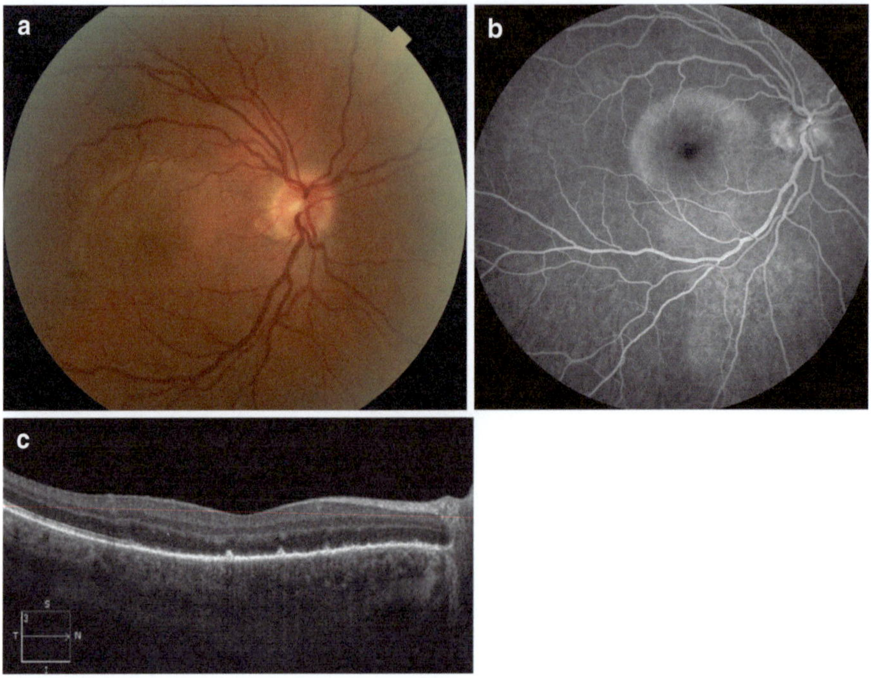

Fig. 6.11 Acute syphilitic posterior placoid chorioretinitis. Diagnosis confirmed with serologic testing and histopathology of skin lesion. (**a**) A discrete nummular area of outer retinal and inner choroidal inflammation in the posterior pole is evident. (**b**) Fluorescein angiography reveals early hyperfluorescence with late leakage in the region of retinitis. (**c**) Optical coherence tomography reveals irregularities of the retinal pigment epithelium and disruptions of the ellipsoid zone

new unexplained ophthalmic abnormalities also warrant further investigation with examination of the cerebrospinal fluid [79]. VDRL is less sensitive than treponema-specific testing in the cerebrospinal fluid. Occasionally, only leukocytosis or elevated protein is present in neurosyphilis [74].

Treatment

Ocular syphilis is typically considered secondary syphilis as well as neurologic syphilis. It is treated in the same manner as neurosyphilis according to CDC guidelines. Subsequent fourfold decrease in titer by the nontreponemal test (RPR or VDRL) is evidence of a response to treatment [79]. Treatment should be given with guidance of an infectious disease specialist.

Intravenous or intramuscular penicillin is the drug of choice for ocular syphilis. The recommended adult regimen is intravenous penicillin G administered either in q4 hour doses or by continuous infusion for 10–14 days. The alternative regimen, if access to therapy can be ensured, is procaine penicillin intramuscularly once daily plus oral probenecid four times a day, both for 10–14 days. An extended course of benzathine penicillin intramuscularly once per week for up to 3 weeks can be considered to provide longer duration of therapy [74]. Generally, the inflammation subsides with penicillin treatment with visual improvement within 1 month [78].

Oral corticosteroid may be used to decrease ocular inflammation and to avoid the Jarisch–Herxheimer reaction, a febrile inflammatory reaction caused by release of antigens from lysis of *Treponema pallidum* or other infectious organisms after initiation of treatment. Corticosteroids should only be given after systemic antibiotic treatment has been initiated [80].

Lyme Disease

Lyme disease is an arthropod-borne zoonosis prevalent in North America and Europe and is transmitted by the Ixodes tick. Lyme disease is caused by infection with the spirochete *Borrelia burgdorferi* in the USA, but other forms of *Borrelia* may cause the disease in European countries [81]. As in syphilis, there are three clinical stages of Lyme disease. Stage one occurs between 1 and 4 weeks after inoculation and is typified by an expanding circular rash (erythema migrans) and nonspecific flu-like symptoms. Stage 2 occurs after 4 weeks and involves hematogenous dissemination of the infection to other parts of the body. Symptoms can be varied but may include more diffuse skin rash, neurologic symptoms, arthritis, and/or carditis [81]. Stage 3 may occur months or years after initial infection and often is associated with central nervous system manifestations. Ocular manifestations are most common in stage 2 or 3 of the disease [82].

Incidence of Lyme disease in the USA has been increasing since national surveillance was instituted in 1991. Lyme disease is regional, with most cases occurring in New England and the mid-Atlantic states and less commonly in parts of the Northern Midwest and Pacific states. The natural reservoirs for *B. burgdorferi* are small mammals and birds. Deer are not competent hosts for the spirochete but are important in sustaining the life cycle of the Ixodes ticks. Because of the mode of transmission, spring and summer months are the most common times for primary infection with *Borrelia* [81].

Presentation

As with syphilis, ocular manifestations of infection with *Borrelia burgdorferi* can be highly variable. The most common manifestation in the eye is conjunctivitis, which is usually self-limited and often does not represent true infection but is rather part of a flu-like syndrome in the first or early second stage of the disease [83]. As part of ocular infection, anterior manifestations may include keratitis, scleritis/episcleritis, and anterior uveitis. Intermediate uveitis is the most common form of uveitis associated with Lyme disease. Posterior involvement commonly may include macular edema, retinal vasculitis, and papillopathy and less commonly retinal venular occlusions or multifocal chorioretinitis [84]. In cases of optic neuritis, concomitant presence of cranial nerve palsies is common (mostly VI or VII) [82].

Diagnostic Testing

Serologic testing for Lyme disease is typically performed to confirm the diagnosis of ocular Lyme. Two-tier serologic testing for antibodies to *B. burgdorferi* is recommended. A quantitative test, usually an enzyme-linked immunosorbent assay [ELISA] of the concentration of antibodies to *B. burgdorferi*, is first performed, and if results are positive or equivocal, a Western blot is performed. Testing is often falsely negative in primary infection; therefore presence of the classic rash of erythema migrans may alone be diagnostic in early cases. The sensitivity of two-tier testing is much better in patients either with second- or third-stage Lyme disease (80–100 %). Although tests for antibodies have good sensitivity and specificity in patients who have had untreated infection for a month or longer, these tests should not be used for screening persons with a low probability of infection because of the poor positive predictive value in such patients [85].

Treatment

Treatment often involves a 2- to 4-week course of systemic antibiotics and should be guided by an infectious disease specialist. Early manifestations of Lyme may be treated with a course of oral doxycycline, amoxicillin, or cefuroxime, while late or neurologic Lyme may require intravenous administration of ceftriaxone or cefotaxime. Rates of cure with oral agents alone are in the 90 % range [81]. About 15 % of patients have a reaction similar to the Jarisch–Herxheimer reaction (increased temperature, myalgia, and arthralgia) within 24 h after treatment is begun with any of the above antimicrobial agents, as a result of an increase in circulating toxins associated with lysis of spirochetes [85].

Cat Scratch Disease

Cat scratch disease is prevalent worldwide and is a zoonosis caused by infection by *Bartonella henselae. Bartonella* are small gram-negative rods and are facultative intracellular bacteria within the class *Proteobacteria* [86]. The primary host reservoir for *B. henselae* is the domestic cat; more than 90 % of all cases of cat scratch disease are associated with a history of contact with cats less than 1 year old [87]. Infection of cats with *B. henselae* is common, but the transmission of the infection to humans is rare [88]. The cat flea, *Ctenocephalides felis*, has been established as the transmission vector from cat to cat and is thought to be a possible human vector as well [88].

Presentation

In most cases, cat scratch disease is a benign and self-limited condition. A localized skin lesion is usually seen at the inoculation site, sometimes accompanied by mild flu-like symptoms. These symptoms are typically followed by regional lymphadenopathy that will slowly resolve over weeks to months. Ocular involvement has been estimated to occur in up to 10 % of patients with cat scratch disease [89].

The most common ocular complication of cat scratch disease is Parinaud's oculoglandular syndrome, a self-limited condition typified by follicular conjunctivitis, regional lymphadenopathy, and fever. Posterior segment manifestations of cat scratch disease include neuroretinitis, focal retinitis, focal choroiditis, multifocal retinitis or choroiditis, vasculitis, intermediate uveitis, and vascular occlusions. Though only 1–2 % of patients infected with *B. henselae* develop neuroretinitis, among all patients with neuroretinitis, nearly two-thirds are seropositive for *B. henselae*, making cat scratch disease the most common cause of this condition. Neuroretinitis is typified by unilateral optic nerve head swelling with an associated exudative macular response, often in the pattern of a macular star (Fig. 6.8). Most patients with focal retinochoroiditis or neuroretinitis will have some degree of vitreous and/or anterior chamber inflammation [88].

Diagnostic Testing

Serologic testing is commonly used in the diagnosis of cat scratch disease. Culture or PCR-based analysis of tissue and/or fluid samples is uncommon but can occasionally be of use. There are two different serologic tests for the diagnosis of cat scratch disease. One involves an indirect immunofluorescent assay for the detection of serum anti-*B. henselae* antibodies. Sensitivity and specificity of this test are high in immunocompetent patients. The other is an ELISA directed toward serum antibodies, but this test is more variable in sensitivity and specificity, resulting in greater false-negative reporting [88].

Treatment

Cat scratch disease is often self-limited, so antibiotics are generally reserved for only the most severe infections. Immunocompromised patients affected with cat scratch disease tend to have a more protracted course and often require antibiotics. The most commonly used antibiotics are oral erythromycin or doxycycline. Doxycycline is typically preferred over erythromycin due to greater intraocular penetration. Both medications can be given intravenously or combined with oral rifampin in more severe infections. The duration of treatment is usually 2–4 weeks for immunocompetent patients and up to 4 months for immunocompromised patients [88].

Rickettsioses

Rickettsioses are a group of arthropod-borne zoonoses due to obligate intracellular small gram-negative bacteria. They are rare diseases, but intraocular involvement has been described. Most of them are transmitted to humans by the bite of contaminated ticks. Rickettsial agents are classified into three major categories: the spotted fever group, the typhus group, and scrub typhus. The spotted fever group includes Mediterranean spotted fever (MSF) and Rocky Mountain spotted fever (RMSF), among others. MSF is caused by the organism *Rickettsia conorii* and is prevalent in

Mediterranean countries and Central Asia. RMSF is caused by *Rickettsia rickettsii* and is endemic in parts of the Americas, especially in the South-Eastern and South-Central USA. Epidemic typhus is caused by the *Rickettsia prowazekii* and is usually found in crowded areas in populations with poor hygiene, such as during wars and natural disasters. Murine typhus, which is caused by *R. typhi*, is found worldwide in warm-climate countries. Scrub typhus, which is caused by *Orientia tsutsugamushi*, is found in East Asian countries [90–94]. See Table 6.2 for additional information on this unusual infection.

Whipple's Disease

Whipple's disease is a rare, multivisceral, and chronic infection typically presenting by a symptom triad of diarrhea, weight loss, and malabsorption. The digestive symptoms are often preceded for months or years by other symptoms, the most common being arthralgia, although cardiovascular, neurologic, or pulmonary involvement may be more prominent at times. Although the source of transmission is unknown, direct bacterial invasion has been found in numerous cases in various sites, including the eye. The bacteria *Tropheryma whipplei* most commonly invades the intestinal lamina propria and the vacuoles of "foamy" macrophages; less frequently, they are found in other intestinal mucosal structures, such as polymorphonuclear cells, smooth muscle, capillaries, lymphocytes, plasma cells, and mast cells. All of the clinical eye manifestations are nonspecific, including glaucoma, chemosis, retinal hemorrhage, papilledema, corneal ulcers, optic atrophy, and epiphora [95, 96]. Other patients have minimal intestinal symptoms with predominant ocular manifestations, leading to unfortunate delays in establishing a diagnosis. See Table 6.2 for additional information.

Viral Infections

Acute Retinal Necrosis

Acute retinal necrosis (ARN) is a rare and severe syndrome caused by intraocular infection by one of the herpes virus family. Although historically thought to affect otherwise healthy adults, more recently certain underlying immune characteristics, including certain human leukocyte antigen (HLA) subtypes, have been found that put patients at higher risk for the infection [97]. Immunosuppressive medications such as corticosteroids have been shown to predispose to infection [98]. Patients who are severely immunocompromised may present with a subtype of ARN called progressive outer retinal necrosis (PORN), described below.

The infectious agents associated with ARN and PORN are members of the herpes virus family. Varicella zoster virus (VZV) is most common, and most of the remaining cases are caused by infection by the herpes simplex virus (HSV)-1 or HSV-2.

Table 6.2 Unusual intraocular infections

Disease	Causative organisms	Epidemiology	Common history and symptoms	Ocular manifestations	Diagnostic testing	Treatment	Prognosis
Bacteria							
Rickettsioses	1. Mediterranean Spotted fever: *Rickettsia conorii* 2. Rocky Mountain Spotted fever: *Rickettsia rickettsii* 3. Epidemic typhus: *Rickettsia prowazekii* 4. Murine typhus: *Rickettsia typhi* 5. Scrub typhus: *Orientia tsutsugamushi*	1. Mediterranean countries and Central Asia 2. Parts of Americas, especially South-Eastern and South-Central USA 3. Crowded areas with poor hygiene 4. Worldwide in warm-climate countries 5. East Asia Transmitted to humans by tick bite	Present in spring or summer History of outdoor activities in endemic area Triad of high fever, headache, and general malaise Characteristic skin rash Local skin lesion (*tache noire*) at site of inoculation	Ocular involvement frequently asymptomatic and self-limited Retinitis common in MSF: perivascular white retinal lesions Multifocal deep retinitis seen in other forms of rickettsiosis Other retinal manifestations include serous retinal detachment, macular edema, macular exudates, and multifocal choroiditis Other ocular manifestations include optic disk edema, ischemic optic neuropathy, conjunctivitis, subretinal hemorrhage, keratitis, non-granulomatous anterior uveitis, and panuveitis	Typical clinical features can be diagnostic Usually confirmed by antibody testing of serum PCR may be useful	Drug of choice: doxycycline (oral or IV) Early systemic treatment advisable Other tetracyclines, chloramphenicol, fluoroquinolones also effective Consider systemic corticosteroids later	Usually good Severe cases may be lethal Ophthalmic manifestations usually self-limited Ocular involvement may cause permanent visual loss due to macular scarring or optic atrophy

(continued)

Table 6.2 (continued)

Disease	Causative organisms	Epidemiology	Common history and symptoms	Ocular manifestations	Diagnostic testing	Treatment	Prognosis
Whipple's disease	*Tropheryma whipplei*	Very rare Ubiquitous in environment, rarely cause of infection >75 % in males Patients usually middle aged and Caucasian	Causes chronic and multisystemic involvement, including GI tract, CNS, joints, and lymph nodes	Ocular manifestations rare and occur late in disease course Usually accompanied by GI symptoms Uveitis, retinitis, retinal hemorrhages, choroiditis, keratitis, optic nerve edema, or optic nerve atrophy	Cytologic diagnosis: (PAS)–positive macrophages 16S ribosomal DNA gene amplification in vitreous specimens or cerebrospinal fluid (CSF) PCR of aqueous or vitreous	TMP-SMX most widely used Third-generation cephalosporins and rifampin also commonly used in conjunction	Variable, worse if optic nerve involved Disease can relapse once treatment stopped
Viruses							
Rift Valley fever	*Bunyaviridae*	Sub-Saharan and North Africa, Arabian Peninsula Virus primarily infects domesticated cattle Transmitted to humans by mosquito bite or contact with infected animals Occurs in epidemics	Incubation: 3–7 days Flu-like febrile illness lasting 2–4 days Other manifestations include hepatitis, thrombocytopenia, bleeding tendencies, rarely encephalitis Death infrequent but can have neurological sequelae	Up to 20 % of patients Presents 4–15 days after systemic symptoms begin Most common ocular manifestation: macular retinitis Other ophthalmic lesions included retinal hemorrhages, vitritis, optic disk edema, and retinal vasculitis Anterior uveitis present in up to 1/3 of patients	Detection of outbreaks helpful Serum IGM and IGG testing CSF IGM testing in encephalitis Virus isolation by specialized virus labs PCR may be helpful	Supportive Prevention of exposure to halt outbreaks	Usually mild and self-limited Ocular involvement may cause permanent visual loss due to macular scarring or optic atrophy

Dengue fever	Dengue virus (*Flavivirus*)	Very common worldwide 100 million people annually Tropical and subtropical regions Transmitted by *Aedes aegypti* mosquito	Characterized by high fevers Other symptoms include headaches, myalgia, and bleeding manifestations (due to thrombocytopenia) Hypotension may occur in *dengue shock syndrome*, which carries high mortality rate	Ocular involvement in up to 10 % of patients hospitalized Subconjunctival hemorrhage common Characteristic "dengue maculopathy" usually bilateral and involves both retina and choroid Dengue maculopathy presents 1 week after onset of fever Other posterior manifestations include retinal hemorrhage, retinal vascular sheathing, yellow subretinal dots, RPE mottling, macular edema, disk edema	Typical clinical presentation often diagnostic Dengue IGM can be measured Dengue maculopathy diagnosis based on clinical features and retinal imaging	Supportive Systemic corticosteroids and immunoglobulin infusion has used with varying success	Ocular involvement may cause permanent visual loss due to macular scarring or optic atrophy Amount of visual loss likely depends on amount of large retinal vessel involvement

(continued)

Table 6.2 (continued)

Disease	Causative organisms	Epidemiology	Common history and symptoms	Ocular manifestations	Diagnostic testing	Treatment	Prognosis
Chikungunya	Chikungunya virus (*Alphavirus*)	Originally endemic in parts of Africa More infectious strains spread from Kenya in 2004 to islands in Indian Ocean and then through Asia and parts of Europe In 2013, large outbreak spread through Americas Transmitted via several mosquito species, usually *Aedes aegypti*	Incubation: 2–5 days Usually self-limiting febrile illness lasting days to weeks Most patients recover without consequences Increased morbidity seen with more recent strains Other features include headache, fatigue, myalgia, diffuse maculopapular rash, bleeding from nose or gums, peripheral edema, joint pain, hepatitis, multi organ failure Main distinguishing clinical feature is prolonged fatigue, lethargy, and depression lasting weeks Severe polyarthralgia may persist for months or years	May be unilateral or bilateral May present acutely or after resolution of systemic manifestations Acute anterior uveitis and retinitis most common Anterior uveitis can mimic herpetic uveitis Chikungunya retinitis, often associated with retinal vasculitis, usually affects the posterior pole Other ocular manifestations include panuveitis, panophthalmitis, optic neuritis, keratitis, episcleritis, neuroretinitis, and central retinal artery occlusion	Complete blood counts early in disease may reveal leukopenia, lymphocytosis, thrombocytopenia Virus isolation and PCR may be used in acute phase (7 days), while IGM testing useful after 10 days	Supportive For ocular disease, local corticosteroids, topical antihypertensives Systemic corticosteroids may be used Systemic acyclovir or valacyclovir may be considered for severe retinitis, although no evidence to support efficacy	Infection thought to confer lifelong immunity Typically benign and self-limiting Ocular involvement may cause permanent visual loss due to macular scarring or optic atrophy

Coxsackievirus	Coxsackievirus (enterovirus)	Grouped as "type A" and "type B" serotypes Hand, foot, and mouth disease most well known (usually type A16) Usually brief and benign Most common in children	Systemic symptoms highly variable, usually nonspecific flu-like symptoms Group A viruses tend to cause skin and mucous membrane eruptions Group B viruses may cause respiratory and GI symptoms, meningoencephalitis, myocarditis, pericarditis, and myositis	Rare Coxsackievirus B3, B4, and hand-foot-mouth disease Retinitis or chorioretinitis may occur, usually deep retinal white lesions similar to other white dot syndromes Occlusive retinal vasculitis may be visualized Cases of unilateral acute idiopathic maculopathy reported	Serological antibody testing	Supportive Topical or periocular corticosteroids may be considered for intraocular inflammation	Findings resolve spontaneously, usually without severe visual sequelae

(continued)

Table 6.2 (continued)

Disease	Causative organisms	Epidemiology	Common history and symptoms	Ocular manifestations	Diagnostic testing	Treatment	Prognosis
Protozoa							
Malaria	*Plasmodium* species (*P. falciparum, P. vivax, P. malariae, P. ovale, P. knowlesi*)	Worldwide health problem resulting in death of over 1 million people annually Caused by infection of erythrocytes Protozoa transmitted by mosquito bite, most commonly *Anopheles* mosquito Endemic to parts of Africa, Asia, and Latin America (species vary regionally) Most US cases imported from endemic regions	High fevers and flu-like illness common Appears weeks to months after inoculation During incubation, organism goes through number of morphologic changes affecting liver and erythrocytes Severe malaria may manifest as coma (cerebral malaria), metabolic acidosis, severe anemia, hypoglycemia, acute renal failure, or acute pulmonary edema Severe complications often fatal	Retinal changes in severe malaria can be of pathophysiological, prognostic, and diagnostic significance Malaria retinopathy: retinal whitening (macular or peripheral), vascular discoloration (white or orange), retinal hemorrhages (particularly with white centers), and papilledema Retinal findings in up to 1/3 of patients with severe malaria	Should be suspected in patients with extremely high fevers and from or recently visited an endemic area Hematopathology may show malaria parasites Serum antigen testing	Systemic treatment for malaria complex if resistant strains Treatment of P. falciparum involves combination of artemisinin derivative with a longer-acting partner drug Chloroquine may be used for other species Supportive treatment with antipyretic medications (e.g., acetaminophen)	Malaria retinopathy indicator of risk of severe organ damage or death Retinal findings resolve over 4–8 weeks, usually with visual improvement Vision may continue to be poor with severe retinal vascular occlusion or optic neuropathy

Parasites							
Onchocerciasis "river blindness"	*Onchocerca volvulus*	Transmitted by *Simulium* blackfly, which lives and breeds in rivers Affects over 35 million people worldwide Most abundant in Africa, but also Mediterranean, Central and South America	Complex life cycle of organism: Female blackfly ingests microfilariae from human blood Microfilariae develop into larva in the fly, then transmitted to humans via blackfly bite Larvae develop into adult worms, which settle in subcutaneous tissue and form fibrous nodules Adult worms then give rise to microfilariae Microfilariae spread throughout the skin, often causing intense skin itching and depigmentation Death of microfilariae causes severe inflammation	Caused by migration of microfilariae to the eye and the subsequent inflammatory response caused by their death Can cause limbal edema, hyperemia, conjunctival nodules, punctate keratitis, sclerosing keratitis, uveitis Less commonly, chorioretinitis, geographic retinal atrophy, optic atrophy Blindness due to corneal vascularization, glaucoma, complicated cataract, chronic chorioretinitis, optic atrophy	Skin biopsy and demonstration of microfilaria (sensitivity low unless palpable skin nodule) The Mazzotti test: a skin patch of diethylcarbamazine (DEC) causes localized microfilarial death Antibody tests may aid in diagnosis	Ivermectin most commonly used, but does not eliminate adult worm Doxycycline can sterilize or kill adult worms as it targets endosymbiotic bacteria in the worm Moxidectin is a new drug, maybe better than ivermectin	Variable depending on location and severity
Gnathostomiasis	*Gnathostoma spinigerum* or *Gnathostoma hispidum* (nematode)	Tropical and subtropical regions Endemic in parts of Asia and Latin America Caused by exposure to raw meat	Classic triad of symptoms: recurrent migratory swellings, eosinophilia, and travel to endemic area Symptoms usually occur in evening because of increasing motility of the worms at that time	Ocular involvement includes visualization of the worm in the eye Secondary effects include lid swelling, iritis, iris atrophy, iris holes, intraocular hemorrhage, retinal scarring, retinal detachment, glaucoma	Definitive diagnosis depends on isolation of the worm	Surgical removal of the worm necessary	Variable depending on location and severity

(continued)

Table 6.2 (continued)

Disease	Causative organisms	Epidemiology	Common history and symptoms	Ocular manifestations	Diagnostic testing	Treatment	Prognosis
Cysticercosis	*Cysticercus cellulosae* (larval form of *Taenia solium* or *Taenia saginata*)	Caused by ingestion of undercooked meat (usually pork) Affects 50 million people worldwide Endemic areas include Mexico and Latin America, sub-Saharan Africa, India, and East Asia	Neurocysticercosis is most common manifestation and causes substantial human morbidity and mortality CNS involvement manifests as neurological defects, hydrocephalus, and meningitis	Ocular findings: inflammation and cyst formation at infection site Inflammation of eyelids, subconjunctival tissue, extraocular muscles, orbit, anterior chamber, vitreous, or subretinal space Translucent cyst with visible undulating movements gives the nickname "living pearl" Rupture of cyst causes severe intraocular inflammation	Neuroimaging required to rule out CNS involvement Histopathological testing is confirmatory	Oral albendazole and prednisolone Surgical removal of parasite	Variable depending on location and severity

GI gastrointestinal, *CNS* central nervous system, *IGM* immunoglobulin M, *IGG* immunoglobulin G, *PCR* polymerase chain reaction

Rarely, cytomegalovirus (CMV) or Epstein–Barr virus (EBV) may be the etiological agent. VZV and HSV-1 are more likely in older patients, while HSV-2 is more common in young adults and children [99]. In patients with concomitant encephalitis or meningitis, the most likely pathogenic agents are HSV-1 and HSV-2, respectively.

Presentation

ARN is characterized by multifocal patches of retinal necrosis with discrete borders, usually starting in the peripheral retina, rapid progression of disease, circumferential spread, occlusive retinal vasculitis affecting arterioles preferentially, and moderate to severe inflammation in the vitreous and anterior chamber [100]. ARN is usually unilateral but can be bilateral (10–30 %) [101, 102]. PORN is characterized by a similar appearance of multifocal necrotizing retinitis with relatively little vitreous inflammation. PORN often involves the posterior pole on presentation but can involve any portion of the retina [103]. PORN is more rapidly progressive than ARN, and bilateral involvement is more common (up to 80 %) [104, 105].

Patients with ARN may present with eye redness, achy pain, photophobia, and/or vision loss. Anterior segment examination may demonstrate conjunctival and episcleral inflammation and either granulomatous or non-granulomatous inflammation. Examination of the posterior segment may reveal vitreous inflammation, retinal arteriolar sheathing, multifocal necrotizing retinitis, and/or optic nerve head edema

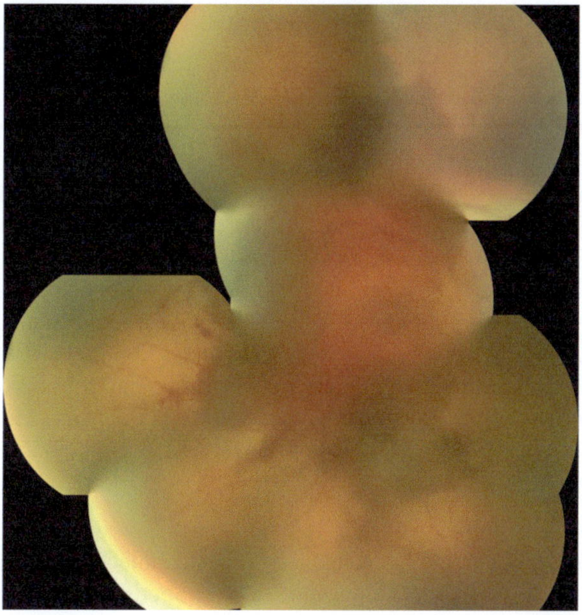

Fig. 6.12 Acute retinal necrosis. PCR was positive for herpes simplex type 1 in the right eye. There was severe vitritis, and retinal examination revealed extensive and confluent chalky retinitis and severe occlusive retinal vasculitis. The optic disk was moderately edematous, and there was a small lesion of retinitis in the papillomacular bundle

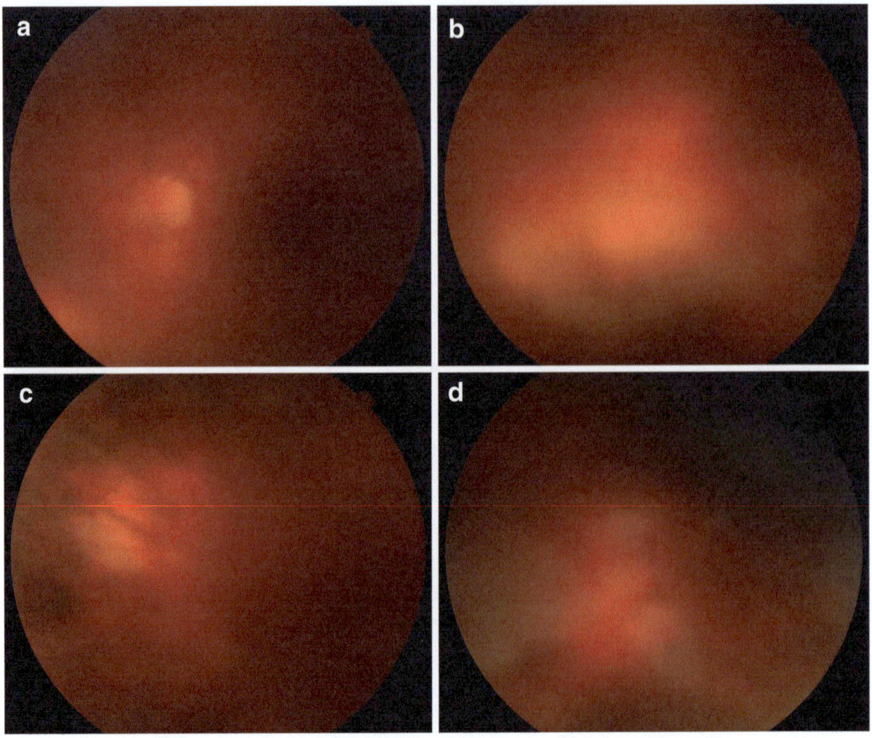

Fig. 6.13 Acute retinal necrosis. An anterior chamber paracentesis was positive for VZV. (**a–d**) Posterior examination revealed moderate vitritis and multifocal peripheral patchy retinitis lesions with discrete borders

(Figs. 6.12 and 6.13). Second eye involvement typically occurs within 6 weeks of presentation of the infection in the first eye but can occur months or years later [97].

As the active retinal infection resolves with treatment, affected areas develop pigmentary changes and retinal atrophy, often with a scalloped appearance at the junction of involved and uninvolved retina. Rhegmatogenous retinal detachment is a common consequence of infection and occurs in up to three-quarters of the eyes with ARN; retinal detachment may develop weeks to months after initial presentation of infection [106]. Other late complications of ARN may include chronic vitritis, macular edema, optic atrophy, epiretinal membrane formation, and recurrence of infection in the same or fellow eye [97].

Diagnostic Testing

Laboratory testing of intraocular samples is often valuable in the diagnosis of ARN and PORN. Past diagnostic techniques included antibody-based analysis of serum or intraocular fluid, viral culture, and pathological examination of retinal specimens [97]. More recently, PCR analysis of intraocular fluid has become the most commonly used test and may influence treatment in a portion of cases. A small sample of aqueous fluid is usually sufficient to detect VZV, HSV, or CMV DNA, and results are typically available within 1 week. Specificity and sensitivity of these tests are high [107]. PCR testing for the herpes viruses is often done in conjunction with PCR testing for toxoplasmosis, which may mimic ARN in some cases [97].

Treatment

The mainstay of treatment in ARN and PORN is systemic antiviral medication, which can stop the progression of the disease and reduce the risk of bilateral involvement [102]. Historically, acyclovir has been the systemic drug of choice, and because the bioavailability of oral acyclovir is relatively low, patients treated with this agent typically undergo induction therapy with intravenous acyclovir, requiring hospitalization. The typical induction dose for acyclovir is 10 to 15 mg/kg divided three times a day for 7 days, followed by oral acyclovir 800 mg five times a day for 3–4 months [108]. With the advent of the newer oral agents valacyclovir and famciclovir, which have much greater bioavailability than oral acyclovir and can produce systemic concentrations nearly equal to those obtained with intravenous acyclovir, patients with ARN may be treated on an outpatient basis in some cases [109]. More specifically, oral agents may be considered in immunocompetent and compliant patients with relatively good vision. The initiating oral dose of valacyclovir is 1–2 g three times daily, and the initiating oral dose of famciclovir is 500 mg three times daily. Of note, these agents may cause renal toxicity; therefore renal function should be monitored.

Depending on treatment response and the type of virus involved, other systemic agents may be considered, including intravenous ganciclovir, intravenous foscarnet, and oral valganciclovir [97]. In cases of CMV, oral valganciclovir has good bioavailability and may be used similarly to valacyclovir for the other herpes viruses. The standard dose of valganciclovir is 900 mg twice daily for 3 weeks followed by 450 mg twice daily for maintenance. Although rare, some strains of HSV and VZV are resistant to acyclovir, and some strains of CMV are resistant to ganciclovir; most of these resistant cases respond to intravenous or intravitreal foscarnet [110]. Notably, ganciclovir may cause bone marrow suppression, and foscarnet may cause renal and central nervous system toxicity.

For certain severe cases, intravitreal injection of the antiviral medications foscarnet and/or ganciclovir may be considered for supplemental treatment of ARN or PORN, in conjunction with systemic antiviral therapy. Intravitreal foscarnet can be administered at a dose of 2.4 mg/0.1 ml, which requires no dilution from the commercially available intravenous solution. The typical dose of intravitreal ganciclovir is 2 mg/0.1 ml, which can be given two or three times weekly [97].

Prophylactic laser retinopexy to prevent retinal detachment has been advocated by some authors, although the recommendation for prophylactic laser as standard treatment has remained controversial [111]. In cases of retinal detachment, often there are both tractional and rhegmatogenous components, and vitrectomy is necessary to obtain anatomic reattachment of the retina. Some believe that early vitrectomy lowers the risk of retinal detachment, while others do not [97, 101].

In cases where significant inflammation is contributing to the vision loss, a course of oral corticosteroids may be considered. Corticosteroids should only be used in conjunction with systemic antiviral medication. A loading dose of 0.5 mg/kg/day of prednisone for the first 7–10 days of treatment is typical [97]. The use of oral aspirin to prevent retinal vascular occlusion has been suggested as well, but its use has not been standard [112].

Prognosis
Prognosis in ARN is guarded, and poor prognostic indicators include immunosuppressed state, bilateral involvement, macular involvement, optic nerve involvement, and retinal detachment. In one series, 50 % of patients had 20/200 or worse visual acuity at 6 months follow-up [106].

Human Immunodeficiency Virus and Opportunistic Infections

Opportunistic infections manifest when the immune system is compromised for any reason. Immunodeficiencies may arise from a host of causes, including acquired immune deficiency syndrome (AIDS), malignancy, pharmacologic immunosuppression, uncontrolled diabetes mellitus, and other illnesses. Much of the study of opportunistic infections in the eye has occurred through research of patients with AIDS, but much of the discussion of opportunistic infections in this section may pertain to other causes of immunodeficiency.

AIDS is an expanding cause of morbidity and mortality worldwide, affecting over 30 million people [113]. It is caused by infection by the human immunodeficiency virus (HIV) retrovirus, which preferentially attacks CD4+ T-lymphocytes. The resultant immunodeficiency, termed AIDS, is caused by destruction of these cells and leads to the development of opportunistic infections, the main cause of illness and death in HIV-infected patients. HIV may be transmitted by sexual intercourse, blood-to-blood contact, transplacentally, or during breastfeeding.

Over 90 % of people with AIDS live in developing countries. Worldwide, the highest number of HIV-infected individuals is in sub-Saharan Africa, but the number of new cases is increasing rapidly in other areas of the world, including India and Southeast Asia. The demographics in the USA have shifted, although men who have sex with men remain the highest risk group. Racial and ethnic minorities represent a disproportionately high portion of those affected in the USA [114]. In the majority of cases in underdeveloped parts of the world, HIV transmission occurs through heterosexual contact [113].

The advent of highly active antiretroviral therapy (HAART) in the late 1990s has resulted in a marked reduction in mortality and a decreased incidence of associated opportunistic infections and neoplasms, including those of the eye. However, despite development of HAART, many patients in underdeveloped countries do not have access to these medications, and ocular manifestations of AIDS may affect 50–75 % of infected persons at some point in their disease course if left untreated with HAART. Ocular manifestations may be caused by extraocular (e.g., neuro-ophthalmic) and intraocular infection. Ocular manifestations caused by intraocular infection will be discussed in this section and may be divided into three categories: HIV retinopathy, opportunistic malignancies, and opportunistic infections [115].

HIV Retinopathy

Retinal microvasculopathy, termed *HIV retinopathy*, is the most common ocular manifestation of HIV. It affects up to 60 % of HIV-positive patients at some point during their disease if untreated with HAART. The prevalence of retinal microvascular changes increases as CD4 counts decrease. Forty-five percent of HIV-positive patients with CD4 count less than 50 cells/μl will have clinically evident microvasculopathy, versus only 16 % who have CD4 counts greater than 50 cells/μl [116].

HIV retinopathy manifests as cotton-wool spots, usually in the posterior pole. Microaneurysms may also be apparent. Cotton-wool spots are usually small and can be distinguished from CMV retinitis by their typically smaller size, a lack of associated retinal hemorrhage, and lack of enlargement over time. Most patients with retinal microvasculopathy are asymptomatic, although larger cotton-wool spots in the posterior pole may cause small scotomata [117]. Rarely, macular edema due to microvascular disease may cause blurred central vision [118]. The pathophysiology of HIV retinopathy is unclear; histopathologic findings resemble those in diabetic retinopathy [119]. Treatment of HIV retinopathy is not typically indicated, but its presence is a marker of severe immunodeficiency [115].

Opportunistic Lymphoma

Non-Hodgkin B-cell lymphoma (NHL) is a malignancy associated with Epstein–Barr virus infection in patients with HIV/AIDS. Intraocular involvement may rarely occur and is usually associated with central nervous system and/or systemic involvement in the AIDS population [120]. Intraocular manifestations of NHL include vitritis, retinitis, retinal vasculitis and vascular occlusion, multifocal choroiditis, subretinal mass, and anterior uveitis. NHL should be considered in cases of retinitis unresponsive to antiviral and other antibiotic medications. If the diagnosis is unknown, a diagnostic vitrectomy may be performed; cytological examination of the vitreous will show neoplastic cells characteristic of large cell lymphoma [115]. Magnetic resonance imaging is warranted to determine presence of central nervous system involvement. Treatment options include radiation and chemotherapy. Prognosis for survival in AIDS patients with central nervous system lymphoma is poor [121].

Opportunistic Infections

A variety of systemic opportunistic infections associated with HIV/AIDS may cause intraocular infection. Because systemic treatment often cannot fully eradicate these infections, treatment typically begins with an "induction" phase and is then continued in a "maintenance" phase. Maintenance treatment may sometimes be stopped once immunosuppression improves with induction of HAART therapy. Posterior segment opportunistic infections typically present as either necrotizing retinitis or multifocal choroiditis. When retinitis is associated with significant vitritis and anterior chamber inflammation, there is usually a higher CD4 count, and ARN, toxoplasmosis, syphilis, or cryptococcosis may be considered. If there is little intraocular inflammation, there is usually a lower CD4 count, and CMV retinitis and PORN are higher on the differential. Toxoplasmosis, cryptococcosis, tuberculosis, and syphilis may present as retinitis or choroiditis, while *Pneumocystis* infection presents as choroiditis [115]. Discussion of many of these intraocular infections is discussed elsewhere in this chapter, but *Pneumocystis* infection, cryptococcosis, and CMV retinitis will be discussed here.

Pneumocystis

Pneumocystis carinii pneumonia was once one of the most common systemic opportunistic infections in AIDS patients in the industrialized world but is much less common in the era of HAART. Extrapulmonary infection is uncommon in patients with AIDS, but ocular involvement may occur. Ocular manifestations of *P. carinii* include conjunctivitis, orbital mass, optic neuropathy, and choroiditis. Choroidal infection is the most common ocular manifestation and is typically bilateral and multifocal; lesions are yellow and well-demarcated, usually located in the posterior pole, and are not associated with intraocular inflammation or retinal vasculitis [122]. Prior to HAART, pneumocystis choroiditis was an indication of disseminated infection in severely immunocompromised patients, and median survival following diagnosis was less than 1 year [123]. Ocular lesions respond in most cases to induction and subsequent maintenance treatment with systemic pentamidine, trimethoprim and sulfamethoxazole, or dapsone [123].

Cryptococcus

Cryptococcus in HIV/AIDS typically causes meningitis; therefore the most common ocular manifestations are neuro-ophthalmic. Cryptococcal choroiditis is the most common intraocular manifestation, and the source may be hematogenous spread from the lungs or direct extension from cryptococcal meningitis. Choroidal lesions may be multifocal, solitary, or confluent (Fig. 6.14) [124]. Other ophthalmic manifestations include eyelid nodules, conjunctival mass, granulomatous iritis, iris mass, vitritis, necrotizing retinitis, endophthalmitis, and optic neuritis [115]. Treatment of cryptococcal choroiditis is systemic intravenous antifungal medication; therapy should be determined by an infectious disease specialist. Although infection may respond to therapy, visual outcome is often limited by optic atrophy, which may be due to the infection itself or secondary to high intracranial pressure and resulting optic nerve damage [115].

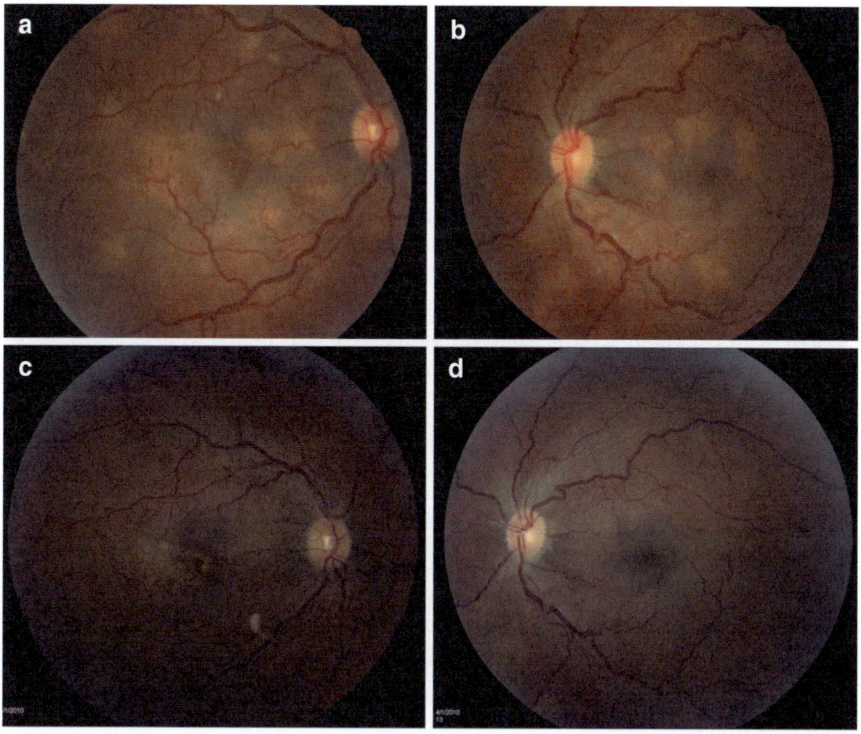

Fig. 6.14 Cryptococcus chorioretinitis. *Cryptococcus* antigen in the spinal fluid was highly positive (1:256). Blood cultures were eventually positive for *Cryptococcus*. The patient was HIV-positive with poor follow-up. (**a**, **b**) Fundus examination revealed no intraocular inflammation and multiple choroidal yellow plaque-like lesions, involving the macula in the right eye and sparing the macula in the left eye. (**c**, **d**) Visual acuity and fundus findings improved with antifungal treatment

Cytomegalovirus Retinitis

CMV retinitis was extremely common in the USA in the era before HAART therapy; around one-third of patients with AIDS in the USA would develop CMV retinitis [125]. CMV retinitis occurs only in severely immunodeficient patients, nearly always with CD4 counts of less than 50 cells/μl. In the era preceding HAART, therefore, life expectancies of patients who presented with CMV retinitis were extremely low, usually less than 1–2 years. In underdeveloped countries, the relatively low incidence of CMV retinitis is likely due to low life expectancy, i.e., patients die before developing CMV retinitis [113].

The clinical appearance of CMV retinitis is usually distinctive. Infection usually starts as a solitary lesion, in contrast to the retinitis in ARN and PORN. Advancement of infection into normal retina is characterized by a dry granular border with multiple dot-like satellite lesions. Other than the retinitis, intraocular inflammation is typically minimal. Spread of the infection is relentless without treatment with antiviral medication and HAART [113]. Patients may present with either a more fulminant form, characterized by retinal necrosis with hemorrhage that develops in the posterior retina, or a more indolent form, seen as a granular lesion in the peripheral retina, often with little or no associated hemorrhage. An uncommon presentation is frosted branch angiitis [115]. Because a sizeable minority of patients with CMV retinopathy are asymptomatic, routine ophthalmoscopic screening has been recommended at 3-month intervals in severely immunocompromised individuals with CD4 counts less than 50 cells/ul [126].

For treatment of CMV retinitis in AIDS patients, intravenous ganciclovir, foscarnet, or cidofovir may be used. More recently, oral valganciclovir, a prodrug of ganciclovir with excellent bioavailability, has been used to treat CMV. Notably, all of these drugs only inactivate and do not eradicate the infection; therefore they must be continued until the patient is no longer severely immunocompromised. In many cases, signs of disease activity persist despite treatment with these drugs, especially late in the course of disease; therefore additional initiation with HAART is critical to eradicate the disease [113].

In combination with systemic therapy, local intravitreal injections of either ganciclovir or foscarnet may be used to achieve high drug levels (as discussed in the Sect. 6.1). To achieve adequate dosage, injections must be given 2–3 times weekly; for this reason, the ganciclovir implant was developed, which released relatively high intraocular drug levels for approximately 8 months [113]. However, because of the rapid decline in incidence of CMV retinitis with the advent of HAART, the ganciclovir implant is no longer in production, and its use is now historical.

Besides systemic treatment with anti-CMV medication, the most important treatment of newly diagnosed CMV retinitis is to start HAART in patients who have not yet started HIV treatment or to reestablish immune recovery by switching medications in patients who are already receiving HAART medication. In some practices, HAART therapy initiation may be delayed until treatment for CMV is started to reduce the risk of systemic inflammatory reactions against the pathogens released during immune recovery [113]. Once immune recovery has been achieved, meaning sustained CD4 counts of greater than 100 cells/uL for 6 months, treatment for CMV may be stopped as long as there are no signs of persistent infection [127]. CMV retinitis can reactivate after anti-CMV drugs are stopped; therefore patients must be monitored for recurrence. The most helpful laboratory indicators are CD4 count and HIV viral load [128].

Immune recovery uveitis is a complication of treatment of CMV retinitis patients with HAART; it is caused by immune reaction to CMV antigens made worse by recovery of the immune system with treatment of HIV/AIDS [129]. The most severe inflammatory response usually begins within several weeks after starting HAART, and complications include macular edema, epiretinal membrane, retinal neovascularization, and a host of other complications of severe uveitis. Patients with immune recovery uveitis may require local or systemic corticosteroids to treat inflammation; systemic CMV infection is usually eradicated once immune recovery is achieved, and systemic anti-CMV medications may often be stopped [113].

Although not as common as in ARN, retinal detachment is a common complication of CMV retinitis. In the era before HAART, retinal detachments occurred in more than one-third of patients with CMV retinitis who survived 1 year or longer. More recently, the risk of detachment is substantially less among patients receiving HAART, perhaps because of better infection control resulting in smaller lesions and more adherent scars [130]. As in ARN, retinal detachment is often due to a combination of tractional and rhegmatogenous components, and treatment requires vitrectomy with laser and either gas, or more commonly, silicone oil tamponade.

West Nile Virus

West Nile virus (WNV) infection is caused by an enveloped single-stranded RNA *Flavivirus*, passed to humans by the *Culex* mosquito, with wild birds serving as the reservoir. Much more rarely, blood-to-blood or transplacental transmission may occur [131]. It is present in many parts of the world including Africa, Europe, Australia, and Asia, and, since 1999, it has spread rapidly throughout many parts of the Western hemisphere, including the USA [132]. Peak season for contraction of the disease is in the summer months.

Presentation

Incubation lasts between 2 and 14 days. About 80 % of human infections are asymptomatic; only 20 % of people develop symptoms. Symptomatic patients usually have a self-limited febrile flu-like illness, which usually lasts less than a week. Fever is often high grade (>39 °C). Severe neurologic disease (meningoencephalitis) is rare, occurring in approximately 1 % of patients, and is associated with advanced age and diabetes mellitus [131]. Patients with WNV meningoencephalitis may present with a wide variety of neurological symptoms following more typical systemic complaints earlier in the disease.

Several ophthalmologic findings have been recognized, including chorioretinitis, anterior uveitis, retinal vasculitis, and optic neuritis. Multifocal chorioretinitis is the most common finding, occurring in almost 80 % of patients with acute WNV infection and associated neurologic illness [133]. An associated mild to moderate vitritis is frequently observed. Most patients have minimal or no ocular symptoms. Active chorioretinal lesions appear as small circular deep creamy lesions, while inactive chorioretinal lesions are atrophic and partially pigmented with a “target-like” appearance. Chorioretinal lesions nearly always involve the periphery but also often involve the posterior pole. Linear clustering of chorioretinal lesions is common, sometimes mirroring the course of retinal nerve fibers [134]. Other ophthalmic manifestations include anterior uveitis, vitritis, retinal hemorrhages, optic nerve edema, and retinal vascular sheathing.

Diagnostic Testing

Serum testing may be helpful in diagnosis of infection with WNV. The most common serum test is detection of WNV IgM antibodies in serum with an enzyme-linked immunosorbent assay (ELISA). Testing for IgM antibodies may also be performed on cerebrospinal fluid to confirm infection of the central nervous system; positive testing confirms WNV meningoencephalitis [131, 135]. Cross-reactivity may occur with other similar viruses, and special testing may be necessary to differentiate WNV from infection with one of these other viruses [131].

Treatment

There is, at present, no proven treatment for WNV infection, but supportive therapy is indicated in severe cases. Prevention of mosquito bites is the mainstay in reducing possibility of infection. Topical corticosteroids may be helpful for cases of anterior uveitis, and various ophthalmic treatments may be indicated for secondary ophthalmic complications (e.g., panretinal photocoagulation for retinal neovascularization) [90].

Prognosis

The outcome of WNV systemic disease is good in most patients, but neurologic sequelae or even death may occur in severe cases of WNV meningoencephalitis [135]. Ocular manifestations are usually self-limited. Inactive choroidal lesions may leave behind pigmented scars and can sometimes cause visual impairment if involving the macula or optic nerve. Rarely, severe occlusive retinal vasculitis may result in retinal neovascularization and its sequelae [90].

Rift Valley Fever

Rift Valley fever (RVF) is an arthropod-borne viral zoonosis caused by Bunyaviridae. The virus primarily infects domesticated cattle. It is transmitted to humans by either mosquito bite or through contact with infected animals, and the disease can occur in epidemics. RVF has been found in sub-Saharan and North Africa and more recently in the Arabian Peninsula [90, 136–138]. For additional information, see Table 6.2.

Dengue Fever

Dengue fever is the most common mosquito-borne viral zoonosis in humans. It is caused by the dengue virus, a *Flavivirus*, and is transmitted by the *Aedes aegypti* mosquito. It is common in tropical and subtropical regions and afflicts 100 million people annually [139]. See Table 6.2 for additional information.

Chikungunya

Chikungunya virus is an arthropod-borne *Alphavirus* that causes epidemics of human disease by transmission via several mosquito species, usually *Aedes aegypti*. It was originally endemic in parts of west, central, and southern Africa. In 2004, novel and highly contagious strains emerged in Kenya, which then spread to several islands in the Indian Ocean, most notably La Reunion. These more infectious strains continued to spread throughout Asia, and subsequently a few outbreaks were seen in Europe. In 2013, a large outbreak began to spread through the Americas, and the virus has now been noted in the Caribbean, Central America, South America, and Mexico [90, 138, 140–146]. See Table 6.2 for additional information.

Coxsackievirus

Coxsackievirus is a type of enterovirus that may cause a variety of syndromes in humans. A number of different serotypes are known, grouped into "type A" and "type B," some of which have been reported to rarely cause ocular symptoms in addition to systemic disease. The most well-known syndrome related to the virus is hand, foot, and mouth disease, which is frequently associated with Coxsackievirus type A16 [147–151]. The disease is usually brief and benign and most common in children. For additional information, see Table 6.2.

Protozoa and Parasites

Ocular Toxoplasmosis

Toxoplasma gondii is an obligate intracellular protozoan parasite and is the most common cause of infectious posterior uveitis in the world. It is most prevalent in South and Latin America as well as Africa and parts of Asia, where seropositivity may be over 80 %, but the organism is found in many other parts of the world, including the USA (seropositivity around 10 %) [152].

T. gondii exists in three states: oocysts, tachyzoites, and bradyzoites. Oocysts are the product of the parasite's sexual cycle in the intestine of felines and release infectious sporozoites in cat feces. Tachyzoites are asexual forms that arise after ingestion of sporozoites by the new host that damage host tissue through rapid replication. Tachyzoites transform into bradyzoites after the host immune system begins attacking the parasite. Bradyzoites are cysts that reside dormant in tissues and replicate slowly without causing significant disease unless they reactivate into the tachyzoite state again. In humans, bradyzoites are often harbored in the central nervous system, including the eye.

Humans become infected by ingestion of undercooked cyst-contaminated meat products or by sporulated oocysts from cat feces, which can be found in contaminated water, soil, or on vegetables [153]. Toxoplasmosis is a well-known cause of congenital infection; however, most cases are contracted after birth [154].

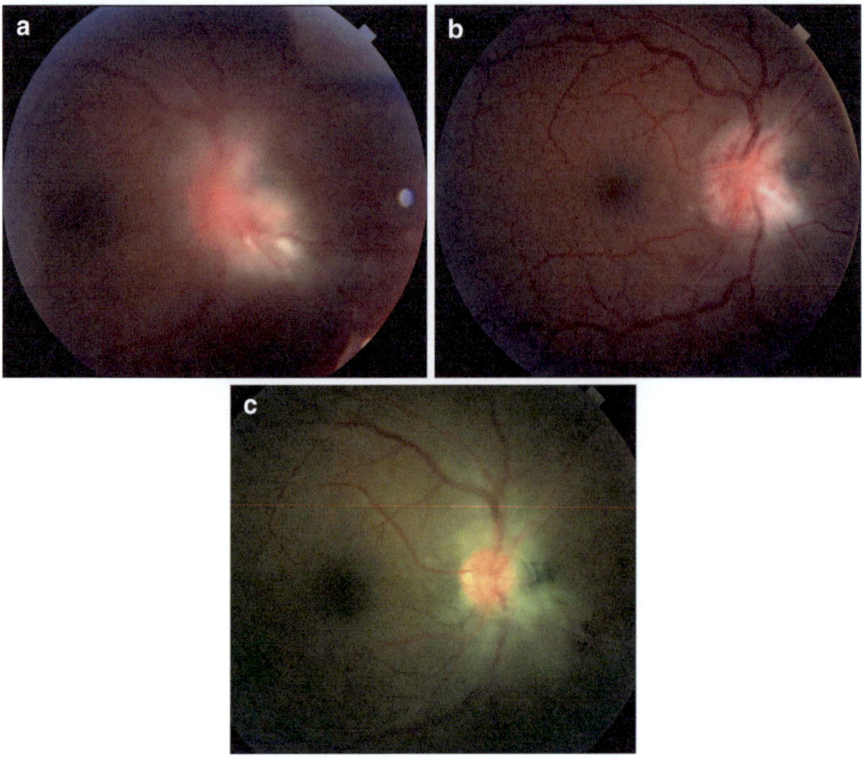

Fig. 6.15 Ocular toxoplasmosis. An anterior chamber paracentesis was negative for toxoplasmosis via PCR. Serum testing was positive for toxoplasmosis IgG. (**a**) Moderate vitritis and severe optic nerve inflammation, with fluffy white chorioretinal infiltrates evident on the nasal border of the optic disk, and sheathing of the peripapillary retinal vessels. (**b**) Over 2 weeks, inflammation improved with trimethoprim/sulfamethoxazole. (**c**) By 2 months, a peripapillary chorioretinal scar became evident, suggesting secondary retinitis and papillitis secondary to prior ocular toxoplasmosis

Presentation

Necrotizing focal chorioretinitis with overlying vitritis, the classic "headlight in fog" if vitritis is dense, is the typical ocular presentation of toxoplasmosis, but a variety of other presentations may be manifest. However, intraocular inflammation does not occur in the absence of a retinal lesion. In secondary infection, the infection is reactivated at the site of a preexisting chorioretinal scar, and retinitis appears adjacent to the scar; 70 % of cases that present to ophthalmologists are due to secondary infection (Fig. 6.15) [155]. In primary infection, no chorioretinal scar has yet developed. The retinitis in toxoplasmosis may be difficult to distinguish from ARN secondary to viral infection, and testing and treatment for both conditions may be warranted initially (Fig. 6.16). Congenital toxoplasmosis may be difficult to distinguish from acquired toxoplasmosis, but congenital lesions are more commonly found in the macula and are more likely to be bilateral [155].

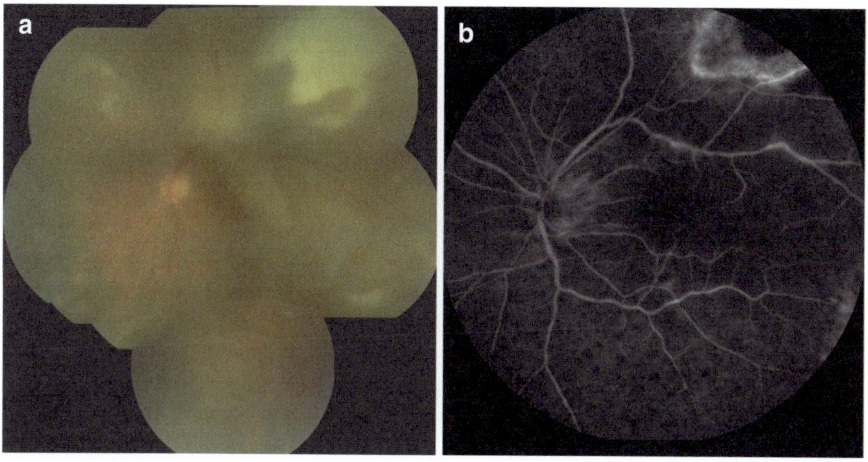

Fig. 6.16 Retinitis secondary to toxoplasmosis. Vitreous paracentesis was positive for toxoplasmosis via PCR. (**a**) Moderate vitritis is evident. There is diffuse preretinal fibrosis over the posterior pole. There are multifocal patches of discrete retinitis, most notably superotemporally. No chorioretinal scar suggestive of toxoplasmosis is evident. (**b**) Fluorescein angiography demonstrates staining of the retinal veins and early hyperfluorescence with late leakage at the border of retinitis superotemporally. The optic nerve is hyperfluorescent

An unusual but well-described presentation of primary or secondary intraocular toxoplasmosis is punctate outer retinal toxoplasmosis (PORT), characterized by multifocal small lesions in the deep retina and RPE. Because the inflammation is focal and deep, there is usually minimal associated vitritis. After resolution of PORT, granular white lesions may remain, and often patients are left with visual loss due to optic neuropathy [156]. Patients with PORT are usually in the pediatric age group and may arise from either congenital or acquired infection [153].

Other presentations may include neuroretinitis with a macular scar, scleritis, granulomatous anterior uveitis, trabeculitis, retinal vasculitis, proliferative vitreoretinopathy, and vitreous hemorrhage and tractional retinal detachment due to secondary retinal neovascularization [153]. Retinal arteriolar plaques, or Kyrieleis plaques, may occur adjacent to the active toxoplasmosis retinitis but are not characteristic of toxoplasmosis.

Patients who present with secondary infection are usually young adults between the ages of 20 and 40 years, while those that present with primary toxoplasmosis infections are usually older, between 40 and 60 years [155]. Recurrence is common, occurring in up to 80 % of patients followed for at least 5 years [155, 157]. Severe presentations of ocular toxoplasmosis may be associated with older age or immunocompromised states, including HIV/AIDS [153].

Diagnostic Testing

Serum testing, usually ELISA, may be helpful in distinguishing primary toxoplasmosis, in which IgM or IgA antibodies may be present, from cases of reactivation. Presence of IgG antibodies is a sign of prior infection; a positive toxoplasma IgG may be of little diagnostic benefit in populations with high seropositivity rates [158].

Testing of intraocular specimens, whether aqueous or vitreous humor, may be helpful in diagnosis of ocular toxoplasmosis. Both PCR testing and detection of intraocular toxoplasma-specific antibodies may be utilized. Intraocular antibody synthesis is determined by the Goldmann–Witmer coefficient (GWC), which is based on the comparison of the *T. gondii*-specific antibodies in the aqueous humor and in the serum in relation to the globulin titers in the same fluids. A high coefficient indicates active toxoplasmosis infection [159]. However, the time interval before activation of local antibody production may vary, and false negatives may occur when using the GWC alone; therefore more recently DNA amplification using PCR has become the test of choice when examining intraocular fluid specimens, either alone or in combination with antibody testing [153].

Treatment

Treatment of toxoplasmosis remains controversial, as there is disagreement regarding indications for treatment as well as ideal treatment regimen. In most immunocompetent patients with ocular toxoplasmosis, the intraocular inflammation is self-limited; therefore treatment may not be indicated if the active lesion is small and peripheral. Common indications for treatment include active retinitis with posterior lesions near the optic nerve or macula, large lesions >2 disk diameters, or lesions in immunocompromised individuals.

Antibiotic therapy is usually given for a 6–8-week course. Classic antibiotic therapy consists of three-drug combination therapy including pyrimethamine, sulfadiazine, and folinic acid. More recently, less toxic medications have become popular in the treatment of toxoplasmosis, including clindamycin, azithromycin, atovaquone, and trimethoprim/sulfamethoxazole. These medications have been used in combination or alone to treat ocular toxoplasmosis. However, there have been no definitive clinical trials examining the efficacy of these medications in improving visual outcomes or in decreasing rates of recurrence [160]. Alternatively, clindamycin (450 ug/0.1 ml) may be injected directly intravitreally, which provides more targeted antibiotic treatment for severe cases [161].

Corticosteroid therapy, either oral, periocular, or topical, may be administered in conjunction with antibiotic therapy in cases of severe vitritis or anterior chamber reaction. It is not recommended unless antibiotic therapy is given in conjunction, as the resultant immunosuppression caused by these medications may lead to fulminant and progressive infection [162].

Prognosis

Most cases of ocular toxoplasmosis are self-limited. Inflammation usually improves between 2 and 4 months after presentation. However, the macula and optic nerve may be involved, particularly in cases of congenital toxoplasmosis. Approximately 25 % of ocular toxoplasmosis cases may result in visual acuity of 20/200 or worse. In addition, recurrences are common; nearly 80 % of patients who were followed for more than 5 years had an episode of recurrence in one study [155].

Malaria

Malaria is a worldwide health problem, resulting in death of over 1 million people annually. It is caused by infection of erythrocytes by *Plasmodium*, which are protozoa transmitted to humans by mosquito bite, most commonly the *Anopheles* mosquito. There are five species of *Plasmodium*, the prevalence of which varies regionally: P. *falciparum*, *P. vivax*, *P. malariae*, *P. ovale*, and *P. knowlesi*. The disease is endemic to parts of Africa, Asia, and Latin America. New cases have been reported in the USA, although most cases in the USA are imported after travel to more endemic regions of the world [145, 163–166]. See Table 6.2 for additional information.

Toxocariasis

Toxocariasis is an infection caused by larvae of *Toxocara canis* (dog roundworm) and less frequently by *Toxocara cati* (cat roundworm). It is contracted by ingestion of soil or food products contaminated with embryonated eggs. Once ingested, larvae hatch in the small intestine and then migrate to tissues, most notably the lungs, muscle, and eyes. Larvae resident in human tissue never develop into adult organisms capable of reproduction [167]. The organism is common in many parts of the world, including the USA, but symptomatic *Toxocara* infection is comparatively rare [167].

Presentation

The systemic form of toxocariasis is termed "viscera larva migrans," which is characterized by fever, malaise, hepatosplenomegaly, rash, and leukocytosis. Ocular toxocariasis, or "ocular larva migrans," is the most common localized manifestation of *Toxocara*. Ocular toxocariasis lesions are unilateral 90 % of the time and appear as a whitish mass involving the retina and peripheral vitreous. A fibrovascular band often runs between the lesion and the posterior pole or optic nerve (Fig. 6.17). The lesions may be associated with vitritis or vitreous haze early in the infection. Other manifestations include panuveitis, posterior pole granuloma, optic nerve granuloma, and vitreous lesions. It is one of the conditions that may cause leukocoria in the pediatric population [168].

Diagnostic Testing

Serologic testing is often inconclusive in ocular toxocariasis, and diagnosis may be difficult. Although eosinophilia is often present in systemic infection, this is often not the case in ocular toxocariasis. ELISA and calculation of Goldmann–Witmer coefficients may be performed on intraocular fluids to aid in diagnosis; PCR may be negative as *Toxocara* DNA is not often shed into intraocular fluids [167]. Vitreous biopsy and cytology may be helpful in difficult cases [169].

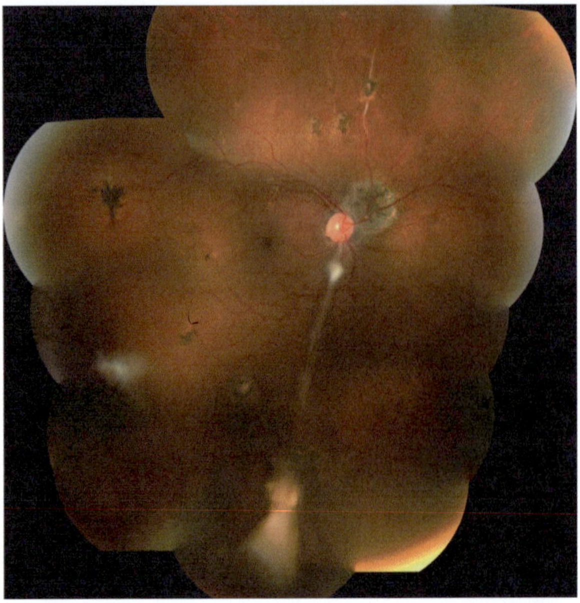

Fig. 6.17 Ocular toxocariasis. Fundus examination revealed findings suggestive of ocular toxocariasis: a whitish mass involving the retina and peripheral vitreous inferiorly, with a fibrovascular band running between the peripheral lesion and the optic nerve. There were a number of multifocal chorioretinal scars but no active inflammation

Treatment
Corticosteroids are the mainstay in treatment of intraocular inflammation and can be administered topically, periocularly, or systemically. Treatment with oral albendazole in ocular toxocariasis is controversial, as it is thought to increase inflammatory response in some cases as organism antigens are released [170]. There have been several reports of pars plana vitrectomy for ocular toxocariasis, which is indicated in cases of tractional or rhegmatogenous retinal detachment, endophthalmitis, or vitreous hemorrhage secondary to retinal neovascularization [167].

Prognosis
Visual prognosis in ocular toxocariasis is often poor and is often due to retinal scarring, detachment, or other sequelae from long-standing intraocular inflammation. In one report, one-third of patients had visual acuity of 20/200 or worse [171].

Diffuse Unilateral Subacute Neuroretinitis

The term *diffuse unilateral subacute neuroretinitis* (DUSN) was first used by Gass and Scelfo in 1978 [177]. They described a syndrome which included insidious severe loss of peripheral and central vision with associated findings of vitreous inflammation, diffuse RPE changes with relative sparing of the macula, narrowing of the retinal vessels, optic atrophy, increased retinal circulation time, and subnormal electroretinographic findings. Dr. Gass then observed a nematode in two patients with similar presentation, and it became clear that the condition was due to migration of a nematode in the subretinal space [178].

Although nematodes are the causative organisms of DUSN, the exact etiological agent is often not clear. Parasites of different sizes and several species of nematodes have been reported as the possible etiologic agent of DUSN, including *Toxocara canis*, *Baylisascaris procyonis*, and *Ancylostoma caninum*, but most reports do not present conclusive evidence about the specific agent. The type of nematode likely varies depending on geographic region, as the average size of observed nematodes varies depending on region [179].

Presentation

The disease often presents in children or young adults. In the early stage, patients may present with scotomas or decreased visual acuity. Ocular findings include mild to moderate vitritis, mild optic disk edema, and multifocal evanescent whitish-yellow deep retinal and choroidal lesions [180]. The patchy choroidal lesions resolve spontaneously but may reappear along with migration of the worm. In the later stage, which is the more common presentation, diffuse degeneration and depigmentation of the RPE, usually most prominent in the peripapillary and peripheral retina, occur along with progressive optic nerve atrophy and arteriolar narrowing [181]. An intraocular worm may be seen in 25–40 % of cases and appears as a motile, white, glistening nematode that varies in length from 400 to 2,000 μm. The worms may sometimes leave tract-like RPE changes in the wake of movement [182].

Diagnostic Testing

Serologic testing, stool samples, and blood smears are often not helpful in DUSN. Eosinophilia may be seen in some cases and can aid in diagnosis. In both the early and late stages, electroretinograms are often diminished but not extinguished and can be helpful in making the diagnosis [179].

Treatment

If a worm is seen, it can be treated with laser photocoagulation without causing significant intraocular inflammation. In a series of 70 patients diagnosed with DUSN, Garcia and colleagues found a live worm in 4 patients in the early stage and in 22 in the late stage. After photocoagulation treatment, all the patients in the early stage but none in the late stage had improved visual acuity [180, 181]. Oral antihelminthic medications, most notable albendazole, may also be used, but the medications do not always kill the subretinal nematode [183, 184].

Prognosis

If caught early and treated, visual acuity often is minimally affected. Visual prognosis in late stages is poor, with 80 % of cases resulting in visual acuity of 20/200 or worse [181].

Onchocerciasis

Onchocerciasis, or "river blindness," is caused by infection of *Onchocerca volvulus*, which is transmitted by the *Simulium* blackfly, a species that lives and breeds in rivers and streams. The disease affects over 35 million people worldwide and is most abundant in Africa, but it may also be found in the Mediterranean and Central and South America [95, 172–176]. The life cycle of *Onchocerca volvulus* begins when the female blackfly ingests microfilariae from infected human blood. The microfilariae develop into larvae in the blackfly and are then transmitted to humans via blackfly bite. The larvae then develop into adult worms, which often settle in subcutaneous tissue and form fibrous nodules called onchocercomas. The adult worms within these nodules then give rise to microfilariae, which spread throughout the skin, often causing intense skin itching and depigmentation. Death of microfilariae often causes a severe inflammatory response [172–176]. See Table 6.2 for additional information.

Gnathostomiasis

Gnathostomiasis is caused by infection by the nematode *Gnathostoma spinigerum* or *Gnathostoma hispidum*. The disease is found in tropical and subtropical regions and is endemic in parts of Asia and Latin America. Humans become accidental hosts by ingesting undercooked or raw meat or through penetration of the skin during preparation of food [174, 185]. See Table 6.2.

Cysticercosis

Cysticercosis is caused by ingestion of undercooked meat (usually pork) containing *Cysticercus cellulosae*, the larval form of *Taenia solium* or *Taenia saginata*. It affects an estimated 50 million people worldwide. Endemic areas include Mexico and Latin America, sub-Saharan Africa, India, and East Asia [174, 186–188]. See Table 6.2.

References

1. Vaziri K, Schwartz SG, Kishor K, Flynn Jr HW. Endophthalmitis: state of the art. Clin Ophthalmol. 2015;9:95–108.
2. Jackson TL, Eykyn SJ, Graham EM, Stanford MR. Endogenous bacterial endophthalmitis: a 17-year prospective series and review of 267 reported cases. Surv Ophthalmol. 2003;48(4):403–23.

3. Jackson TL, Paraskevopoulos T, Georgalas I. Systematic review of 342 cases of endogenous bacterial endophthalmitis. Surv Ophthalmol. 2014;59(6):627–35.
4. Dossarps D, Bron AM, Koehrer P, Aho-Glele LS, Creuzot-Garcher C, FRCR net. Endophthalmitis after intravitreal injections: incidence, presentation, management, and visual outcome. Am J Ophthalmol. 2015;160(1):17–25.
5. Leng T, Miller D, Flynn Jr HW, Jacobs DJ, Gedde SJ. Delayed-onset bleb-associated endophthalmitis (1996–2008): causative organisms and visual acuity outcomes. Retina. 2011;31(2):344–52.
6. Meredith TA, McCannel CA, Barr C, Doft BH, Peskin E, Maguire MG, et al. Postinjection endophthalmitis in the comparison of age-related macular degeneration treatments trials (CATT). Ophthalmology. 2015;122(4):817–21.
7. Results of the Endophthalmitis Vitrectomy Study. A randomized trial of immediate vitrectomy and of intravenous antibiotics for the treatment of postoperative bacterial endophthalmitis. Arch Ophthalmol. 1995;113(12):1479–96.
8. Shirodkar AR, Pathengay A, Flynn Jr HW, Albini TA, Berrocal AM, Davis JL, et al. Delayed-versus acute-onset endophthalmitis after cataract surgery. Am J Ophthalmol. 2012;153(3):391–8.e2.
9. Harris EW, D'Amico DJ, Bhisitkul R, Priebe GP, Petersen R. Bacterial subretinal abscess: a case report and review of the literature. Am J Ophthalmol. 2000;129(6):778–85.
10. Combey de Lambert A, Campolmi N, Cornut PL, Aptel F, Creuzot-Garcher C, Chiquet C, et al. Baseline factors predictive of visual prognosis in acute postoperative bacterial endophthalmitis in patients undergoing cataract surgery. JAMA Ophthalmol. 2013;131(9):1159–66.
11. Bhagat N, Nagori S, Zarbin M. Post-traumatic infectious endophthalmitis. Surv Ophthalmol. 2011;56(3):214–51.
12. Barza M, Pavan PR, Doft BH, Wisniewski SR, Wilson LA, Han DP, et al. Evaluation of microbiological diagnostic techniques in postoperative endophthalmitis in the Endophthalmitis Vitrectomy Study. Arch Ophthalmol. 1997;115(9):1142–50.
13. Wykoff CC, Parrott MB, Flynn Jr HW, Shi W, Miller D, Alfonso EC. Nosocomial acute-onset postoperative endophthalmitis at a university teaching hospital (2002–2009). Am J Ophthalmol. 2010;150(3):392–8.e2.
14. Sandvig KU, Dannevig L. Postoperative endophthalmitis: establishment and results of a national registry. J Cataract Refract Surg. 2003;29(7):1273–80.
15. Fileta JB, Scott IU, Flynn Jr HW. Meta-analysis of infectious endophthalmitis after intravitreal injection of anti-vascular endothelial growth factor agents. Ophthalmic Surg Lasers Imaging Retina. 2014;45(2):143–9.
16. Cutler Peck CM, Brubaker J, Clouser S, Danford C, Edelhauser HE, Mamalis N. Toxic anterior segment syndrome: common causes. J Cataract Refract Surg. 2010;36(7):1073–80.
17. Ciulla TA, Starr MB, Masket S. Bacterial endophthalmitis prophylaxis for cataract surgery: an evidence-based update. Ophthalmology. 2002;109(1):13–24.
18. Schimel AM, Miller D, Flynn Jr HW. Endophthalmitis isolates and antibiotic susceptibilities: a 10-year review of culture-proven cases. Am J Ophthalmol. 2013;156(1):50–2.e1.
19. Gentile RC, Shukla S, Shah M, Ritterband DC, Engelbert M, Davis A, et al. Microbiological spectrum and antibiotic sensitivity in endophthalmitis: a 25-year review. Ophthalmology. 2014;121(8):1634–42.
20. Hariprasad SM, Mieler WF, Holz ER. Vitreous and aqueous penetration of orally administered gatifloxacin in humans. Arch Ophthalmol. 2003;121(3):345–50.
21. Hooper CY, Lightman SL, Pacheco P, Tam PM, Khan A, Taylor SR. Adjunctive antibiotics in the treatment of acute bacterial endophthalmitis following cataract surgery. Acta Ophthalmol. 2012;90(7):e572–3.
22. Prasad N, Latina MA. Blebitis and endophthalmitis after glaucoma filtering surgery. Int Ophthalmol Clin. 2007;47(2):85–97.
23. Pflugfelder SC, Flynn Jr HW, Zwickey TA, Forster RK, Tsiligianni A, Culbertson WW, et al. Exogenous fungal endophthalmitis. Ophthalmology. 1988;95(1):19–30.

24. Kim DY, Moon HI, Joe SG, Kim JG, Yoon YH, Lee JY. Recent clinical manifestation and prognosis of fungal endophthalmitis: a 7-year experience at a tertiary referral center in Korea. J Korean Med Sci. 2015;30(7):960–4.
25. Kernt M, Neubauer AS, De Kaspar HM, Kampik A. Intravitreal voriconazole: in vitro safety-profile for fungal endophthalmitis. Retina. 2009;29(3):362–70.
26. Verbraeken H, Geeroms B, Karemera A. Treatment of endophthalmitis by pars plana vitrectomy. Ophthalmologica. 1988;197(1):19–25.
27. Busbee BG, Recchia FM, Kaiser R, Nagra P, Rosenblatt B, Pearlman RB. Bleb-associated endophthalmitis: clinical characteristics and visual outcomes. Ophthalmology. 2004;111(8):1495–503; discussion 503.
28. Lindstedt EW, Bennebroek CA, van der Werf DJ, Veckeneer M, Norel AO, Nielsen CC, et al. A prospective multicenter randomized placebo-controlled trial of dexamethasone as an adjuvant in the treatment of postoperative bacterial endophthalmitis: interim safety analysis of the study drug and analysis of overall treatment results. Graefes Arch Clin Exp Ophthalmol. 2014;252(10):1631–7.
29. Albrecht E, Richards JC, Pollock T, Cook C, Myers L. Adjunctive use of intravitreal dexamethasone in presumed bacterial endophthalmitis: a randomised trial. Br J Ophthalmol. 2011;95(10):1385–8.
30. Friling E, Lundstrom M, Stenevi U, Montan P. Six-year incidence of endophthalmitis after cataract surgery: Swedish national study. J Cataract Refract Surg. 2013;39(1):15–21.
31. Chaudhry IA, Shamsi FA, Al-Harthi E, Al-Theeb A, Elzaridi E, Riley FC. Incidence and visual outcome of endophthalmitis associated with intraocular foreign bodies. Graefes Arch Clin Exp Ophthalmol. 2008;246(2):181–6.
32. Simunovic MP, Rush RB, Hunyor AP, Chang AA. Endophthalmitis following intravitreal injection versus endophthalmitis following cataract surgery: clinical features, causative organisms and post-treatment outcomes. Br J Ophthalmol. 2012;96(6):862–6.
33. Mamalis N, Edelhauser HF, Dawson DG, Chew J, LeBoyer RM, Werner L. Toxic anterior segment syndrome. J Cataract Refract Surg. 2006;32(2):324–33.
34. Hatch WV, Cernat G, Wong D, Devenyi R, Bell CM. Risk factors for acute endophthalmitis after cataract surgery: a population-based study. Ophthalmology. 2009;116(3):425–30.
35. Cao H, Zhang L, Li L, Lo S. Risk factors for acute endophthalmitis following cataract surgery: a systematic review and meta-analysis. PLoS One. 2013;8(8):e71731.
36. Endophthalmitis Study Group ESoC, Refractive S. Prophylaxis of postoperative endophthalmitis following cataract surgery: results of the ESCRS multicenter study and identification of risk factors. J Cataract Refract Surg. 2007;33(6):978–88.
37. Moloney TP, Park J. Microbiological isolates and antibiotic sensitivities in culture-proven endophthalmitis: a 15-year review. Br J Ophthalmol. 2014;98(11):1492–7.
38. Aldave AJ, Stein JD, Deramo VA, Shah GK, Fischer DH, Maguire JI. Treatment strategies for postoperative Propionibacterium acnes endophthalmitis. Ophthalmology. 1999;106(12): 2395–401.
39. Rai P, Kotecha A, Kaltsos K, Ruddle JB, Murdoch IE, Bunce C, et al. Changing trends in the incidence of bleb-related infection in trabeculectomy. Br J Ophthalmol. 2012;96(7):971–5.
40. VanderBeek BL, Bonaffini SG, Ma L. The association between intravitreal steroids and post-injection endophthalmitis rates. Ophthalmology. 2015;122(11):2311–5.
41. Roth DB, Flynn Jr HW. Distinguishing between infectious and noninfectious endophthalmitis after intravitreal triamcinolone injection. Am J Ophthalmol. 2008;146(3):346–7.
42. Shah CP, Garg SJ, Vander JF, Brown GC, Kaiser RS, Haller JA, et al. Outcomes and risk factors associated with endophthalmitis after intravitreal injection of anti-vascular endothelial growth factor agents. Ophthalmology. 2011;118(10):2028–34.
43. Small KW, Chan CK, Silva-Garcia R, Walsh TJ. Onset of an outbreak of Bipolaris hawaiiensis fungal endophthalmitis after intravitreal injections of triamcinolone. Ophthalmology. 2014;121(4):952–8.
44. Goldberg RA, Flynn Jr HW, Isom RF, Miller D, Gonzalez S. An outbreak of streptococcus endophthalmitis after intravitreal injection of bevacizumab. Am J Ophthalmol. 2012;153(2): 204–8.e1.

45. Essex RW, Yi Q, Charles PG, Allen PJ. Post-traumatic endophthalmitis. Ophthalmology. 2004;111(11):2015–22.
46. Andreoli CM, Andreoli MT, Kloek CE, Ahuero AE, Vavvas D, Durand ML. Low rate of endophthalmitis in a large series of open globe injuries. Am J Ophthalmol. 2009;147(4):601–8. e2.
47. Colyer MH, Chun DW, Bower KS, Dick JS, Weichel ED. Perforating globe injuries during operation Iraqi Freedom. Ophthalmology. 2008;115(11):2087–93.
48. Lit ES, Young LH. Anterior and posterior segment intraocular foreign bodies. Int Ophthalmol Clin. 2002;42(3):107–20.
49. Patel SN, Langer PD, Zarbin MA, Bhagat N. Diagnostic value of clinical examination and radiographic imaging in identification of intraocular foreign bodies in open globe injury. Eur J Ophthalmol. 2012;22(2):259–68.
50. Long C, Liu B, Xu C, Jing Y, Yuan Z, Lin X. Causative organisms of post-traumatic endophthalmitis: a 20-year retrospective study. BMC Ophthalmol. 2014;14:34.
51. Alfaro DV, Roth D, Liggett PE. Posttraumatic endophthalmitis. Causative organisms, treatment, and prevention. Retina. 1994;14(3):206–11.
52. Spalding SC, Sternberg Jr P. Controversies in the management of posterior segment ocular trauma. Retina. 1990;10 Suppl 1:S76–82.
53. Sridhar J, Kuriyan AE, Flynn Jr HW, Miller D. Endophthalmitis caused by Pseudomonas aeruginosa: clinical features, antibiotic susceptibilities, and treatment outcomes. Retina. 2015;35(6):1101–6.
54. Wong JS, Chan TK, Lee HM, Chee SP. Endogenous bacterial endophthalmitis: an east Asian experience and a reappraisal of a severe ocular affliction. Ophthalmology. 2000;107(8):1483–91.
55. Shankar K, Gyanendra L, Hari S, Narayan SD. Culture proven endogenous bacterial endophthalmitis in apparently healthy individuals. Ocul Immunol Inflamm. 2009;17(6):396–9.
56. Chen YJ, Kuo HK, Wu PC, Kuo ML, Tsai HH, Liu CC, et al. A 10-year comparison of endogenous endophthalmitis outcomes: an east Asian experience with Klebsiella pneumoniae infection. Retina. 2004;24(3):383–90.
57. Schiedler V, Scott IU, Flynn Jr HW, Davis JL, Benz MS, Miller D. Culture-proven endogenous endophthalmitis: clinical features and visual acuity outcomes. Am J Ophthalmol. 2004;137(4):725–31.
58. Lingappan A, Wykoff CC, Albini TA, Miller D, Pathengay A, Davis JL, et al. Endogenous fungal endophthalmitis: causative organisms, management strategies, and visual acuity outcomes. Am J Ophthalmol. 2012;153(1):162–6.e1.
59. Sridhar J, Flynn Jr HW, Kuriyan AE, Miller D, Albini T. Endogenous fungal endophthalmitis: risk factors, clinical features, and treatment outcomes in mold and yeast infections. J Ophthalmic Inflamm Infect. 2013;3(1):60.
60. Shen X, Xu G. Vitrectomy for endogenous fungal endophthalmitis. Ocul Immunol Inflamm. 2009;17(3):148–52.
61. Smiddy WE. Treatment outcomes of endogenous fungal endophthalmitis. Curr Opin Ophthalmol. 1998;9(3):66–70.
62. Jolly SS, Brownstein S. Endogenous Nocardia subretinal abscess. Arch Ophthalmol. 1996;114(9):1147–8.
63. Silva RA, Young R, Sridhar J. Nocardia choroidal abscess: risk factors, treatment strategies, and visual outcomes. Retina. 2015;35(10):2137–46.
64. Ness T, Pelz K, Hansen LL. Endogenous endophthalmitis: microorganisms, disposition and prognosis. Acta Ophthalmol Scand. 2007;85(8):852–6.
65. Smith SR, Kroll AJ, Lou PL, Ryan EA. Endogenous bacterial and fungal endophthalmitis. Int Ophthalmol Clin. 2007;47(2):173–83.
66. Gupta V, Gupta A, Rao NA. Intraocular tuberculosis – an update. Surv Ophthalmol. 2007;52(6):561–87.
67. Yeh S, Sen HN, Colyer M, Zapor M, Wroblewski K. Update on ocular tuberculosis. Curr Opin Ophthalmol. 2012;23(6):551–6.
68. Mandelcorn ED. Infectious causes of posterior uveitis. Can J Ophthalmol. 2013;48(1):31–9.

69. Biswas J, Sharma T, Gopal L, Madhavan HN, Sulochana KN, Ramakrishnan S. Eales disease – an update. Surv Ophthalmol. 2002;47(3):197–214.
70. Dheda K, van Zyl Smit R, Badri M, Pai M. T-cell interferon-gamma release assays for the rapid immunodiagnosis of tuberculosis: clinical utility in high-burden vs. low-burden settings. Curr Opin Pulm Med. 2009;15(3):188–200.
71. Kuruvilla A. Ocular tuberculosis. Lancet. 2003;361(9353):260–1; author reply 1.
72. Butler NJ, Thorne JE. Current status of HIV infection and ocular disease. Curr Opin Ophthalmol. 2012;23(6):517–22.
73. Patton ME, Su JR, Nelson R, Weinstock H, Centers for Disease C, Prevention. Primary and secondary syphilis – United States, 2005–2013. MMWR Morb Mortal Wkly Rep. 2014;63(18):402–6.
74. Davis JL. Ocular syphilis. Curr Opin Ophthalmol. 2014;25(6):513–8.
75. Fu EX, Geraets RL, Dodds EM, Echandi LV, Colombero D, McDonald HR, et al. Superficial retinal precipitates in patients with syphilitic retinitis. Retina. 2010;30(7):1135–43.
76. Eandi CM, Neri P, Adelman RA, Yannuzzi LA, Cunningham Jr ET, International Syphilis Study G. Acute syphilitic posterior placoid chorioretinitis: report of a case series and comprehensive review of the literature. Retina. 2012;32(9):1915–41.
77. Gass JD, Braunstein RA, Chenoweth RG. Acute syphilitic posterior placoid chorioretinitis. Ophthalmology. 1990;97(10):1288–97.
78. Pichi F, Ciardella AP, Cunningham Jr ET, Morara M, Veronese C, Jumper JM, et al. Spectral domain optical coherence tomography findings in patients with acute syphilitic posterior placoid chorioretinopathy. Retina. 2014;34(2):373–84.
79. Workowski KA, Berman S, Centers for Disease C, Prevention. Sexually transmitted diseases treatment guidelines, 2010. MMWR Recomm Rep. 2010;59(RR-12):1–110.
80. Pound MW, May DB. Proposed mechanisms and preventative options of Jarisch-Herxheimer reactions. J Clin Pharm Ther. 2005;30(3):291–5.
81. Shapiro ED. Lyme disease. N Engl J Med. 2014;371(7):684.
82. Mora P, Carta A. Ocular manifestations of Lyme borreliosis in Europe. Int J Med Sci. 2009;6(3):124–5.
83. Steere AC, Bartenhagen NH, Craft JE, Hutchinson GJ, Newman JH, Rahn DW, et al. The early clinical manifestations of Lyme disease. Ann Intern Med. 1983;99(1):76–82.
84. Mikkila HO, Seppala IJ, Viljanen MK, Peltomaa MP, Karma A. The expanding clinical spectrum of ocular lyme borreliosis. Ophthalmology. 2000;107(3):581–7.
85. Wormser GP, Dattwyler RJ, Shapiro ED, Halperin JJ, Steere AC, Klempner MS, et al. The clinical assessment, treatment, and prevention of Lyme disease, human granulocytic anaplasmosis, and babesiosis: clinical practice guidelines by the Infectious Diseases Society of America. Clin Infect Dis. 2006;43(9):1089–134.
86. Biancardi AL, Curi AL. Cat-scratch disease. Ocul Immunol Inflamm. 2014;22(2):148–54.
87. Hamilton DH, Zangwill KM, Hadler JL, Cartter ML. Cat-scratch disease – Connecticut, 1992–1993. J Infect Dis. 1995;172(2):570–3.
88. Roe RH, Jumper MJ, Fu AD, Johnson RN, McDonald R, Cunningham ET. Ocular bartonella infections. Int Ophthalmol Clin. 2008;48(3):93–105.
89. Carithers HA. Cat-scratch disease. An overview based on a study of 1,200 patients. Am J Dis Child. 1985;139(11):1124–33.
90. Khairallah M, Chee SP, Rathinam SR, Attia S, Nadella V. Novel infectious agents causing uveitis. Int Ophthalmol. 2010;30(5):465–83.
91. Duffey RJ, Hammer ME. The ocular manifestations of Rocky Mountain spotted fever. Ann Ophthalmol. 1987;19(8):301–3, 6.
92. Lukas JR, Egger S, Parschalk B, Stur M. Bilateral small retinal infiltrates during rickettsial infection. Br J Ophthalmol. 1998;82(10):1217–8.
93. Khairallah M, Ladjimi A, Chakroun M, Messaoud R, Yahia SB, Zaouali S, et al. Posterior segment manifestations of Rickettsia conorii infection. Ophthalmology. 2004;111(3):529–34.
94. Khairallah M, Ben Yahia S, Toumi A, Jelliti B, Loussaief C, Romdhane FB, et al. Ocular manifestations associated with murine typhus. Br J Ophthalmol. 2009;93(7):938–42.

95. Razonable RR, Pulido JS, Deziel PJ, Dev S, Salomao DR, Walker RC. Chorioretinitis and vitritis due to Tropheryma whipplei after transplantation: case report and review. Transpl Infect Dis. 2008;10(6):413–8.
96. Touitou V, Fenollar F, Cassoux N, Merle-Beral H, LeHoang P, Amoura Z, et al. Ocular Whipple's disease: therapeutic strategy and long-term follow-up. Ophthalmology. 2012;119(7):1465–9.
97. Wong RW, Jumper JM, McDonald HR, Johnson RN, Fu A, Lujan BJ, et al. Emerging concepts in the management of acute retinal necrosis. Br J Ophthalmol. 2013;97(5):545–52.
98. Saatci AO, Ayhan Z, Arikan G, Sayiner A, Ada E. Unilateral acute retinal necrosis in a multiple sclerosis patient treated with high-dose systemic steroids. Int Ophthalmol. 2010;30(5): 629–32.
99. Ganatra JB, Chandler D, Santos C, Kuppermann B, Margolis TP. Viral causes of the acute retinal necrosis syndrome. Am J Ophthalmol. 2000;129(2):166–72.
100. Holland GN. Standard diagnostic criteria for the acute retinal necrosis syndrome. Executive Committee of the American Uveitis Society. Am J Ophthalmol. 1994;117(5):663–7.
101. Hillenkamp J, Nolle B, Bruns C, Rautenberg P, Fickenscher H, Roider J. Acute retinal necrosis: clinical features, early vitrectomy, and outcomes. Ophthalmology. 2009;116(10):1971–5.e2.
102. Palay DA, Sternberg Jr P, Davis J, Lewis H, Holland GN, Mieler WF, et al. Decrease in the risk of bilateral acute retinal necrosis by acyclovir therapy. Am J Ophthalmol. 1991;112(3):250–5.
103. Guex-Crosier Y, Rochat C, Herbort CP. Necrotizing herpetic retinopathies. A spectrum of herpes virus-induced diseases determined by the immune state of the host. Ocul Immunol Inflamm. 1997;5(4):259–65.
104. Engstrom Jr RE, Holland GN, Margolis TP, Muccioli C, Lindley JI, Belfort Jr R, et al. The progressive outer retinal necrosis syndrome. A variant of necrotizing herpetic retinopathy in patients with AIDS. Ophthalmology. 1994;101(9):1488–502.
105. Gore DM, Gore SK, Visser L. Progressive outer retinal necrosis: outcomes in the intravitreal era. Arch Ophthalmol. 2012;130(6):700–6.
106. Lau CH, Missotten T, Salzmann J, Lightman SL. Acute retinal necrosis features, management, and outcomes. Ophthalmology. 2007;114(4):756–62.
107. Rothova A, de Boer JH, Ten Dam-van Loon NH, Postma G, de Visser L, Zuurveen SJ, et al. Usefulness of aqueous humor analysis for the diagnosis of posterior uveitis. Ophthalmology. 2008;115(2):306–11.
108. Blumenkranz MS, Culbertson WW, Clarkson JG, Dix R. Treatment of the acute retinal necrosis syndrome with intravenous acyclovir. Ophthalmology. 1986;93(3):296–300.
109. Aizman A, Johnson MW, Elner SG. Treatment of acute retinal necrosis syndrome with oral antiviral medications. Ophthalmology. 2007;114(2):307–12.
110. Balfour HH, Benson C, James B, Cassens B, Erice A, Friedman-Kien A, Klein T, Polsky B, Sabrin S. Management of acyclovir-resistant Herpes simplex and Varicella-Zoster virus infections. J Acquir Immune Defic Syndr. 1994;7(3):254–60.
111. Park JJ, Pavesio C. Prophylactic laser photocoagulation for acute retinal necrosis. Does it raise more questions than answers? Br J Ophthalmol. 2008;92(9):1161–2.
112. Kawaguchi T, Spencer DB, Mochizuki M. Therapy for acute retinal necrosis. Semin Ophthalmol. 2008;23(4):285–90.
113. Holland GN. AIDS and ophthalmology: the first quarter century. Am J Ophthalmol. 2008;145(3):397–408.
114. Centers for Disease C, Prevention. Twenty-five years of HIV/AIDS – United States, 1981–2006. MMWR Morb Mortal Wkly Rep. 2006;55(21):585–9.
115. Vrabec TR. Posterior segment manifestations of HIV/AIDS. Surv Ophthalmol. 2004;49(2):131–57.
116. Kuppermann BD, Petty JG, Richman DD, Mathews WC, Fullerton SC, Rickman LS, et al. Correlation between CD4+ counts and prevalence of cytomegalovirus retinitis and human immunodeficiency virus-related noninfectious retinal vasculopathy in patients with acquired immunodeficiency syndrome. Am J Ophthalmol. 1993;115(5):575–82.

117. Cunningham Jr ET, Levinson RD, Jampol LM, Engstrom Jr RE, Lewis H, Holland GN. Ischemic maculopathy in patients with acquired immunodeficiency syndrome. Am J Ophthalmol. 2001;132(5):727–33.
118. Palestine AG, Frishberg B. Macular edema in acquired immunodeficiency syndrome-related microvasculopathy. Am J Ophthalmol. 1991;111(6):770–1.
119. Newsome DA, Green WR, Miller ED, Kiessling LA, Morgan B, Jabs DA, et al. Microvascular aspects of acquired immune deficiency syndrome retinopathy. Am J Ophthalmol. 1984;98(5):590–601.
120. Rivero ME, Kuppermann BD, Wiley CA, Garcia CR, Smith MD, Dreilinger A, et al. Acquired immunodeficiency syndrome-related intraocular B-cell lymphoma. Arch Ophthalmol. 1999;117(5):616–22.
121. Dore GJ, Li Y, McDonald A, Ree H, Kaldor JM, National HIVSC. Impact of highly active antiretroviral therapy on individual AIDS-defining illness incidence and survival in Australia. J Acquir Immune Defic Syndr. 2002;29(4):388–95.
122. Shami MJ, Freeman W, Friedberg D, Siderides E, Listhaus A, Ai E. A multicenter study of Pneumocystis choroidopathy. Am J Ophthalmol. 1991;112(1):15–22.
123. Sha BE, Benson CA, Deutsch T, Noskin GA, Murphy RL, Pottage Jr JC, et al. Pneumocystis carinii choroiditis in patients with AIDS: clinical features, response to therapy, and outcome. J Acquir Immune Defic Syndr. 1992;5(10):1051–8.
124. Verma S, Graham EM. Cryptococcus presenting as cloudy choroiditis in an AIDS patient. Br J Ophthalmol. 1995;79(6):618–9.
125. Jabs DA. Ocular manifestations of HIV infection. Trans Am Ophthalmol Soc. 1995;93:623–83.
126. Baldassano V, Dunn JP, Feinberg J, Jabs DA. Cytomegalovirus retinitis and low CD4+ T-lymphocyte counts. N Engl J Med. 1995;333(10):670.
127. Benson CA, Kaplan JE, Masur H, Pau A, Holmes KK, CDC, NIH, Inf Dis Soc Am. Treating opportunistic infections among HIV-infected adults and adolescents: recommendations from CDC, the National Institutes of Health, and the HIV Medicine Association/Infectious Diseases Society of America. MMWR Recomm Rep. 2004;53(RR-15):1–112.
128. Lin DY, Warren JF, Lazzeroni LC, Wolitz RA, Mansour SE. Cytomegalovirus retinitis after initiation of highly active antiretroviral therapy in HIV infected patients: natural history and clinical predictors. Retina. 2002;22(3):268–77.
129. Kuppermann BD, Holland GN. Immune recovery uveitis. Am J Ophthalmol. 2000;130(1):103–6.
130. Jabs DA, Van Natta ML, Thorne JE, Weinberg DV, Meredith TA, Kuppermann BD, et al. Course of cytomegalovirus retinitis in the era of highly active antiretroviral therapy: 2. Second eye involvement and retinal detachment. Ophthalmology. 2004;111(12):2232–9.
131. Garg S, Jampol LM. Systemic and intraocular manifestations of West Nile virus infection. Surv Ophthalmol. 2005;50(1):3–13.
132. Nash D, Mostashari F, Fine A, Miller J, O'Leary D, Murray K, et al. The outbreak of West Nile virus infection in the New York City area in 1999. N Engl J Med. 2001;344(24):1807–14.
133. Khairallah M, Ben Yahia S, Ladjimi A, Zeghidi H, Ben Romdhane F, Besbes L, et al. Chorioretinal involvement in patients with West Nile virus infection. Ophthalmology. 2004;111(11):2065–70.
134. Khairallah M, Ben Yahia S, Attia S, Zaouali S, Ladjimi A, Messaoud R. Linear pattern of West Nile virus-associated chorioretinitis is related to retinal nerve fibres organization. Eye (Lond). 2007;21(7):952–5.
135. Petersen LR, Marfin AA. West Nile virus: a primer for the clinician. Ann Intern Med. 2002;137(3):173–9.
136. Garcia S, Crance JM, Billecocq A, Peinnequin A, Jouan A, Bouloy M, et al. Quantitative real-time PCR detection of Rift Valley fever virus and its application to evaluation of antiviral compounds. J Clin Microbiol. 2001;39(12):4456–61.

137. Al-Hazmi A, Al-Rajhi AA, Abboud EB, Ayoola EA, Al-Hazmi M, Saadi R, et al. Ocular complications of Rift Valley fever outbreak in Saudi Arabia. Ophthalmology. 2005;112(2):313–8.
138. Khairallah M, Kahloun R. Ocular manifestations of emerging infectious diseases. Curr Opin Ophthalmol. 2013;24(6):574–80.
139. Bacsal KE, Chee SP, Cheng CL, Flores JV. Dengue-associated maculopathy. Arch Ophthalmol. 2007;125(4):501–10.
140. Weaver SC, Forrester NL. Chikungunya: evolutionary history and recent epidemic spread. Antiviral Res. 2015;120:32–9.
141. Mohan A. Chikungunya fever: clinical manifestations & management. Indian J Med Res. 2006;124(5):471–4.
142. Borgherini G, Poubeau P, Staikowsky F, Lory M, Le Moullec N, Becquart JP, et al. Outbreak of chikungunya on Reunion Island: early clinical and laboratory features in 157 adult patients. Clin Infect Dis. 2007;44(11):1401–7.
143. Taubitz W, Cramer JP, Kapaun A, Pfeffer M, Drosten C, Dobler G, et al. Chikungunya fever in travelers: clinical presentation and course. Clin Infect Dis. 2007;45(1):e1–4.
144. Pialoux G, Gauzere BA, Jaureguiberry S, Strobel M. Chikungunya, an epidemic arbovirosis. Lancet Infect Dis. 2007;7(5):319–27.
145. Mirzaian E, Durham MJ, Hess K, Goad JA. Mosquito-borne illnesses in travelers: a review of risk and prevention. Pharmacotherapy. 2010;30(10):1031–43.
146. Mahendradas P, Avadhani K, Shetty R. Chikungunya and the eye: a review. J Ophthalmic Inflamm Infect. 2013;3(1):35.
147. Haamann P, Kessel L, Larsen M. Monofocal outer retinitis associated with hand, foot, and mouth disease caused by coxsackievirus. Am J Ophthalmol. 2000;129(4):552–3.
148. Forster W, Bialasiewicz AA, Busse H. Coxsackievirus B3-associated panuveitis. Br J Ophthalmol. 1993;77(3):182–3.
149. Takeuchi M, Sakai J, Usui M. Coxsackievirus B4 associated uveoretinitis in an adult. Br J Ophthalmol. 2003;87(4):501–2.
150. Hughes EH, Hunyor AP, Gorbatov M, Ho IV. Acute idiopathic maculopathy with coxsackievirus infection. Retin Cases Brief Rep. 2012;6(1):19–21.
151. Mao Q, Wang Y, Yao X, Bian L, Wu X, Xu M, et al. Coxsackievirus A16: epidemiology, diagnosis, and vaccine. Hum Vaccin Immunother. 2014;10(2):360–7.
152. Robert-Gangneux F, Darde ML. Epidemiology of and diagnostic strategies for toxoplasmosis. Clin Microbiol Rev. 2012;25(2):264–96.
153. Maenz M, Schluter D, Liesenfeld O, Schares G, Gross U, Pleyer U. Ocular toxoplasmosis: past, present and new aspects of an old disease. Prog Retin Eye Res. 2014;39:77–106.
154. Talabani H, Mergey T, Yera H, Delair E, Brezin AP, Langsley G, et al. Factors of occurrence of ocular toxoplasmosis. A review. Parasite. 2010;17(3):177–82.
155. Bosch-Driessen LE, Berendschot TT, Ongkosuwito JV, Rothova A. Ocular toxoplasmosis: clinical features and prognosis of 154 patients. Ophthalmology. 2002;109(5):869–78.
156. de Souza EC, Casella AM. Clinical and tomographic features of macular punctate outer retinal toxoplasmosis. Arch Ophthalmol. 2009;127(10):1390–4.
157. Hovakimyan A, Cunningham Jr ET. Ocular toxoplasmosis. Ophthalmol Clin North Am. 2002;15(3):327–32.
158. Marcolino PT, Silva DA, Leser PG, Camargo ME, Mineo JR. Molecular markers in acute and chronic phases of human toxoplasmosis: determination of immunoglobulin G avidity by Western blotting. Clin Diagn Lab Immunol. 2000;7(3):384–9.
159. Vasconcelos-Santos DV. Ocular manifestations of systemic disease: toxoplasmosis. Curr Opin Ophthalmol. 2012;23(6):543–50.
160. Rajapakse S, Chrishan Shivanthan M, Samaranayake N, Rodrigo C, Deepika Fernando S. Antibiotics for human toxoplasmosis: a systematic review of randomized trials. Pathog Glob Health. 2013;107(4):162–9.

161. Baharivand N, Mahdavifard A, Fouladi RF. Intravitreal clindamycin plus dexamethasone versus classic oral therapy in toxoplasmic retinochoroiditis: a prospective randomized clinical trial. Int Ophthalmol. 2013;33(1):39–46.
162. Garweg JG, Stanford MR. Therapy for ocular toxoplasmosis – the future. Ocul Immunol Inflamm. 2013;21(4):300–5.
163. Beare NA, Taylor TE, Harding SP, Lewallen S, Molyneux ME. Malarial retinopathy: a newly established diagnostic sign in severe malaria. Am J Trop Med Hyg. 2006;75(5):790–7.
164. Beare NA, Lewallen S, Taylor TE, Molyneux ME. Redefining cerebral malaria by including malaria retinopathy. Future Microbiol. 2011;6(3):349–55.
165. Abu Sayeed A, Maude RJ, Hasan MU, Mohammed N, Hoque MG, Dondorp AM, et al. Malarial retinopathy in Bangladeshi adults. Am J Trop Med Hyg. 2011;84(1):141–7.
166. Guidelines for the treatment of malaria. Global Malaria Programme, 3rd ed. Geneva: WHO; 2015, p. 32–44.
167. Schneier AJ, Durand ML. Ocular toxocariasis: advances in diagnosis and treatment. Int Ophthalmol Clin. 2011;51(4):135–44.
168. Shields JA. Ocular toxocariasis. A review. Surv Ophthalmol. 1984;28(5):361–81.
169. Won KY, Kruszon-Moran D, Schantz PM, Jones JL. National seroprevalence and risk factors for Zoonotic Toxocara spp. infection. Am J Trop Med Hyg. 2008;79(4):552–7.
170. Barisani-Asenbauer T, Maca SM, Hauff W, Kaminski SL, Domanovits H, Theyer I, et al. Treatment of ocular toxocariasis with albendazole. J Ocul Pharmacol Ther. 2001;17(3):287–94.
171. Stewart JM, Cubillan LD, Cunningham Jr ET. Prevalence, clinical features, and causes of vision loss among patients with ocular toxocariasis. Retina. 2005;25(8):1005–13.
172. Taylor MJ, Hoerauf A, Bockarie M. Lymphatic filariasis and onchocerciasis. Lancet. 2010;376(9747):1175–85.
173. Murdoch ME, Asuzu MC, Hagan M, Makunde WH, Ngoumou P, Ogbuagu KF, et al. Onchocerciasis: the clinical and epidemiological burden of skin disease in Africa. Ann Trop Med Parasitol. 2002;96(3):283–96.
174. Rathinam SR, Annamalai R, Biswas J. Intraocular parasitic infections. Ocul Immunol Inflamm. 2011;19(5):327–36.
175. Ozoh G, Boussinesq M, Bissek AC, Kobangue L, Kombila M, Mbina JR, et al. Evaluation of the diethylcarbamazine patch to evaluate onchocerciasis endemicity in Central Africa. Trop Med Int Health. 2007;12(1):123–9.
176. Weil GJ, Steel C, Liftis F, Li BW, Mearns G, Lobos E, et al. A rapid-format antibody card test for diagnosis of onchocerciasis. J Infect Dis. 2000;182(6):1796–9.
177. Gass JD, Scelfo R. Diffuse unilateral subacute neuroretinitis. J R Soc Med. 1978;71(2): 95–111.
178. Gass JD, Braunstein RA. Further observations concerning the diffuse unilateral subacute neuroretinitis syndrome. Arch Ophthalmol. 1983;101(11):1689–97.
179. Amorin-Garcia CA, Sabrosa NA, Gomes AB, Segundo P-S, Garcia Filho CA, Sabrosa AS. Diffuse unilateral subacute neuroretinitis – DUSN. Int Ophthalmol Clin. 2008;48(3):119–29.
180. Garcia CA, Gomes AH, Garcia Filho CA, Vianna RN. Early-stage diffuse unilateral subacute neuroretinitis: improvement of vision after photocoagulation of the worm. Eye (Lond). 2004;18(6):624–7.
181. Garcia CA, Gomes AH, Vianna RN, Souza Filho JP, Garcia Filho CA, Orefice F. Late-stage diffuse unilateral subacute neuroretinitis: photocoagulation of the worm does not improve the visual acuity of affected patients. Int Ophthalmol. 2005;26(1–2):39–42.
182. Arevalo JF, Arevalo FA, Garcia RA, de Amorim Garcia Filho CA, de Amorim Garcia CA. Diffuse unilateral subacute neuroretinitis. J Pediatr Ophthalmol Strabismus. 2013;50(4): 204–12.
183. Cortez R, Denny JP, Muci-Mendoza R, Ramirez G, Fuenmayor D, Jaffe GJ. Diffuse unilateral subacute neuroretinitis in Venezuela. Ophthalmology. 2005;112(12):2110–4.

184. Souza EC, Casella AM, Nakashima Y, Monteiro ML. Clinical features and outcomes of patients with diffuse unilateral subacute neuroretinitis treated with oral albendazole. Am J Ophthalmol. 2005;140(3):437–45.
185. Biswas J, Gopal L, Sharma T, Badrinath SS. Intraocular Gnathostoma spinigerum. Clinicopathologic study of two cases with review of literature. Retina. 1994;14(5):438–44.
186. Prasad KN, Prasad A, Verma A, Singh AK. Human cysticercosis and Indian scenario: a review. J Biosci. 2008;33(4):571–82.
187. Del Brutto OH, Rajshekhar V, White Jr AC, Tsang VC, Nash TE, Takayanagui OM, et al. Proposed diagnostic criteria for neurocysticercosis. Neurology. 2001;57(2):177–83.
188. Rath S, Honavar SG, Naik M, Anand R, Agarwal B, Krishnaiah S, et al. Orbital cysticercosis: clinical manifestations, diagnosis, management, and outcome. Ophthalmology. 2010;117(3): 600–5, 5 e1.

Chapter 7
Infections of the Eyelids, Orbit, and Ocular Adnexa

Guneet Sodhi, Erica Liu, Jennifer Renz, Katrinka Heher, and Mitesh Kapadia

Introduction

This chapter provides an overview of the diagnosis and treatment of infections of the periocular soft tissues and orbit. Common infections in this area include preseptal and orbital cellulitis and infections of the lacrimal outflow system. Cellulitis commonly originates in the paranasal sinuses and spreads to the orbits by direct extension. It is imperative to distinguish between a superficial infection of the eyelids (preseptal cellulitis) and a deeper infection in the orbit (orbital cellulitis), which can lead to cavernous sinus thrombosis and morbidity affecting multiple organ systems. It is also important to recognize inflammatory conditions which may mimic infection but require different treatments.

G. Sodhi, MD
Ophthalmology, Eastern Virginia Medical School-Sentara Norfolk General Hospital Lions Center for Sight, Tufts University Medical Center-New England Eye Center, 600 Gresham Drive, Norfolk, Virginia 23507, USA
e-mail: guneet.s.sodhi@gmail.com

E. Liu, MD
Ophthalmology, Tufts Medical Center-New England Eye Center,
Biewend Building, 9-11th Floor, 260 Tremont Street, Boston, MA 02111, USA
e-mail: ericaliu11@gmail.com

J. Renz, MD, MA
Ophthalmology, Dartmouth-Hitchcock Medical Center, One Medical Center Drive, Lebanon, New Hampshire 03756, USA

Tufts Medical Center-New England Eye Center, Boston, MA, USA
e-mail: jenrenz@me.com

K. Heher, MD • M. Kapadia, MD, PhD (✉)
Ophthalmology-Oculoplastic Surgery, Tufts Medical Center-New England Eye Center,
Biewend Building, 11th Floor, 260 Tremont Street, Boston, MA 02116, USA
e-mail: kheher@tuftsmedicalcenter.org; doctorkapadia@gmail.com;
mkapadia@tuftsmedicalcenter.org

N.V. Laver, C.S. Specht (eds.), *The Infected Eye*,
DOI 10.1007/978-3-319-42840-6_7

Cellulitis

Preseptal Cellulitis

Background Preseptal cellulitis is a common infection of the eyelid soft tissue anterior to the orbital septum. Preseptal cellulitis typically presents with unilateral periorbital erythema and edema (Fig. 7.1). Preseptal cellulitis must be distinguished from orbital cellulitis, a deeper and more serious infection.

Etiology Preseptal cellulitis is most often preceded by an upper respiratory infection. Prior to widespread usage of the *Haemophilus influenzae* type B (HiB) vaccine in 2000, HiB was the most common and devastating culprit and was sometimes associated with septicemia and meningitis [1, 2]. Since the incidence of HiB infections has decreased dramatically, the most common organisms involved now are *Staphylococcus* and *Streptococcus species* with a notable rise in methicillin-resistant *Staphylococcus aureus* (MRSA) [1, 3]. Inoculation can be direct, such as from eyelid trauma, insect bites, or infection of hordeola, or it can be subsequent to contiguous spread from paranasal sinusitis or lacrimal system infections. Less commonly, preseptal cellulitis can be caused by hematogenous spread from infections elsewhere in the body.

Diagnosis and workup Workup starts with a thorough history with focused attention to potential orbital involvement, type of infectious organism, and sources of infection. Symptoms such as double vision, pain with eye movements, or sinus pain suggest a diagnosis of orbital cellulitis over preseptal cellulitis. Medical conditions including poorly controlled diabetes and immunocompromised states require

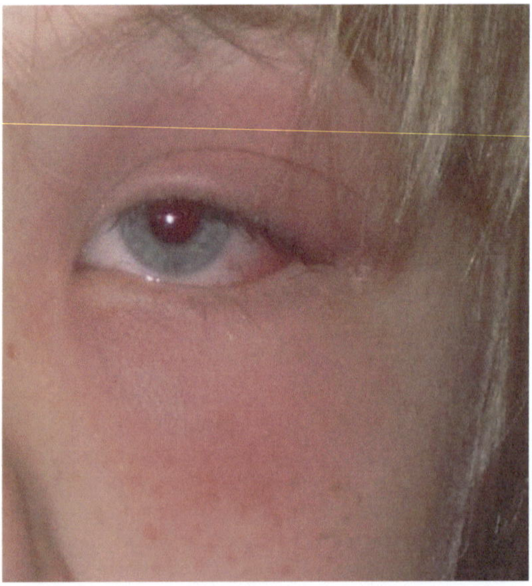

Fig. 7.1 Child with preseptal cellulitis of the left eye. Note mild erythema and swelling of eyelids

consideration for fungal organisms. Recent facial trauma, surgery or injury, sinusitis, or IV drug use may suggest possible sources of infection.

A full ocular exam should be performed looking for signs of orbital involvement. An afferent pupillary defect, pain or limitation of extraocular movements, conjunctival chemosis and injection, resistance to retropulsion, proptosis, a decline in visual acuity, or dyschromatopsia should raise suspicion for orbital involvement. Discharge from the conjunctiva, eyelid lesions, or puncta can be sent for culture but is often contaminated by normal ocular surface flora and may not correlate with blood or abscess cultures [4]. If systemic symptoms of fever, headache, or malaise are present, it may be prudent to send blood cultures to assess for hematogenous dissemination and possible sepsis.

Imaging studies, ideally a CT scan of the orbits and sinuses with contrast, should be considered for all cases where there is no obvious source of infection. Patients with mild preseptal cellulitis with an obvious source such as a bug bite or minor eyelid trauma can be treated without imaging studies. Imaging in these cases can be reserved for a poor response or progression in spite of appropriate initial treatment. There is now evidence that the radiation from CT scans is related to an increased risk of solid tumors and leukemia, so clinical judgment of the risks and benefits should always be considered prior to ordering imaging studies [5]. The goal of imaging studies is to identify the presence of sinusitis as a source of infection and to look for radiologic evidence of orbital involvement.

Differential Clinical signs are often used to distinguish between preseptal and orbital cellulitis, but radiographic studies can be helpful when the diagnosis is uncertain. The presence of an orbital fat stranding or a subperiosteal abscess confirms orbital involvement.

Other entities which cause periorbital swelling and can mimic cellulitis include idiopathic orbital inflammation, rhabdomyosarcoma, ruptured dermoid cyst, and allergic dermatitis. Viral conjunctivitis can also sometimes cause impressive eyelid swelling and be mistaken for cellulitis. Chalazia can provoke an inflammatory response leading to diffuse eyelid swelling.

Treatment Most cases of orbital cellulitis can be treated on an outpatient basis with oral antibiotics. We recommend daily monitoring until there is significant improvement to confirm that the choice of antibiotics is appropriate. Cephalexin and amoxicillin/clavulanic acid are good choices which provide coverage against common skin and sinus pathogens. Methicillin-resistant *Staphylococcus aureus* (MRSA) infections were usually acquired in hospitals and nursing homes in the past but are now frequently encountered in the community setting. If MRSA is suspected, initial antibiotic treatment should include double-strength Bactrim. In the setting of eyelid trauma, there should be a suspicion for MRSA and anaerobic involvement, in which case Bactrim with clindamycin or metronidazole should be added. If a patient does not respond to oral antibiotics in 24–48 h, or in children younger than 2 years old, the patient should be admitted for IV antibiotics. Common choices include vancomycin and cephalosporins. Any fluid collection in the eyelids is a potential abscess and requires surgical drainage. In cooperative, adult patients, this can be performed at the bedside using local anesthesia. Cultures and sensitivities should always be sent when purulent material is encountered in order to help narrow antibiotic coverage.

Prognosis and complications Preseptal cellulitis diagnosed and treated promptly has an excellent prognosis. Most patients have complete resolution and no long-term sequelae.

Orbital Cellulitis

Background Orbital cellulitis is an infection of the soft tissues posterior to the orbital septum and requires more aggressive management and surveillance than its more superficial counterpart, preseptal cellulitis. Orbital cellulitis typically presents with unilateral eyelid erythema and edema, often with conjunctival chemosis, ophthalmoplegia, and pain with extraocular movement. Systemic findings may include fever, leukocytosis, and malaise. More ominous findings include decreased visual acuity, dyschromatopsia, restricted visual fields, afferent pupillary defect, and optic nerve edema. Bilateral symptoms should raise suspicion for posterior extension (Fig. 7.2).

Etiology Orbital cellulitis most frequently arises from bacterial upper respiratory infections that spread from the paranasal sinuses, most often from the ethmoid sinus through the thin lamina papyracea of the medial orbital wall. Other causes include posterior extension from an overlying skin infection, dacryocystitis, direct inoculation by trauma, and endophthalmitis [6–8]. Less commonly, orbital cellulitis may arise from hematogenous spread from more distant infections. Similar to preseptal cellulitis, the most common organisms are *Staphylococcus, Streptococcus*, and anaerobes spread from upper respiratory tract.

For children less than 9 years old, infections are typically from one aerobic organism, and for children over 9 years old and adults, infections are typically polymicrobial with both aerobic and anaerobic bacteria. In immunocompromised and diabetic patients, fungal infections such as *Mucor* and *Aspergillus* should be considered [9].

Diagnosis and workup Orbital cellulitis is distinguished from preseptal cellulitis by the presence of clinical orbital signs and radiographic evidence of orbital disease.

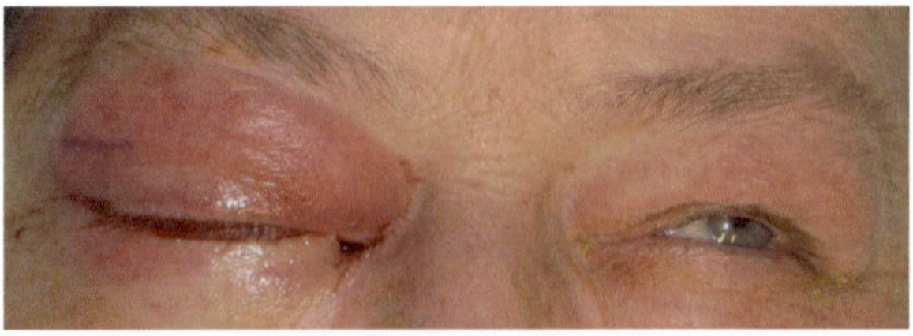

Fig. 7.2 Orbital cellulitis of the right eye. Note significant swelling and inability to open the eye

A CT scan of the orbits and sinuses with contrast is an essential part of the workup whenever orbital signs are present and should be performed quickly after presentation. Findings may include proptosis, orbital fat stranding, or orbital abscess (Figs. 7.3 and 7.4).

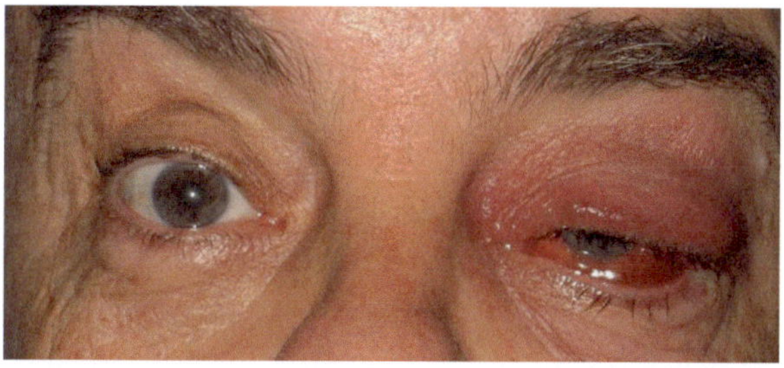

Fig. 7.3 Idiopathic inflammatory orbital disease of the left eye. Note significant eyelid redness and conjunctival chemosis. Patient can still open the eye at least partially

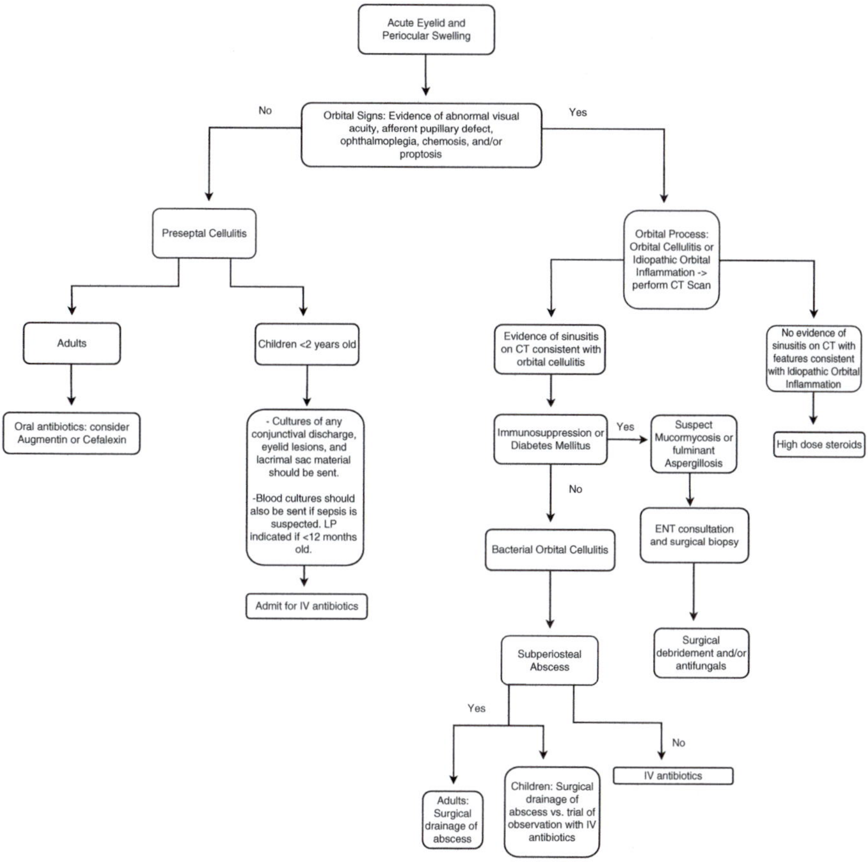

Fig. 7.4 Preseptal cellulitis versus orbital cellulitis diagnostic and treatment algorithm

Differential Idiopathic orbital inflammatory disease (or orbital pseudotumor) is commonly misdiagnosed as orbital cellulitis because of a very similar presentation. Both present with periocular swelling and often have pain, proptosis, diplopia, or chemosis. However, in contrast to orbital cellulitis, the paranasal sinuses are usually clear. Treatment is with corticosteroids and a rapid improvement in symptoms within 24–48 h is pathognomonic for this disease. We manage most patients with a slow 3-month taper of oral steroids, which help reduce the high recurrence rate when patients are tapered more quickly.

Other entities which may mimic orbital cellulitis include Wegener's granulomatosis, sarcoidosis, ruptured dermoid cyst, carotid cavernous fistula, rhabdomyosarcoma, scleritis, and sickle cell disease. In children, Langerhans cell histiocytosis may present with symptoms suggestive of orbital cellulitis [10].

Treatment Patients with orbital cellulitis should be admitted and treated with IV antibiotics. In addition to an ophthalmologist, otolaryngologist consultation is recommended for management of sinusitis and an infectious disease consultant to help guide antibiotic treatment. Empiric broad-spectrum antibiotics such as piperacillin-tazobactam or ampicillin-sulbactam are frequently used as first-line treatment. With the rise in methicillin resistance even in community-acquired *Staphylococcus* infections, vancomycin may be added if MRSA is suspected. Metronidazole or clindamycin can be added for anaerobic coverage [11]. Antibiotic selection may later be modified once culture and sensitivity results become available. Patients should be monitored closely until definitive improvement is seen. If no improvement is observed after 48 h on IV antibiotics, repeat imaging and changes to antibiotic coverage should be considered. After significant clinical improvement is noted, patients are usually transitioned to oral antibiotics in preparation for hospital discharge and outpatient management.

Prognosis and complications Complications of orbital cellulitis include optic neuropathy, retinal vein occlusion, cavernous sinus thrombosis, brain abscesses, meningitis, and death [9, 12].

Subperiosteal abscesses must be ruled out in all cases of orbital cellulitis, as this condition often warrants surgical intervention. In adults, subperiosteal and orbital abscesses require urgent incision and drainage through either a cutaneous or endoscopic approach. In children, subperiosteal abscesses can sometimes be watched closely to see if there is a response to IV antibiotics before pursuing surgical intervention (Table 7.1, Fig. 7.5).

Cavernous sinus thrombosis (CST) is a potentially life-threatening complication of orbital cellulitis. The cavernous sinuses receive venous blood from the facial veins via the superior and inferior ophthalmic veins, as well as the sphenoid and middle cerebral veins, providing a conduit for infections from the orbit, sinuses, nose, ears, and teeth. Cranial nerves III–VI course through the cavernous sinus and are often affected. CST typically presents with onset of periorbital edema, chemosis, dilated ocular vessels, ophthalmoplegia, ptosis, and proptosis abruptly or over

Table 7.1 Garcia and Harris criteria for medical management of subperiosteal abscesses of the orbit

Observation with IV antibiotics
Age less than 9 years old
No frontal sinus involvement
Medial wall abscess
Small-to-moderate size of abscess (less than 4 cm in width)
No suspicion of anaerobic infection
No recurrence after previous drainage
No chronic sinusitis
No evidence of optic nerve or retinal compromise
No dental abscess

Oxford and McClay [13], Garcia [14]

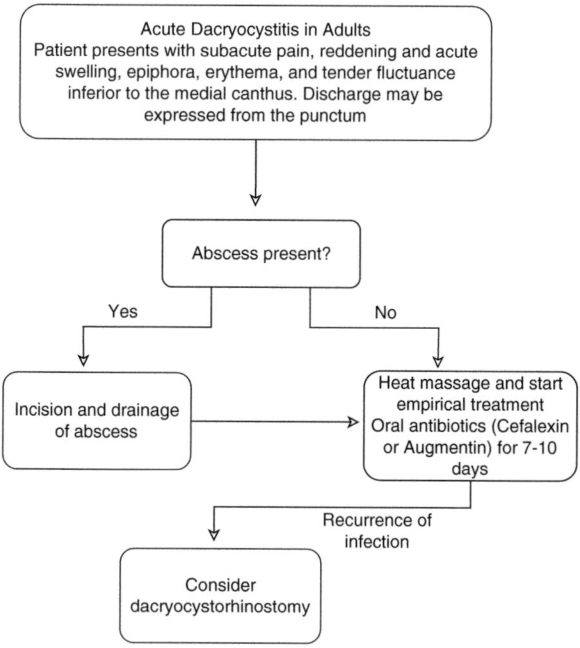

Fig. 7.5 Acute dacryocystitis in adults

the course of a few days. Unilateral to bilateral spread is common. The most frequently identified pathogen is *Staphylococcus aureus* with less frequent reports of *Streptococcus*, gram-negative bacilli, anaerobes, and fungi. Magnetic resonance venogram (MRV) is the most sensitive imaging study for diagnosing and monitoring CST treatment [15]. CT angiography is also useful and most often the first study performed if unable to perform an MRI due to availability or time. Imaging will show irregular filling defects in an enhancing cavernous sinus. Treatment is directed at the primary infection, with IV antibiotics recommended for a minimum of 3–4 weeks. Heparin use is controversial given the increased potential for bleeding weighed against the possible suppressive role of anticoagulation on the extension of infectious thrombophlebitis. Though no randomized controlled studies have been conducted, there is evidence that early anticoagulation therapy may have a beneficial effect on mortality and morbidity, reducing oculomotor sequelae, blindness, and motor sequelae, as well as the risk of hypopituitarism [16].

Fungal Orbital Cellulitis

Background Fungal orbital cellulitis is a rare but sometimes devastating diagnosis. Presentation is varied and depends on the species involved. Mucormycosis tends to present as a fulminant, rapidly progressive course, while aspergillosis is typically a chronic, indolent infection [17, 18]. Diagnosis may be delayed if the suspicion for fungal disease is not considered. In addition, patients are often immunocompromised, contributing to poor outcomes.

Etiology Orbital fungal infection is most often via direct extension from the paranasal sinuses. Traumatic inoculation and hematogenous spread are also possible [17, 19]. The main risk factors for orbital fungal infections are poorly controlled diabetes and immunosuppression, but these diseases may also be seen in seemingly healthy hosts without risk factors [20]. The most common fungal pathogens are both ubiquitous molds found in the soil and decaying vegetation: *Mucorales Rhizopus* is a nonseptate filamentous fungus and *Aspergillus flavus* is a septate filamentous mold [18, 21].

Mucormycosis often progresses rapidly with soft tissue and bony destruction by vascular spread, thrombosis, and tissue necrosis. Cranial neuropathy is seen early in the disease due to involvement of the orbital apex. Mucormycosis is most often seen in diabetics, often in the setting of ketoacidosis [22].

Aspergillosis can be an indolent disease of the sinuses or present in a more fulminant manner.

Diagnosis and workup A high index of suspicion is required for fungal infection in high-risk individuals as listed above. Diagnosis is frequently delayed due to nonspecific symptoms and low clinical suspicion, resulting in a worse prognosis and possible potentiation of disease [21].

As with bacterial orbital cellulitis, a complete history and ocular exam should be undertaken. If *Mucor* is suspected, the oral and nasal cavities should be examined for ulceration or black necrotic eschars that are classic for this disease [18].

Imaging of fungal lesions is often nonspecific with heterogenous enhancement on CT and subtle enhancement and hypointensity on T1-weighted MRI but may also include dense sinusitis with bony erosion [20]. Definitive diagnosis is by tissue biopsy. Fine needle aspiration may be sufficient in some cases, but fungal organisms are often difficult to find on pathology, so larger tissue samples are more likely to help with the diagnosis. *Mucor* has broad, irregular, nonseptate hyphae that branch at right angles and *Aspergillus* has septate hyphae that branch at 45°. The specimen can be fixed in formalin and stained with Gomori's methenamine silver (GMS) and periodic acid-Schiff (PAS) to identify *Mucor* and other fungi. The specimen can be sent fresh if a frozen section diagnosis is needed. Calcofluor-white can be used to diagnose Acanthamoeba keratitis.

Differential Fungal orbital cellulitis is frequently misdiagnosed initially as bacterial orbital cellulitis, neoplasm, idiopathic inflammation of the orbit, or giant cell temporal arteritis. Fungal infection should be excluded prior to treatment with steroids for any of the previously named conditions, especially in high-risk immunocompromised individuals, as steroids can temporarily improve symptoms of fungal infection but worsen the outcome [20].

Treatment Surgical removal and debridement of affected tissues along with systemic administration of antifungals, most commonly amphotericin B, is considered first-line treatment. In many cases, preservation of the globe can be accomplished, but advanced cases may require orbital exenteration to control infection [23]. Risk factors such as hyperglycemia and neutropenia should be addressed. Newer antifungals such as voriconazole or itraconazole can be considered in patients who cannot tolerate amphotericin B [20].

Prognosis and complications Morbidity and mortality are high with fungal orbital infections. For *Mucor* infections specifically, permanent vision loss and cranial nerve palsies are common, and mortality is above 50 %, particularly with misdiagnosis and delayed treatment [18, 24]. Extension of infection can cause central retinal artery or ophthalmic artery occlusion. Spread to the cavernous sinus can lead to cavernous sinus thrombosis and may lead to carotid artery invasion, aneurysm, stroke, and death (Table 7.2).

Table 7.2 *Mucor* versus *Aspergillus* infections

	Mucor	Aspergillus
Risk factors	Diabetic	Immunocompromised
Time course	Acute	Chronic or acute
Presentation	Proptosis, ophthalmoplegia, diplopia	Proptosis, ophthalmoplegia, diplopia
Pathology	Broad irregular nonseptate hyphae that branch at 90°	Septate hyphae that branch at 45°
Treatment	Aggressive debridement, systemic antifungal, correction of underlying metabolic imbalance	Surgical excision, systemic antifungal
Prognosis	Poor	Fair

The Lacrimal Apparatus

Dacryocystitis

Background Dacryocystitis is an infection of the nasolacrimal sac and can be acute or chronic. It is the most common infection of the lacrimal apparatus. Acute dacryocystitis often presents with swelling, epiphora, erythema, and tender fluctuance inferior to the medial canthus. Discharge may be present and can often be expressed from the punctum with pressure. Frequently there will be accompanying preseptal cellulitis [25]. Chronic dacryocystitis is more common than acute and presents with the same symptoms as acute dacryocystitis with a more indolent course. Often times, mild discharge is the only symptom, and the diagnosis may be difficult to make without lacrimal irrigation. If the infection becomes closed off and purulent material cannot be expressed from the punctum, a lacrimal sac abscess may develop.

Etiology Dacryocystitis is thought to be precipitated by obstruction of the nasolacrimal duct with stasis of tears and debris leading to eventual bacterial proliferation and overgrowth. In adults nasolacrimal duct obstruction is usually acquired, while in children it is usually congenital [4, 26].

Diagnosis and workup A full history and exam should be performed with particular focus on previous nasal pathology, surgeries, or trauma. Dacryocystitis is diagnosed clinically. Most patients are empirically treated as outpatients with oral antibiotics, as cultures are often difficult to obtain without surgical drainage. Imaging studies are not typically needed for most cases.

Differential Mucocele, granulomatous diseases such as sarcoid or granulomatosis polyangiitis (Wegener's), and malignancies may rarely present as dacryocystitis [27].

Treatment and prognosis Topical antibiotics are rarely helpful. Most patients can be treated with oral antibiotics and monitored, but recurrence is common after antibiotics are stopped. Definitive treatment is surgical with endoscopic or external dacryocystorhinostomy surgery to relieve the nasolacrimal duct obstruction [11]. Infants should be admitted and monitored very closely given their propensity for bacteremia and rapid escalation to systemic involvement. They can often be treated successfully with IV antibiotics and probing of the nasolacrimal duct [28]. The development of a lacrimal sac abscess is a common feature of this disease. Low-grade abscesses without surrounding cellulitis can often be observed, but large or progressive abscess requires surgical drainage (Fig. 7.6).

Canaliculitis

Background Canaliculitis is an infection of the superficial portions of the lacrimal outflow system. The infection may occur primarily or be related to an infected punctal plug. It is an uncommon, often misdiagnosed disease more prevalent in females. Canaliculitis typically occurs after age 40 with increasing incidence with age.

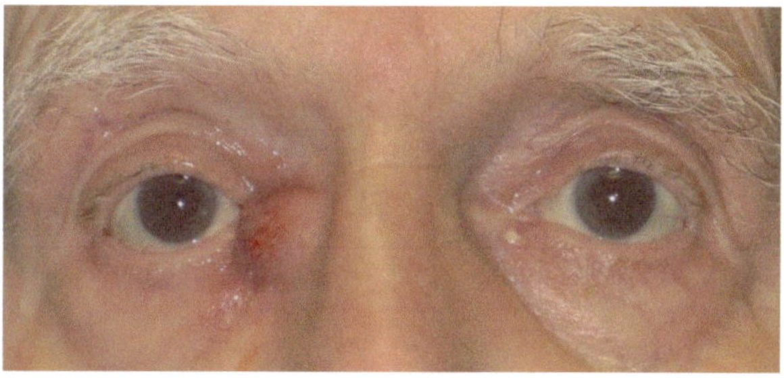

Fig. 7.6 Lacrimal sac abscess of the right eye (OD)

Canaliculitis presents unilaterally with irritation, epiphora, punctal pouting, and mucopurulent conjunctivitis. There can be swelling, erythema, and tenderness of the lid margin and conjunctival injection. About 25 % will have lacrimal stones [29, 30]. Pressure often precipitates mucopurulent exudates or lacrimal stones from the punctum.

Etiology The most common pathogen is often reported as *Actinomyces israelii* but varies depending on the study and whether primary or secondary to punctal plugs. Additional common pathogens include *Pseudomonas aeruginosa*, *Propionibacterium acnes*, and *Staphylococcus* species in punctal plug-associated canaliculitis and *Streptococcus* species, *Propionibacterium acnes*, and *Staphylococcus* species in primary canaliculitis. Infection is frequently polymicrobial and is more common after placement of intracanalicular plugs, usually presenting over 3 years after placement of plugs [29]. Fungal and viral causes have also been reported [31].

Diagnosis and workup Diagnosis is made by clinical exam and history. History of chronic discharge and conjunctivitis refractory to treatment should prompt more thorough examination of the lacrimal system. There is often focal erythema and swelling centered adjacent to the affected canaliculus with pouting of the punctum. Discharge from punctal pressure is the most common exam finding. Unlike dacryocystitis, the lacrimal outflow system is patent to irrigation.

Treatment Conservative management with topical medications can improve symptoms. If symptoms recur on cessation of antibiotics, a canaliculotomy procedure including removal of the infected punctal plug, if present, is usually curative. Canaliculotomy involves incision of the canaliculus along the lid margin and curettage/removal of infected tissues and debris including lacrimal stones and punctal plugs. Complex cases may require dacryocystorhinostomy surgery [32].

Prognosis and complications Without a canaliculotomy procedure, recurrence is common, with increased risk for males and with presence of stones. Potential complications of treatment include scarring and dysfunction of the canaliculus [29].

References

1. Donahue S, Schwartz G. Preseptal and orbital cellulitis in childhood. Ophthalmology. 1998;105(10):1902–6.

2. Sharma A, Liu E, Le T, Adatia F, Buncic J, Blaser S, et al. Pediatric orbital cellulitis in the Haemophilus influenzae vaccine era. J AAPOS. 2015;19(3):206–10.
3. Atfeh M, Khalil H. Orbital infections: five-year case series, literature review and guideline development. J Laryngol Otol. 2015;129(07):670–6.
4. Mills R. Orbital and periorbital sepsis. J Laryngol Otol. 1987;101:1242–7.
5. Miglioretti D, Johnson E, Williams A, Greenlee R, Weinmann S, Solberg L, et al. The use of computed tomography in pediatrics and the associated radiation exposure and estimated cancer risk. JAMA Pediatr. 2013;167(8):700.
6. Howe L, Jones N. Guidelines for the management of periorbital cellulitis/abscess. Clin Otolaryngol Allied Sci. 2004;29(6):725–8.
7. Bergin D, Wright J. Orbital cellulitis. Br J Ophthalmol. 1986;70(3):174–8.
8. Lee S, Yen MT. Management of preseptal and orbital cellulitis. Saudi J Ophthalmol. 2011;25(1):21–9.
9. Reynolds D, Kodsi S, Rubin S, Rodgers I. Intracranial infection associated with preseptal and orbital cellulitis in the pediatric patient. J AAPOS. 2003;7(6):413–7.
10. Rubin P, Foster C. Etiology and management of idiopathic orbital inflammation. Am J Ophthalmol. 2004;138(6):1041–3.
11. Lee D, Chai C, Loon S. Primary external dacryocystorhinostomy versus primary endonasal dacryocystorhinostomy: a review. Clin Experiment Ophthalmol. 2010;38(4):418–26.
12. Chaudhry I, Shamsi F, Elzaridi E, Al-Rashed W, Al-Amri A, Al-Anezi F, et al. Outcome of treated orbital cellulitis in a tertiary eye care center in the Middle East. Ophthalmology. 2007;114(2):345–54.
13. Oxford L, McClay J. Medical and surgical management of subperiosteal orbital abscess secondary to acute sinusitis in children. Int J Pediatr Otorhinolaryngol. 2006;70(11):1853–61.
14. Garcia G. Criteria for nonsurgical management of subperiosteal abscess of the orbit analysis of outcomes 1988–1998. Ophthalmology. 2000;107(8):1454–6.
15. Gulati D, Strbian D, Sundararajan S. Cerebral venous thrombosis: diagnosis and management. Stroke. 2013;45(2):e16–8.
16. Ebright J, Pace M, Niazi A. Septic thrombosis of the cavernous sinuses. Arch Intern Med. 2001;161(22):2671.
17. Zafar M, Waheed S, Enam S. Orbital aspergillus infection mimicking a tumour: a case report. Cases J. 2009;2(1):7860.
18. Warwar R, Bullock J. Rhino-orbital-cerebral mucormycosis: a review. Orbit. 1998;17(4):237–45.
19. Li S, Perlman J, Edward D, Weiss R. Unilateral Blastomyces dermatitidis endophthalmitis and orbital cellulitis. Ophthalmology. 1998;105(8):1466–70.
20. Pushker N, Meel R, Kashyap S, Bajaj M, Sen S. Invasive aspergillosis of orbit in immunocompetent patients: treatment and outcome. Ophthalmology. 2011;118(9):1886–91.
21. Levin L, Avery R, Shore J, Woog J, Sullivan BA. The spectrum of orbital aspergillosis: a clinicopathological review. Surv Ophthal. 1996;41(2):142–54.
22. Ibrahim AS, Kontoyiannis DP. Update on mucormycosis pathogenesis. Curr Opin Infect Dis. 2013;26(6):508–15.
23. Kohn R, Hepler R. Management of limited rhino-orbital mucormycosis without exenteration. Ophthalmology. 1985;92(10):1440–4.
24. Marcet M. Aspergillus infection of the orbital apex masquerading as tolosa-hunt syndrome. Arch Ophthalmol. 2007;125(4):563.
25. Campolattaro B, Lueder G, Tychsen L. Spectrum of pediatric dacryocystitis: medical and surgical management of 54 cases. J Pediatr Ophthalmol Strabismus. 2016;34(3):143–53.
26. Bale R. Dacryocystitis: bacteriological study and its relation with nasal pathology. Indian J Ophthalmol. 2016;35(4):178–82.
27. Asheim J, Spickler E. CT demonstration of dacryolithiasis complicated by dacryocystitis. AJNR Am J Neuroradiol. 2016;26(10):2640–1.

28. Baskin D, Reddy A, Chu Y, Coats D. The timing of antibiotic administration in the management of infant dacryocystitis. J AAPOS. 2008;12(5):456–9.
29. Mohan E, Kabra S, Udhay P, Madhavan H. Intracanalicular antibiotics may obviate the need for surgical management of chronic suppurative canaliculitis. Indian J Ophthalmol. 2008;56(4):338.
30. Lin S, Kao S, Tsai C, Cheng C, Kau H, Hsu W, et al. Clinical characteristics and factors associated the outcome of lacrimal canaliculitis. Acta Ophthalmol. 2010;89(8):759–63.
31. Varma B, Chang D, Musaad S. A case series on chronic canaliculitis. Orbit. 2016;25(11):4.
32. Huang Y, Yu W, Tsai C, Kao S, Kau H, Liu C. Clinical features, microbiological profiles and treatment outcome of lacrimal plug-related canaliculitis compared with those of primary canaliculitis. Br J Ophthalmol. 2015 [Epub ahead of print].

Chapter 8
Ocular Infection in Children

Mitchell B. Strominger

Introduction

Throughout the life of a child, from conception to adulthood, the human organism is consistently being exposed to organisms that may lead to an infection of the eye and ocular adnexa. To some extent these infections are related to environmental factors and exposures that are age and developmentally dependent. Thus the site of infection may vary and be tissue dependent, whether it involves the orbit, conjunctiva, cornea, or retina, all giving clues to the etiology and time of primary inoculation. Age of presentation along with the site of infection helps to determine the most likely cause and location. Primarily, infectious ocular diseases in children can be divided in four broad categories. These include intrauterine and perinatal infections, ophthalmia neonatorum, conjunctivitis, and orbital and adnexal infections.

Intrauterine and Perinatal Infections

Very early on, intrauterine infections are the fetus's first exposure to potential pathogens. Classically, these maternally transmitted congenital infections are remembered by the acronym TORCHES (toxoplasmosis; rubella; cytomegalovirus (CMV); herpes viruses, including Epstein-Barr; syphilis). Lymphocytic choriomeningitis virus is also included in the differential. While all can affect the developing eye and cause ongoing damage, they tend to do so in three major different ways: (1) direct tissue damage from the infecting organism, (2) interference in embryogenesis by a

M.B. Strominger, MD
Pediatric Ophthalmology Service Director, Tufts Medical Center-New England Eye Center, Tufts University School of Medicine, Boston, MA, USA
e-mail: mstrominger@tuftsmedicalcenter.org

N.V. Laver, C.S. Specht (eds.), *The Infected Eye*,
DOI 10.1007/978-3-319-42840-6_8

teratogenic effect, and (3) reactivation postconception leading to further organ damage later on in life and into adulthood. Thus the specific organism has a predilection for specific sites and potential reactivation giving clues as to its type that is dependent on the site and presentation (Tables 8.1 and 8.2).

Rubella

First trimester exposure to rubella (German measles) primarily affects the developing eye leading to microphthalmia, keratitis, cataracts, glaucoma, and a retinal pigmentary disturbance. Other organ systems are notably involved that can lead to sensorineural hearing loss, hepatosplenomegaly, mental retardation, osteopathy,

Table 8.1 Intrauterine and perinatal infection

TORCHES – intrauterine and perinatal infections
Toxoplasmosis
Rubella
Cytomegalovirus (CMV)
Herpes virus including Epstein-Barr
Syphilis
Lymphocytic choriomeningitis virus

Table 8.2 Intrauterine and perinatal infections

Causative organism	Ocular abnormalities
Toxoplasmosis	Microphthalmos
	Cataracts
	Panuveitis
	Optic atrophy
	Chorioretinitis
Rubella	Microphthalmos
	Keratitis
	Cataracts
	Glaucoma
	Pigmentary retinopathy
Cytomegalovirus	Microphthalmos
	Keratitis
	Cataracts
	Chorioretinitis
Herpes virus including Epstein-Barr	Conjunctivitis
	Keratitis
	Anterior uveitis
	Cataracts
Syphilis	Interstitial keratitis
	Iridocyclitis
	Iris atrophy
	Pigmentary retinopathy
Lymphocytic choriomeningitis virus	Chorioretinitis/pigmentary retinopathy

lymphadenopathy, thrombocytopenia purpura, and diabetes [1]. Intracerebral calcification of the white matter and basal ganglion can be seen on computed tomography (CT). Overall, its incidence has decreased substantially in the developed world since the introduction of the attenuated rubella virus vaccine in 1969. Corneal involvement presents with clouding from a keratitis. However in combination with microphthalmia and anterior segment dysgenesis, this can lead to glaucoma with secondary corneal haze or abnormal development of the endothelium (Fig. 8.1) [2]. Cataracts are more commonly present and are typically bilateral and diffusely involved [3]. This is thought to be due to viral load within the lens itself, and virus has been cultured at the time of lens extraction [4]. Most often a pigmentary retinopathy is present and characterized as fine, granular, or powdery discrete deposits that are typically limited to the posterior pole (Fig. 8.2). Vision is preserved other than in those cases that develop subretinal neovascularization [5].

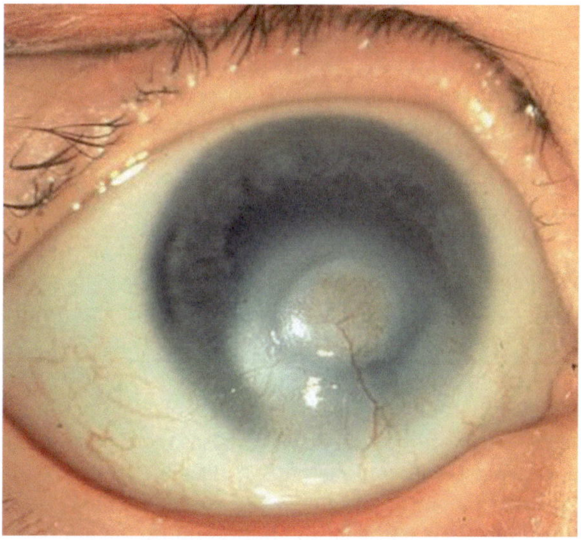

Fig. 8.1 Corneal keratitis with neovascularization from rubella

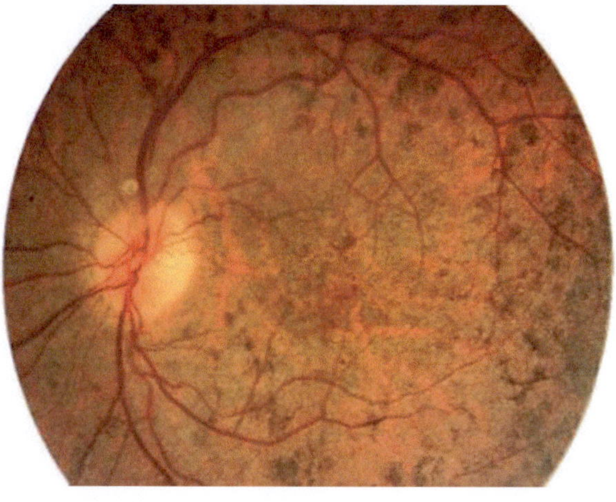

Fig. 8.2 Pigmentary retinopathy from rubella

Herpes Virus Family

The herpes virus family includes two types of simplex virus (HSV-1 and HSV-2), herpes zoster, Epstein-Barr virus, and cytomegalovirus.

Cytomegalovirus

Cytomegalovirus (CMV) is a member of the herpes virus family and is the most common intrauterine infection in the United States occurring in 1 % of all newborns, of which the majority remains asymptomatic [6]. Transmissions transplacentally and early in gestation affect the developing eye and are less common than systemic organ involvement. Ocular findings include keratitis, microphthalmos, cataracts, and chorioretinitis. The typical chorioretinitis presents with focal areas of retinal pigment epithelium atrophy, whitish areas of ischemia, and retinal hemorrhages [7]. Because CMV can also be transmitted from contact while passing through the birth canal or from breast milk, it is often difficult to determine the age at which the infection occurred. CMV can lead to periventricular calcification and hydrocephalus along with generalized cerebral atrophy and associated optic atrophy.

Herpes Simplex

Congenital herpes simplex virus (HSV) is usually acquired via passage through the birth canal in mothers who have active infection either with HSV-1 (labialis) or HSV-2 (vulvovaginitis) [8]. Primary infection is more likely to result in transmission versus secondary reactivation. HSV-2 is the most common culprit and can also occur following premature rupture of the membranes with ascending uterine involvement. Localized disease causes the typical vesicular skin lesions, oral ulceration, and keratoconjunctivitis (Fig. 8.3). However disseminated disease involves the viscera and central nervous system which portends a high mortality rate. Systemic HSV can lead to chorioretinitis, pneumonia, hepatitis, encephalitis, and disseminated intravascular coagulation.

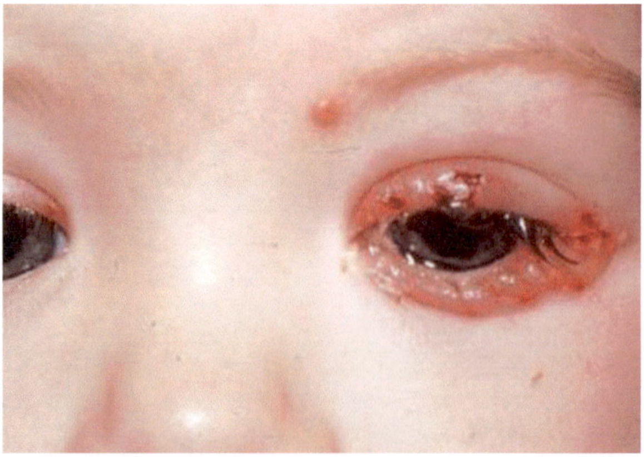

Fig. 8.3 Vesicular lid lesions from herpes simplex

Localized ocular involvement typically consists of eyelid vesicles, conjunctivitis, and a keratitis. Corneal infection may present as dendritic with epithelial involvement or as stromal infiltrates. This can be associated with anterior uveitis and lead to the development of cataracts. In neonates with disseminated disease, especially central nervous system involvement, chorioretinitis can occur with accompanying vitritis and optic atrophy. The chorioretinitis typically involves the retinal periphery and results in hyperpigmented scars that are well circumscribed. Acute retinal necrosis can occur later on in life with reactivation of the virus [9].

Epstein-Barr

Epstein-Barr virus (EBV) (infectious mononucleosis) can lead to toxic and teratogenic effects on ocular development via transplacental transmission. The case reports are limited which is thought to be due to a mild illness in the mother. This makes the diagnosis more difficult and the likelihood of clinical manifestations reduced. Anomalies are multiple and include microphthalmos, cataracts, micrognathia, cleft palate, hypotonia, hepatosplenomegaly, and cardiovascular malformations [10–12].

Varicella Zoster

Varicella and herpes zoster virus (HZV) is the same virus with the initial response considered chicken pox and reactivation herpes zoster. Varicella is not a potent teratogen. It leads to abnormalities in only 12 % of infants exposed and before 20 weeks of gestation. Maternal infection is also exceedingly low since the introduction of immunization programs against chicken pox. Clinical features of congenital varicella infection are primarily skin lesions in a dermatomal distribution and limb hypoplasia. Microcephaly, cortical atrophy, hydrocephalus, mental retardation, and abnormalities of the gastrointestinal, genitourinary, and cardiovascular systems have all been reported. The primary ocular disorders include microphthalmia, cataracts, and chorioretinitis [13]. Theoretically if the varicella virus is reactivated during pregnancy causing herpes zoster in the T10 to L4 root ganglion, intrauterine shedding could occur. However this mode of transmission to the fetus has not been reported and only in a case from a mother with disseminated herpes zoster at 12 weeks of gestation [14]. Neonatal chicken pox can develop if the mother is infected late in pregnancy. This can be transmitted either transplacental or ascending from the uterus. The mortality rate is low except in those born either premature or with low birth weight.

Toxoplasmosis

Toxoplasmosis is caused by *Toxoplasma gondii* which is an obligate intracellular parasite. Human infection occurs from exposure to cat feces, eating undercooked meat, or poorly washed vegetables. Cats are the definitive host and the parasite lives in the intestinal mucosa. When the unsporulated oocyst is excreted into the environment, it can then be ingested by humans. The oocysts then transform into tachyzoites. They then migrate into cardiac, muscular, neural, and retinal tissue and develop into tissue cyst bradyzoites. Disease reactivation can occur with rupture of the cysts or can remain dormant indefinitely. The stimulus for cyst rupture and reactivation is unknown.

The majority of human disease was thought to result primarily from congenital infection by transplacental transmission; however, postnatal infection also occurs. From the ocular standpoint, chorioretinitis is the most recognized feature. Other findings include microphthalmos, cataracts, panuveitis, and optic atrophy [15]. The chorioretinal scarring is usually heavily pigmented with associated areas of chorioretinal atrophy. It is usually bilateral and often involves the macula (Fig. 8.4) [16]. The primary active infection or reactivation is characterized by retinal inflammation that is thickened and cream colored with overlying vitritis. This vitreous inflammation has been classically described as a "headlight in the fog."

The common systemic findings of first trimester transplacental transmission include intracranial calcification with resultant seizures, hydrocephalus, microcephaly, hepatosplenomegaly, jaundice, anemia, and fever. Second or third trimester infection is associated with mild generalized disease during the first few months of life. Some of these children can then develop central nervous system involvement and chorioretinitis later in life [17]. From the ocular standpoint, the diagnosis is often clinical, based on the typical chorioretinal findings. However, a positive enzyme-linked immunosorbent assay (ELISA) supports the diagnosis. Finding toxoplasma-specific IgM is also specific since maternal IgM does not cross the placenta.

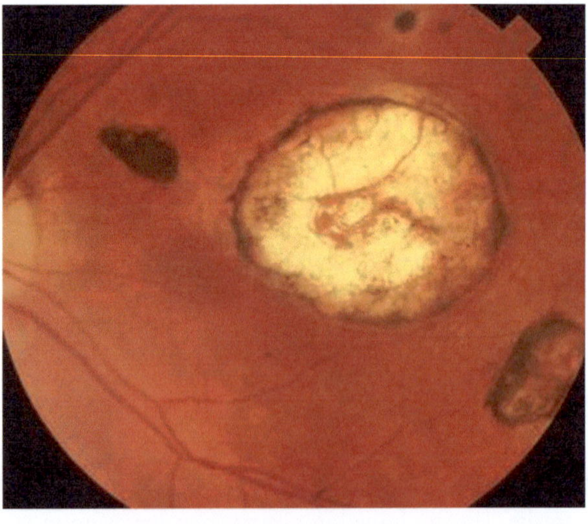

Fig. 8.4 Chorioretinal atrophy from toxoplasmosis

Syphilis

Syphilis is caused by the spirochete *Treponema pallidum*. Exposure leading to signs and symptoms of congenital syphilis typically occurs following maternal primary infection after the first trimester. The incidence of transmission decreases to 90 % in secondary syphilis and approximately 30 % in tertiary disease. Manifestations can be early or late. Early findings include skeletal abnormalities because of metaphyseal involvement or periostitis, maculopapular rash, hepatosplenomegaly with jaundice, pneumonia, anemia, and lymphadenopathy. The typical late manifestations are sensorineural hearing loss, dental abnormalities, and the ocular manifestations. Interstitial keratitis, deafness, and malformed incisors are known as Hutchinson's triad.

The interstitial keratitis is typically bilateral with associated iridocyclitis and iris atrophy. It is a hypersensitivity reaction that occurs in 10–40 % of untreated congenital syphilis cases and most commonly presents at 5–20 years of age [18]. It can be sectorial or diffuse and consists of corneal inflammation with interstitial vessels. These become "ghost vessels" that along with scarring lead to visual loss. Chorioretinitis may develop in the peripheral retina and cause pigment mottling. The primary findings are that of a salt and pepper granularity. However, pigmentation can become heavier leading to a pseudoretinitis pigmentosa-type appearance.

Diagnosis of congenital syphilis is dependent upon identification of the organism by direct-field microscopy from a scraping of a lesion or serologic testing. A positive VDRL (Venereal Disease Research Laboratory) greater than the mothers', with systemic findings, or a positive FTA-ABS (fluorescent treponemal antibody absorption) test, supports the diagnosis.

Lymphocytic Choriomeningitis Virus

Lymphocytic choriomeningitis virus (LCMV) is an arenavirus that is transmitted by exposure to infected rodents. Hydrocephalus, microcephaly, and periventricular calcifications are the most common neurologic manifestations. Ocular findings can be similar in appearance to toxoplasmosis with chorioretinal scars that may involve the entire macula, although peripheral chorioretinitis is most commonly present [19]. The retinal lesions can occur without the systemic findings. Positive antibodies to LCMV support the diagnosis since it is uncommon in the general population.

Ophthalmia Neonatorum

Conjunctivitis that occurs during the first month of life is referred to as ophthalmia neonatorum. In addition to bacterial agents which will be discussed, it can also be caused by viruses and chemicals. Prior to the worldwide institution of prophylaxis

Table 8.3 Ophthalmia neonatorum

Ophthalmia neonatorum – causative agents
Neisseria gonorrhoeae – 2–5 days of age
Chlamydia trachomatis – 7 days of age
Staphylococcus aureus
Streptococcus pneumoniae
Haemophilus
Pseudomonas aeruginosa – rarely

programs, the incidence exceeded 10 % of live births in some areas. If untreated, ocular morbidity is high leading to corneal damage and blindness. Inoculation typically occurs during passage through an infected birth canal, although inoculation can also result from ascending infection of the uterus especially as it may occur following premature rupture of membranes. The two most common organisms are *Neisseria gonorrhoeae* and *Chlamydia trachomatis*. Other etiologic agents include *Staphylococcus aureus*, *Streptococcus pneumoniae*, *Haemophilus influenzae*, and rarely *Pseudomonas aeruginosa* (Table 8.3).

Neisseria gonorrhoeae

Neisseria gonorrhoeae is the most serious of causative agents and typically occurs 2–5 days after birth. It begins as a mild conjunctival hyperemia with serosanguinous discharge that can rapidly progress to a thick purulent yellowish exudate with chemosis and eyelid edema. Corneal ulceration and perforation can quickly occur since the bacterium has a propensity to penetrate the cornea and replicate rapidly. Although the clinical course and findings are typical for *Neisseria gonorrhoeae*, conjunctival culture and Gram stain are paramount in making the diagnosis. Classic gram-negative intracellular diplococci are seen on Gram stain, although *Neisseria gonorrhoeae* cannot be differentiated from *Neisseria meningitidis*. Systemic infection can also occur including meningitis and sepsis [20, 21].

Chlamydia trachomatis

In the industrialized world, *Chlamydia trachomatis*, an obligate intracellular organism, is the most common cause of ophthalmia neonatorum. Also known as trachoma-inclusion conjunctivitis (TRIC), it usually occurs at around 1 week of age and often begins in one eye and then becomes bilateral. Clinically there is a mild mucopurulent discharge with moderate lid swelling and chemosis. Pseudomembranes can develop and if untreated this leads to scarring of the tarsal conjunctiva and corneal micropannus. The concern with *Chlamydia* is systemic involvement of the pharynx and lungs which can be fatal [22]. The diagnosis is made by conjunctival culture and scrapings. The culture material must include epithelial cells. Testing with polymerase chain reaction, direct fluorescent antibody staining, and enzyme immunoassay is also available to identify the organism.

Conjunctivitis

Conjunctivitis – red or pink eye – has a number of causative agents including bacterial, viral, allergic, and chlamydial. Common clinical features and symptoms in addition to redness include pain, burning, and stinging. Often they can be differentiated by other features including type of discharge, degree of itching, involvement of the lashes, and associated conjunctival response [23]. Five morphological conjunctival forms can occur: papillary, follicular, membranous/pseudomembranous, cicatrizing, and granulomatous. Papillae are characterized by a central fibrovascular core that arborizes on the conjunctival surface. They are a nonspecific finding of polymorphonuclear cell infiltration, but classically occur in bacterial conjunctivitis. Follicular conjunctivitis is most commonly caused by viral infections. Follicles are discrete round elevations of the conjunctiva from a lymphocytic response. The central portion is avascular with blood vessels sweeping up and over from the base. In membranous bacterial conjunctivitis, a fibrinous adherent exudate forms that bleeds with attempted removal. It occurs with *Corynebacterium diphtheria* and *Streptococcus pyogenes* infections. Pseudomembranous conjunctivitis has a less severe inflammatory response without necrosis where the thick exudate can be removed. It is somewhat nonspecific and can occur in conjunctivitis caused by *Neisseria gonorrhoeae*, *Haemophilus influenzae*, *Streptococcus pyogenes*, *Staphylococcus aureus*, *Candida*, adenovirus, and herpes simplex virus. Cicatrizing conjunctivitis is primarily an autoimmune process that develops in mucus membrane pemphigoid and Stevens-Johnson syndrome. Conjunctival scarring develops from progressive subepithelial fibrosis leading to severe dry eye from loss of goblet cells and obliteration of lacrimal gland ductules along with forniceal foreshortening and symblepharon formation. Granulomatous conjunctivitis describes nodular conjunctival elevations that are typically associated with preauricular adenopathy. Infectious causes include *Bartonella henselae* (cat scratch), *Francisella tularensis* (tularemia), *Mycobacterium tuberculosis*, and *Treponema pallidum* (syphilis). Biopsy of the conjunctival nodules demonstrates central caseation. This is in contrast to noncaseating causes for granulomatous conjunctivitis which include sarcoidosis and a foreign body reaction. Types of discharge include serous, mucopurulent, or purulent. Purulent discharge occurs more with bacterial infection while watery or serous in viral conjunctivitis.

Bacterial Conjunctivitis

Acute bacterial conjunctivitis occurs in school-age children and is most often caused by *Streptococcus pneumoniae*, *Haemophilus influenzae*, and *Moraxella* spp. [24, 25]. Most cases are self-limited with symptoms subsiding in around 14 days even without treatment. However, because of the morbidity involved and its contagious nature, topical antibiotics are recommended. Treatment shortens the course to a few days and decreases the contagion. The recent widespread immunization against some subspecies of *Streptococcus* and *Haemophilus* has decreased the incidence of these causative agents. Clinically children with bacterial conjunctivitis present with hyperemia of the bulbar conjunctiva, matting of the lashes, and discharge. It can be unilateral or bilateral. Concomitant otitis media can occur with associated low-grade fever, cough, sore throat, and nasal discharge. In these instances systemic antibiotics are warranted.

Membranous bacterial conjunctivitis is primarily caused by *Corynebacterium diphtheria* and *Streptococcus pyogenes*. It is seen uncommonly in developed countries because of vaccination programs. Adherent membranes are formed primarily to the palpebral conjunctiva because of a necrotic inflammatory response leading to a fibrinous adherent exudate. The membrane is thick and gray yellow in color. It bleeds on attempted removal. The membrane ultimately sloughs and is replaced by granulation tissue. Cicatrization may develop leading to trichiasis and xerosis. In the acute phase, corneal ulceration can occur and the bacterial can penetrate intact epithelium

Viral Conjunctivitis

Adenovirus is the most common pathogen in viral conjunctivitis. The severity of the disease can be mild to severe and is often associated with upper respiratory tract infection. Mild symptoms include a clear watery discharge. Preauricular adenopathy is often present. The usual source of the infection is via droplet and person to person. Thus viral conjunctivitis can be highly contagious. More severe forms include epidemic keratoconjunctivitis (EKC) and pharyngoconjunctival fever.

Epidemic keratoconjunctivitis tends to occur in outbreaks. It is most often caused by adenovirus serotypes 8, 19, and 37. Presenting symptoms include discomfort, photophobia, conjunctival chemosis, small subconjunctival hemorrhages, and preauricular adenopathy. A focal corneal epithelial keratitis ensues within 3–5 days followed by subepithelial focal infiltrates. Although the epithelial component is self-limited, the subepithelial opacities may persist for years. In severe infections there is marked swelling of the eyelids that is often confused with primary preseptal or orbital cellulitis. Conjunctival membranes can also develop, especially in infants.

Pharyngoconjunctival fever is associated with type 3 and 7 adenovirus. The presenting symptoms are similar to EKC, but without the subepithelial infiltrates or membrane formation. Corneal involvement is usually limited to punctate keratitis.

Herpes simplex virus conjunctivitis presents with similar viral symptoms of discomfort, redness, watery discharge, and preauricular adenopathy. Periocular and eyelid vesicles develop and help identify the disease. It is commonly unilateral and caused by both HSV-1 and HSV-2. There often is a history of recurrent cold sores. 50 % of patients with HSV conjunctivitis develop corneal epithelial manifestations

Table 8.4 Infectious conjunctivitis

Infectious conjunctivitis Causative agent	Ophthalmic findings	Systemic findings
Bacterial conjunctivitis *Streptococcus pneumoniae* *Haemophilus influenzae* *Moraxella*	Bulbar conjunctival hyperemia Matting of the lashes Mucopurulent discharge	Otitis media Low-grade fever Cough Sore throat Nasal discharge
Viral conjunctivitis Adenovirus	Clear watery discharge	Preauricular adenopathy

that range from fine punctate epithelial staining to the classic dendrites. Anterior uveitis can be present, but is usually mild (Table 8.4).

Blepharitis

Blepharitis is a common cause of chronic conjunctivitis in children. Disease anterior to the gray line of the lid margin is often caused by *Staphylococcus aureus* and *Staphylococcus epidermidis*. Symptoms include irritation, crusting, erythema, photophobia, and rubbing. It can be associated with atopic eczema and styes. Collarettes can be present. These are fibrinous scales centered on a lash. Tear film instability and inferior keratitis may develop. This can be severe with resultant peripheral corneal scarring and phlyctenules [26]. Involvement posterior to the gray line of the lid margin is more consistent with Meibomian dysfunction. Inspissated secretions are present with the development of chalazion [27].

Orbital and Adnexal Infections

Preseptal Cellulitis

Preseptal cellulitis is an inflammation or infection that is confined to the tissues anterior to the orbital septum. It primarily involves the eyelid, but can extend to surrounding areas such as the brow and forehead. Symptoms include redness, swelling, and pain. Preseptal cellulitis must be differentiated from secondary involvement of the orbit. In these cases, pain on eye movements, proptosis, and optic neuropathy would be consistent with orbital cellulitis [28]. Causes of preseptal cellulitis are multiple and historical data can help in its elucidation. Secondary infection of a chalazion can spread to involve the whole lid. In this case the child may have a history of prior chalazion or have noticed a small bump prior to the more severe lid swelling. Trauma with a small puncture wound or laceration is not uncommon with secondary staphylococcal infection. Insect bites can cause a significant allergic reaction with lid swelling or become secondarily infected. Association with a severe conjunctivitis can also develop from herpes zoster or impetigo. If bilateral, adenoviral infection leading to epidemic keratoconjunctivitis or pharyngoconjunctival fever should be suspected. This is a not uncommon scenario where a younger child might get admitted to the hospital for presumed bilateral orbital cellulitis because of difficulty in examination for orbital signs from severe conjunctival chemosis and lid swelling, only to discover that there is no sinus involvement on imaging and the causative agent is severe adenoviral conjunctivitis [29]. Clues to the diagnosis include other family members with conjunctivitis, large preauricular nodes, and whitish membranes on the palpebral conjunctiva. Finally, preseptal cellulitis can occur in association with an upper respiratory tract infection from *Haemophilus influenzae* especially in children under age 2 where the sinuses are not developed. This incidence has diminished, however, with the widespread use of Hib vaccine.

Orbital Cellulitis

The vast majority of orbital cellulitis occurs in children over age 5 (average 7 years) from contiguous spread of infection from the ethmoid or frontal sinuses [28]. This is because the bones separating the orbit and sinuses are thin at this age allowing for easy spread of infection. Less commonly it develops with associated penetrating orbital trauma or dental infections. Signs and symptoms of orbital cellulitis include progressive ocular pain, fever, lid edema, rhinorrhea, lethargy, and headache. Progressive proptosis and limited extraocular movement are of concern since this can lead to increased intraocular pressure and a compressive or infiltrative optic neuropathy (Fig. 8.5). Delay in treatment can also allow intracranial spread of the infection, especially via the venous drainage system of the orbit. This can cause septic cavernous sinus thrombosis, subdural empyema, and intracranial abscesses. Orbital cellulitis is therefore sight and life threatening. These patients should be admitted to the hospital for workup to include imaging of the sinuses. Identification of the extent of sinus involvement is important as well as the possible presence of a subperiosteal abscess or foreign body. Blood, nasal, and throat cultures can help with identifying the causative agent. Consultation with otolaryngology and infectious disease is important as a multidisciplinary approach to treatment is often needed.

The most common etiologic agents causing orbital cellulitis vary with age. *Staphylococcus aureus* and gram-negative bacilli are more common in the neonate. In children under age 9, a single aerobic pathogen such as *Streptococcus pneumoniae*, *Moraxella catarrhalis*, and *Haemophilus influenzae* is more common. This mirrors the microbiology of sinusitis. Older children have more complex infections with multiple pathogens both aerobic and anaerobic. Anaerobic organisms include *Fusobacterium* and *Bacteroides. Streptococcus pyogenes* may cause erysipelas, necrotizing fasciitis, or toxic shock, which requires aggressive treatment. Fungal infections are rare, but must be excluded in diabetic or immunocompromised patients (Table 8.5).

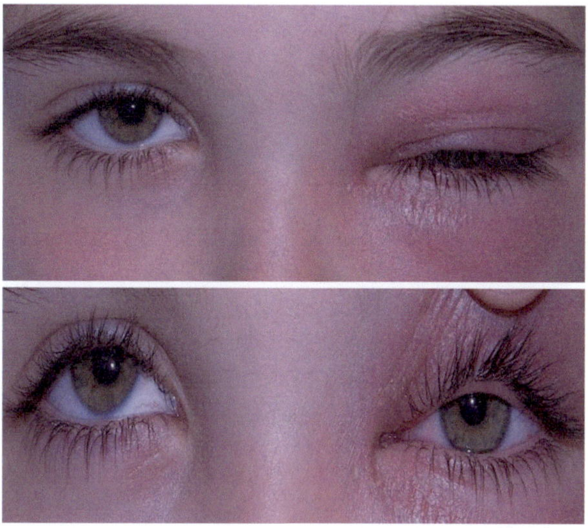

Fig. 8.5 Orbital cellulitis left eye with associated elevation deficit

Table 8.5 Preseptal vs. orbital sinusitis

Cellulitis	Site of infection	Signs and symptoms	Causative agents
Preseptal	Tissue anterior to the orbital septum, eyelid, brow, forehead	Redness, pain, and swelling of preseptal tissues	Chalazion, trauma, insect bite, viral
Orbital	Orbit and preseptum	Lid edema, proptosis, pain, and limitation of eye movements, optic neuropathy	Spread of infection from ethmoid, maxillary, or frontal sinus

Recommended Therapy for Common Clinical Conditions

Treatment of infectious ocular disorders in children in most cases is antibiotic driven, but the choice of therapeutic approach is dependent on the age of the patient, the site of the disorder, and the underlying natural history. Thus with some congenital or acquired infections, there may be no specific treatment, or the disorder may resolve without intervention.

Intrauterine or Perinatal Infections

Intrauterine infections that cause ocular anomalies typically do so by disturbing embryogenesis with associated organ damage that can extend into postnatal life. Most common ocular anomalies occur during the first trimester of gestation. However, ocular damage can also occur due to infection with varicella or CMV during the second trimester or with postnatal syphilitic infection. Thus the treatment of these disorders includes (1) primary prevention by eliminating exposure or through maternal vaccination, (2) treatment of the mother or the neonate with appropriate antibiotics or antivirals, and (3) treatment of the underlying ocular damage, i.e., cataract extraction, refractive error, and visual rehabilitation.

Rubella

Treatment of rubella has primarily been directed toward its prevention with the introduction of the attenuated vaccine in 1969 [30]. Since that time its incidence has been dramatically reduced; however it is still prevalent in those areas of the world that do not have robust vaccination programs. Thus the primary intervention in these children is lensectomy for cataractous changes which most often occur bilaterally [31]. An intense postoperative inflammatory process can develop that is thought to be due to sequestered virus [4]. Unfortunately there is no specific treatment for the pigmentary retinopathy and it may be slowly progressive. The rare development of subretinal neovascularization is an additional concern with these patients.

Herpes Virus Family

Cytomegalovirus

The mainstay of treatment of infants with cytomegalovirus causing systemic or ocular disease is ganciclovir. Administration may reduce the severity of sensorineural hearing loss although its effect on neurodevelopmental outcomes is still to be determined [32]. Treatment in older immunocompromised children includes ganciclovir, valganciclovir, foscarnet, cidofovir, and fomivirsen. The use of intraocular ganciclovir implants in children has been reported [33].

Herpes Simplex

Neonatal herpes simplex viral infections are often initially detected by a vesicular eruption. Dissemination leads to multisystemic involvement and a high mortality rate. Treatment is with systemic acyclovir [34].

Varicella Zoster

Maternal vaccination is the mainstay of prevention of chicken pox. It also has been shown to be effective following exposure if given within 3 days of maternal exposure [35]. Maternal treatment includes the antivirals, acyclovir, valacyclovir, and famciclovir. They can also be combined with VZIG. Despite a theoretical risk of teratogenesis with fetal exposure to acyclovir especially in the first trimester, this has not been demonstrated. Neonates with chicken pox may benefit from the use of intravenous acyclovir. VZIG may also reduce the severity of infection if given to neonates whose mothers develop chicken pox from 5 days before delivery to 2 days after delivery.

Toxoplasmosis

Treatment of toxoplasmosis is to some extent dependent on the age of detection. In those neonates who develop intrauterine infection detected serologically with or without systemic findings, it is recommended that they be treated with pyrimethamine and sulfadiazine. Folic acid should be given with this regimen to prevent leukopenia and thrombocytopenia associated with the use of pyrimethamine [36]. From the ophthalmic standpoint, treatment in cases of reactivation is determined by the degree of vision-threatening ocular involvement. Reactivation or acute chorioretinitis is typically self-limited. Thus peripheral lesions can be observed without treatment. However in cases of severe visual loss or with lesions that threaten the optic nerve or macula, treatment is indicated. Regimens include pyrimethamine and sulfadiazine with folic acid, sulfonamides, clindamycin, Bactrim, or doxycycline. With severe inflammation corticosteroids are used cautiously with antibiotics [37].

Syphilis

Treatment of congenital syphilis is with intravenous aqueous crystalline penicillin G. In order to ensure adequate treatment, serologic tests are repeated. Persistent positive titers require retreatment [38].

Lymphocytic Choriomeningitis Virus

Unfortunately there is no effective antiviral treatment for LCMV at this time and no vaccine exists. Since the manifestations are developmental anomalies including the peripheral chorioretinitis, the primary intervention is in prevention. Since a significant number of women who contract LCMV do so because of exposure to rodents, this contact should be minimized [39].

Ophthalmia Neonatorum

Treatment of ophthalmia neonatorum is dependent on early recognition, the time course of presentation, and isolation or detection of the offending organisms. The two most common organisms are *Neisseria* and *Chlamydia*. Prophylaxis for gonorrheal ophthalmia neonatorum was introduced in the 1880s with the use of 2 % silver nitrate.

With the increased incidence of *Chlamydia*, erythromycin ointment became the agent of choice. In the last decade, povidone-iodine drops have been shown to be equally effective, less toxic, and less costly. Now povidone-iodine is playing an important role in developing countries [40]. Treatment of *Neisseria* and *Chlamydia* conjunctivitis is with a directed appropriate antibiotic regimen. In addition to treatment of the neonates, it is equally important to treat their mothers and all of their contacts.

Neisseria gonorrhoeae

The mainstay of treatment for *Neisseria gonorrhoeae* conjunctivitis is intravenous penicillin G. However because of widespread resistance in many urban areas, a third-generation cephalosporin is recommended. Both intramuscular and intravenous administration appears to be equally effective. In addition frequent ocular irrigation with saline as well as the addition of topical antibiotics is typically recommended. Because concomitant infection with *Chlamydia* often occurs, treatment for inclusion conjunctivitis should be instituted until ruled out [41].

Chlamydia trachomatis

Treatment of neonatal conjunctivitis due to *Chlamydia trachomatis* is with oral erythromycin. This is because of the high incidence of pneumonitis and nasopharyngeal colonization. Although there is no evidence that it is necessary, supplemental topical erythromycin ophthalmic ointment is often recommended [22, 41].

Conjunctivitis

Treatment of conjunctivitis truly depends upon the offending agent, whether bacterial, viral, allergic, or associated with blepharitis. The diagnosis is often made on the clinical signs and symptoms, as well as findings of papillae, follicles, membranes, or granuloma to support a diagnosis. Gram stain and culture are needed to definitively confirm the offending agent, but this is often impractical. Thus broad-spectrum treatment directed at the most likely pathogens is typically employed.

Bacterial Conjunctivitis

Treatment of bacterial conjunctivitis is directed toward the most likely offending organisms, that being *Streptococcus*, *Staphylococcus*, *Haemophilus*, and *Moraxella* [25]. Because in many instances the infection is self-limited, especially if the child is being treated with systemic antibiotics for concomitant otitis, there is great debate about the efficacy of any particular antibiotic agent. Issues to take into consideration include whether the antibiotic is bacteriostatic vs. bactericidal, parental compliance regarding the dosage regimen, the contagiousness, and the overall cost. Most clinicians do recommend treatment because it leads to a more rapid clinical resolution and a higher eradication rate of bacteria [42]. Systemic treatment is necessary for membranous conjunctivitis and in immunocompromised patients. This often requires hospital admission as the majority of these patients are often toxic and febrile. In addition prevention of symblepharon by sweeping the fornices with a lubricated glass rod or the placement of contact shell is required.

Viral Conjunctivitis

Unfortunately there are no antiviral treatments directed toward the adenoviruses that cause viral conjunctivitis, epidemic keratoconjunctivitis, or pharyngoconjunctival fever. Intervention is primarily supportive with ocular lubricants, cool compresses, and occasionally topical antihistamines. Since viral conjunctivitis is very contagious, discussion with patients regarding proper hygiene is important to eradicate spread to others. Topical steroids potentiate viral replication. However in cases where the keratopathy is symptomatic and vision threatening, topical steroids can rapidly improve the keratopathy at the risk of difficulty in its taper with reactivation.

In contrast to adenoviral infections, treatment is available for conjunctivitis or keratitis secondary to herpes simplex. Although treatment of the conjunctivitis does not seem to alter the course of the disease, if the cornea is involved, intervention is warranted. Oral acyclovir has been shown to be effective for treating herpetic epithelial keratitis and for reducing the rate of recurrence when used prophylactically [43]. However, more recently the introduction of topical ganciclovir gel 0.15 % is increasingly being shown to be equally effective for the acute keratitis [44].

Blepharitis

Treatment of blepharitis is multifactorial. The primary goals are to treat any acute infection, reduce bacterial load at the lid margin, and manage the hypersensitivity response that can cause keratopathy. Thus the mainstays of therapy include topical antibiotics, lid hygiene with warm compresses and eyelid scrubs, flaxseed oil supplementation, and topical steroids. Persistent cases may benefit from oral antibiotics. Because tetracyclines can lead to dental staining, erythromycin is the preferred agent [45, 46].

Orbital and Adnexal Infections

Preseptal Cellulitis

Preseptal cellulitis is most often caused by *Staphylococcus aureus*, *Streptococcus pneumoniae*, *Haemophilus influenzae*, and *Streptococcus epidermidis*. Thus treatment consists of intravenous or oral antibiotics directed toward the suspected organism. Typically intravenous antibiotics are used in cases where the infection is severe and could spread into the orbit. Oral antibiotics on the other hand are reserved for more local infections. If the preseptal cellulitis is associated with a chalazion, incision and drainage might be required. Suspicion should also be high for occult trauma. If so, any retained foreign body must be identified and removed. Also any wound discharge should be cultured and tetanus prophylaxis provided. Of concern would be the development of necrotizing fasciitis and septic shock from beta-hemolytic *Streptococcus* [47].

Orbital Cellulitis

All patients with orbital cellulitis require immediate hospitalization for intravenous antibiotics and imaging to evaluate the extent of sinusitis and subperiosteal abscess [48]. In most instances pediatric otolaryngological consultation should be considered. Although many subperiosteal abscesses will resolve with intravenous antibiotics, drainage should be undertaken if there is progressive enlargement, optic nerve involvement, or risk of cavernous sinus thrombosis [49]. In addition, drainage of the offending sinus is often required.

References

1. Wolff SM. The ocular manifestations of congenital rubella. Trans Am Ophthalmol Soc. 1972;70:577–614.
2. Sears ML. Congenital glaucoma in neonatal rubella. Br J Ophthalmol. 1967;51:744–8.
3. Givens KT, Lee DA, Jones T, Ilstrup DM. Congenital Rubella syndrome: ophthalmic manifestations and associated systemic disorders. Br J Ophthalmol. 1993;77:358–63.
4. Cotlier E, Fox J, Smith M. Rubella virus in the cataractous lens of congenital rubella syndrome. Am J Ophthalmol. 1966;62:233–6.
5. Collis WJ, Cohen DN. Rubella retinopathy. A progressive disorder. Arch Ophthalmol. 1970;84:33–5.
6. Fowler KB, Stagno S, Pass RF. Maternal immunity and prevention of congenital cytomegalovirus infection. JAMA. 2003;289:1008–11.
7. Coats DK, Demmler GJ, Paysee EA, et al.; Congenital CMV Longitudinal Study Group. Ophthalmic findings in children with congenital cytomegalovirus infection. J AAPOS. 2000;4:110–16.
8. Riley LE. Herpes simplex virus. Semin Perinatol. 1998;22:284–92.
9. Thompson WS, Culbertson WW, Smiddy WE, et al. Acute retinal necrosis caused by reactivation of herpes simplex virus type 2. Am J Ophthalmol. 1994;118:205–11.
10. Mets MB. Eye manifestations on intrauterine infection and their impact on childhood blindness. Surv Ophthalmol. 2008;53(2):95–111.
11. Goldberg GN, Fulginiti VA, Ray G, et al. In-utero Epstein-Barr virus (infectious mononucleosis) infection. JAMA. 1981;246:1579–81.
12. Brown ZA, Stenchever MA. Infectious mononucleosis and congenital malformations. Am J Obstet Gynecol. 1978;131:108–9.
13. Lamont RF, Sobel JD, Carrington D, Mazaki-Tovi S, Kusanovic JP, Vaisbuch E, Romero R. Varicella zoster virus (chickenpox) infection in pregnancy. BJOG. 2011;118(10):1155–62.

14. Higa K, Dan K, Manabe H. Varicella-zoster virus infections during pregnancy: hypothesis concerning the mechanisms of congenital malformations. Obstet Gynecol. 1987;69(2):214–22.
15. Holland GN. Ocular toxoplasmosis: a global reassessment. Part 1: epidemiology and course of disease. Am J Ophthalmol. 2003;136(6):973–88.
16. Brezin AP, Thulliez P, Couvreur J, Nobre R, McLeod R, Met MB. Ophthalmic outcomes after prenatal and postnatal treatment of congenital toxoplasmosis. Am J Ophthalmol. 2003;135(6):779–84.
17. Koppe JG, Lowewer-Sieger DH, Roever-Bonnet H. Results of 20-year follow-up of congenital toxoplasmosis. Lancet. 1986;1:254–6.
18. Ruusuvaara P, Setala K, Kivela T. Syphilitic interstitial keratitis with bilateral funnel-shaped iridocorneal adhesions. Eur J Ophthalmol. 1996;6:6–10.
19. Mets MB, Barton LL, Khan AS, Ksiazek TG. Lymphocytic choriomeningitis virus: an underdiagnosed cause of congenital chorioretinitis. Am J Ophthalmol. 2000;130(2):209–15.
20. Wood CR. Gonococcal infections in neonates and young children. Semin Pediatr Dis. 2005;16(4):258–70.
21. Hammerschlag MR. Chlamydial and gonococcal infections in infants and children. Clin Infect Dis. 2011;53:S99–102.
22. Harrison HR, Phil D, English MG, et al. Chlamydia trachomatis infant pneumonitis. Comparison with matched controls and other infant pneumonitis. N Engl J Med. 1978;298:702–8.
23. Azai AA, Barney NP. Conjunctivitis: a systematic review of diagnosis and treatment. JAMA. 2013;310(16):1721–9.
24. Epling J, Smucny J. Bacterial conjunctivitis. Clin Evid. 2005;2(14):756–61.
25. Weiss A, Brinser JH, Nazar-Stewart V. Acute conjunctivitis in childhood. J Pediatr. 1993;122:10–4.
26. Jones SM, Weinstein JM, Cumberland P, Klein N, Nischal KK. Visual outcome and corneal changes in children with chronic blepharoconjunctivitis. Ophthalmology. 2007;114(12):2271–80.
27. Viswalingam M, Rauz S, Morlet N, Dart JKG. Blepharitis in children: diagnosis and treatment. Br J Ophthalmol. 2005;89(4):400–3.
28. Weiss A, Friendly D, Eglin K, et al. Bacterial periorbital and orbital cellulitis in children. Ophthalmology. 1983;90:195–203.
29. Ruttum MS, Ogawa G. Adenovirus conjunctivitis mimics preseptal and orbital cellulitis in young children. Pediatr Infect Dis J. 1996;15:266–7.
30. Krugman S, editor. International conference of rubella immunization. Am J Dis Child. 1969;118:1–41.
31. Vijayalakshmi P, Srivastava MK, Poornima B, Nirmalan P. Visual outcome of cataract surgery in children with congenital rubella syndrome. J AAPOS. 2003;7(2):91–5.
32. Mareri A, Lasorella S, Iapadre G, Maresca M, Tambucci R, Nigro G. Antiviral therapy for cytomegalovirus infections: pharmacokinetics, efficacy and side effects. J Matern Fetal Neonatal Med. 2015;29:1–8.
33. Wong IB, Teoh SC, Yeoh AE, Lingam G. Sustained-release ganciclovir implant as prophylaxis for cytomegalovirus retinitis in a child undergoing bone marrow transplantation. Eye (Lond). 2013;27(7):890–1.
34. James SH, Kimberlin DW. Neonatal herpes simplex infection: epidemiology and treatment. Clin Perinatol. 2015;42(1):47–59.
35. Watson B, Seward J, Yang A, Witte P, Lutz J, Chan C, et al. Postexposure effectiveness of varicella vaccine. Pediatrics. 2000;105:84–8.
36. McAuley J, Boyer KM, Patel D, et al. Early and longitudinal evaluations of treated infants and children and untreated historical patients with congenital toxoplasmosis: the Chicago Collaborative Treatment Trial. Clin Infect Dis. 1994;18:38–72.
37. Holland GN, Lewis KG. An update on current practices in the management of ocular toxoplasmosis. Am J Ophthalmol. 2002;134(1):102–14.

38. Phiske MM. Current trends in congenital syphilis. Indian J Sex Dis. 2014;35(1):12–20.
39. Barton LL, Mets MB. Congenital lymphocytic choriomeningitis virus infection: decade of rediscovery. Clin Infect Dis. 2001;33:370–4.
40. Isenberg SJ, Apt L, Wood M. A controlled trial of povidone-iodine as prophylaxis against ophthalmia neonatorum. N Engl J Med. 1995;332(9):562–6.
41. Matejck A, Goldman RD. Treatment and prevention of ophthalmia neonatorum. Can Fam Physician. 2013;59(11):1187–90.
42. Giogliotti F, Williams WT, Hayden FG, et al. Etiology of acute conjunctivitis in children. J Pediatr. 1981;98:531–6.
43. Schwartz GS, Holland EJ. Oral acyclovir for the management of herpes simplex virus keratitis in children. Ophthalmology. 2000;107(2):278–82.
44. Chou TY, Hong BY. Ganciclovir 0.1% gel for the treatment of acute herpetic keratitis: background, effectiveness, tolerability, safety, and future applications. Ther Clin Risk Manag. 2014;10:665–81.
45. McCulley JP, Dougherty JM, Deneau DG. Classification of chronic blepharitis. Ophthalmology. 1982;89:1173–80.
46. Lindsley K, Matsumara S, Hatef E, Akpek E. Intervention for chronic blepharitis. Cochrane Database Syst Rev. 2014;5:CD005559.
47. Rose GE, Howard DJ, Watts MR. Periorbital necrotizing fasciitis. Eye. 1991;5:736–40.
48. Starkey CR, Steele RW. Medical management of orbital cellulitis. Pediatr Infect Dis J. 2001;20:1002–5.
49. Garcia GH, Harris GJ. Criteria for nonsurgical management of subperiosteal abscess of the orbit: analysis of outcomes 1988–1998. Ophthalmology. 2000;107(8):1454–8.

Chapter 9
Anti-infective Therapy for Ocular Infection

Jihye Kim

Early antibiotic administration and ability to penetrate the infected site can be critical in preserving vision when treating various types of ocular infections [1]. An understanding of the pharmacokinetics and pharmacodynamics of antibiotics while acknowledging the bactericidal or bacteriostatic properties of these agents aids in prescribing appropriate therapy. A variety of antibiotic agents are currently available to treat ocular infections. Topical antibiotic agents are most commonly used to treat superficial or external ocular infections, whereas infections that are located farther away from the cornea or within the eye require additional methods of administration (i.e., intravitreal injection or parenteral therapy) to achieve therapeutic concentration at the site of infection [2]. Therefore, early identification of the depth of eye involvement and potential causative microorganisms is essential in choosing the most appropriate mode of medication administration and therapeutic option. This chapter provides the enumeration of relevant antibiotics by class, antimicrobial activity, antibiotic mechanism of action, mode of application, and antibiotic toxicity.

J. Kim, PharmD, BCPS
Department of Pharmacy, Penn State College of Medicine, Penn State Health-Milton S. Hershey Medical Center, 500 University Drive, Hershey, PA 17033, USA
e-mail: jkim6@hmc.psu.edu

N.V. Laver, C.S. Specht (eds.), *The Infected Eye*,
DOI 10.1007/978-3-319-42840-6_9

Overview of Antibiotics: Mechanisms of Action, Spectrum of Activity

Topical Antibiotics

Topical antibiotic agents can provide direct delivery of antibiotic in high concentration at the site of infection when treating bacterial conjunctivitis, keratitis, or uncomplicated blepharitis [1, 3]. Ophthalmic antibiotic solutions are preferred in adults as they do not interfere with vision, although more frequent administration is required due to short contact time with the eye. Antibiotic ointments have prolonged contact time and will be more resistant to medication loss through dilution by tears [4]. Often, ointments are recommended in children or adults who do not have concerns for visual interference.

The most extensively developed topical antibiotic class with a broad spectrum of activity is the fluoroquinolones (Table 9.1) [5–12]. Fluoroquinolones (besifloxacin, ciprofloxacin, gatifloxacin, levofloxacin, moxifloxacin, and ofloxacin) cause rapid bacterial cell death due to inhibition of bacterial DNA synthesis. These agents limit the activity of two key topoisomerase classes of enzymes that play an important role in bacterial DNA replication. DNA gyrase introduces negative supercoils into DNA within the bacterial cell, and topoisomerase IV divides the chromosomal DNA during bacterial cell division [13]. Antibacterial activities of fluoroquinolones vary between the generations. Although the initial generations such as ofloxacin and ciprofloxacin have limited gram-positive activity, especially against streptococci, ciprofloxacin still shows the best activity against *Pseudomonas aeruginosa* [13]. New generations such as levofloxacin, gatifloxacin, moxifloxacin, and besifloxacin have a broader spectrum of activity including methicillin-susceptible *Staphylococcus aureus* (MSSA), methicillin-resistant *S. aureus* (MRSA), and *Streptococcus* species [13]. In a recent surveillance study that reviewed ocular microorganisms and antibiotic activity, ciprofloxacin was the least potent agent against staphylococcal isolates with 80 % resistance to MRSA, whereas besifloxacin was the most potent agent in the class followed by moxifloxacin [14]. All fluoroquinolones have great atypical coverage such as *Chlamydia trachomatis*; however moxifloxacin is the only fluoroquinolone that has additional anaerobic coverage [13].

Macrolides (azithromycin, erythromycin) are generally thought to inhibit RNA-dependent protein synthesis at the chain elongation step; however the ability to bind to the 50S ribosomal subunit differs between azithromycin and erythromycin which results in varying antibacterial activities [15–17]. When compared to erythromycin, azithromycin may have better penetrating ability to the outer envelope of gram-negative organisms such as *Moraxella catarrhalis* and *Haemophilus influenzae*. Also, *C. trachomatis* coverage is much better with azithromycin compared to erythromycin [18]. With regard to gram-negative and atypical coverage, macrolides have great activity against *Neisseria gonorrhoeae* and *M. catarrhalis*. Macrolides also have activity against actinomycetes and mycobacteria which have been identified as causative pathogens in canaliculitis and keratitis [3].

Table 9.1 Topical antibiotic agents of ocular infections

Drug (brand name)	FDA-approved indication(s)	Dosage
Aminoglycosides		
Gentamicin 0.3 % solution	Conjunctivitis Keratitis Keratoconjunctivitis Corneal ulcers Blepharitis Blepharoconjunctivitis Acute meibomianitis Dacryocystitis	1–2 drops every 4 h
Gentamicin 0.3 % ointment (Gentak®)		½ inch ribbon 2–3×/day
Tobramycin 0.3 % solution (Tobrex®)	Superficial ocular infection (conjunctivitis, keratitis)	1–2 drops every 4 h; 2 drops hourly (severe cases)
Tobramycin 0.3 % ointment (Tobrex®)	Treatment of external infections of the eye and its adnexa	½ inch ribbon every 3–4 h up to 2–3×/day (dosing based on severity of infection)
Fluoroquinolones		
Besifloxacin 0.6 % suspension (Besivance®)	Bacterial conjunctivitis	1 drop 3×/day 4–12 h apart for 7 days
Ciprofloxacin 0.3 % solution (Ciloxan®)	Bacterial conjunctivitis	1–2 drops every 2 h while awake for 2 days then 1–2 drops every 4 h while awake for 5 days
	Corneal ulcers	Day 1: 2 drops every 15 min for 6 h, then every 30 min Day 2: 2 drops every hour Day 3–14: 2 drops every 4 h
Ciprofloxacin 0.3 % ointment (Ciloxan®)	Bacterial conjunctivitis	½ inch 3×/day for 2 days then ½ inch 2×/day for 5 days
Gatifloxacin 0.3 % solution (Zymaxid®)	Bacterial conjunctivitis	1 drop every 2 h (up to 8 times) while awake for 2 days then 1 drop up to 4×/day while awake for 5 days
Levofloxacin 0.5 % solution (Quixin®)	Bacterial conjunctivitis	1–2 drops every 2 h (up to 8 times) while awake for 2 days Day 3–7: 1–2 drops every 4 h while awake up to 4×/day
Levofloxacin 1.5 % solution (Iquix®)	Corneal ulcers	Day 1–3: 1–2 drops every 30 min to 2 h while awake and every 4–6 h after retiring Days 4 through treatment completion: 1–2 drops every 1–4 h while awake
Moxifloxacin 0.5 % solution (Vigamox®)	Bacterial conjunctivitis	1 drop 3×/day for 7 days

(continued)

Table 9.1 (continued)

Drug (brand name)	FDA-approved indication(s)	Dosage
Ofloxacin 0.3 % solution (Ocuflox®)	Bacterial conjunctivitis	1–2 drops every 2–4 h for 2 days then 1–2 drops 4×/day for 5 days
	Corneal ulcers	Days 1–2: 1–2 drops every 30 min while awake. Awaken at ~4–6 h after retiring and instill 1–2 drops Days 3–7: 1–2 drops hourly, while awake Days 7 through treatment completion: 1–2 drops 4×/day
Macrolides		
Azithromycin 1 % solution (Azasite™)	Bacterial conjunctivitis	1 drop in the affected eye(s) 2×/day for the first 2 days then 1 drop daily for the next 5 days
Erythromycin 0.5 % ointment (Romycin®)	Superficial ocular infection involving the conjunctiva or cornea	½ inch to affected eye (s) every 4–6 h
Others		
Bacitracin	Superficial ocular infection involving the conjunctiva or cornea	½ inch every 3–4 h for 7–10 days
Sulfacetamide 10 % ointment	Conjunctivitis Superficial ocular infections	½ inch 4×/day and bedtime for 7–10 days
Sulfacetamide solution (Bleph®-10)	Bacterial conjunctivitis Superficial ocular infections Adjunctive therapy with systemic sulfonamide therapy for trachoma	1–2 drops every 1–3 h while awake, less frequently at night for 7–10 days
Combination therapy		
Bacitracin/polymyxin B ointment	Bacterial conjunctivitis Keratitis Keratoconjunctivitis Blepharitis Blepharoconjunctivitis	Thin film every 3–4 h for 7–10 days
Gramicidin/neomycin/ polymyxin B (Neosporin®)		Up to 2 drops every hour then 1–2 drops every 4 h for 7–10 days
Trimethoprim/polymyxin B (Polytrim®)	Bacterial conjunctivitis Blepharoconjunctivitis Superficial ocular infection	1 drop every 3 h up to 6 doses daily for 7–10 days

Macrolides have been highly potent against *S. pneumoniae* and group A streptococcus isolates; however, the prevalence of erythromycin resistance to *S. pneumoniae* is continuously increasing in the United States and worldwide [19–21]. Although group A streptococcus resistance to erythromycin has been reported, the prevalence of resistance is not as high as is seen with *S. pneumoniae* [22, 23]. Erythromycin has activity against viridans group streptococcus; however, Europe and Asia have higher resistance rates than those that occurred in North America

[24]. MRSA is generally resistant to erythromycin; therefore, the use of erythromycin should be based on the local antibiogram or culture result [15].

Aminoglycosides such as gentamicin and tobramycin have limited activity against gram-positive organisms and anaerobic bacteria [25–27]. These agents work by binding to the 30S ribosomal subunit to inhibit protein synthesis and require aerobic metabolism to cause antibacterial effect [28]. In general, aminoglycosides have great activity against gram-negative bacilli such as *Enterobacteriaceae*, *P. aeruginosa*, and *Acinetobacte*r spp.; however, no activity has been shown for *Stenotrophomonas maltophilia* or *Burkholderia cepacia*.

Combination topical antibiotics are typically paired with narrow spectrum antibiotics to expand the overall spectrum of activity. Polymyxin B is a polypeptide with high molecular weight and works by penetrating the cell membrane of bacteria and interacting with phospholipids [29, 30]. The main antibacterial activity of polymyxin B is *P. aeruginosa*, *Acinetobacter baumannii*, and carbapenem-resistant *Enterobacteriaceae* (CRE). Most gram-positive organisms are resistant to polymyxin B; thus it is commonly paired with another antibiotic with good gram-positive coverage such as bacitracin or trimethoprim. Bacitracin inhibits cell wall synthesis by preventing transfer of mucopeptides into the growing cell wall [31]. As a combination agent, bacitracin zinc/polymyxin B sulfate has activity against *S. aureus*, *S. pneumoniae*, *Escherichia coli*, *H. influenzae*, *Klebsiella*/*Enterobacter* species, *Neisseri*a species, and *P. aeruginosa* [32]. Trimethoprim is a synthetic antibacterial agent that blocks the production of tetrahydrofolic acid from dihydrofolic acid by binding to and reversibly inhibiting the enzyme dihydrofolate reductase. It has good activity against gram-positive and gram-negative organisms such as *S. aureus*, *S. epidermidis*, *S. pyogenes*, *S. pneumoniae*, *H. influenzae*, *E. coli*, *Proteus vulgaris*, *E. aerogenes*, and *Serratia marcescens* [33, 34].

Sulfonamides have bacteriostatic properties and inhibit bacterial growth by interfering with folic acid synthesis [35]. The sulfonamides show antibacterial activity against *S. aureus*, *S. pneumoniae*, viridans group streptococcus, *E. coli*, *H. influenzae*, *Klebsiella* species, and *Enterobacter* species. These agents should not be used empirically for *Neisseria* species, *S. marcescens*, *P. aeruginosa*, or resistant *Staphylococcus* species [36].

Topical Antifungal/Antiviral

Natamycin eyedrops (5 % suspension) is the only antifungal agent that is commercially available. Natamycin is a tetraene polyene agent that works by binding to the sterol of the fungal cell membrane, which causes membrane permeability changes [37]. It is used for the treatment of fungal keratitis caused by *Candida* species, *Aspergillus*, *Cephalosporium*, *Fusarium*, and *Penicillium*; however, poor corneal tissue penetration limits its use in intraocular infections [3, 37]. Amphotericin B, nystatin, fluconazole, miconazole, and flucytosine eyedrops have been compounded for use [3, 38], but extemporaneous preparations of these products are not widely used. Furthermore, topical amphotericin B made with a deoxycholate formulation is known to be toxic to the cornea [39].

Commercially available topical antiviral agents are more common than antifungal agents. Trifluridine ophthalmic suspension is used for the treatment of herpes simplex keratitis and keratoconjunctivitis [3]. It inhibits viral DNA synthesis and has activity against herpes simplex virus (HSV) types 1 and 2, cytomegalovirus (CMV), and adenoviruses [40]. Vidarabine ointment is also available for the treatment of HSV keratitis. It has activity against idoxuridine-resistant and acyclovir-resistant HSV; however, it is more toxic and less effective compared to trifluridine for the treatment of HSV keratoconjunctivitis [3, 40]. Idoxuridine is approved for the treatment of HSV keratitis. Its mechanism of action is not completely understood, and it is also inferior to trifluridine and acyclovir for the treatment of HSV epithelial keratitis [40]. Topical 0.15 % ganciclovir ophthalmic gel is indicated for the treatment of acute herpetic keratitis [41]. Finally, topical acyclovir is not available in the United States [3].

Intravitreal/Subconjunctival Injection

Table 9.2 shows a list of commonly used antibiotic agents for intravitreal/subconjunctival injection. These agents are used since topical antibiotics are ineffective in treating endophthalmitis due to their inability to penetrate the intraocular site [42]. Antifungal agents such as voriconazole and conventional amphotericin B are often used for intravitreal infection, which result in rapid achievement of high concentration in the posterior chamber [43, 44].

Systemic Therapy

The data for intraocular penetration of antibiotic therapy delivered via parenteral routes is limited. There are a few antibiotic classes that are used as adjunctive therapy when treating endophthalmitis or when the use of systemic antibiotics is the

Table 9.2 Commonly used anti-infective agents for intravitreal injection

Anti-infective agents	Dose	Concentration
Amphotericin B	5–10 mcg/0.1 mL	50–100 mg/mL
Ampicillin	4 mg	50 mg/mL
Amikacin	0.2–0.1 mg	4 mg/mL
Ceftazidime	2–2.25 mg	22.5 mg/mL
Gentamicin	0.1–0.2 mg	1 mg/mL
Tobramycin	0.1–0.2 mg	1 mg/mL
Vancomycin	1 mg	10 mg/mL
Voriconazole	100 mcg/0.1 mL	1 mg/mL

Data are from Lopez-Carbezas et al. [42] and Pappas et al. [44]

Table 9.3 Pathogens and systemic treatment for ocular infections

Pathogens	Antimicrobial treatment (s)
Gram-positive Methicillin-susceptible *S. epidermidis* (MSSE) *S. aureus* (MSSA)	Nafcillin, cefazolin, vancomycin[a], linezolid[a]
Methicillin-resistant *S. epidermidis* (MRSE) *S. aureus* (MRSA)	Vancomycin, linezolid
Streptococci	Ampicillin/sulbactam, ceftriaxone, vancomycin[a]
Enterococci *E. faecalis. E. faecium*	Ampicillin (if ampicillin susceptible) Linezolid (if resistant to ampicillin and vancomycin)
Bacillus cereus	Carbapenem vancomycin
Propionibacterium acnes	Vancomycin, linezolid
Gram-negative *Enterobacteriaceae* *E. coli* *Klebsiella* spp. *Proteus* spp. *H. influenzae* *Moraxella* spp. *Pseudomonas aeruginosa*[b]	Ceftriaxone, ceftazidime[b], cefepime[b], ampicillin/sulbactam, piperacillin/tazobactam[b], meropenem[b], moxifloxacin, levofloxacin[b], ciprofloxacin[b]

[a]For patients with penicillin and/or cephalosporin allergies
[b]Antibiotics with pseudomonas activity

best treatment option (i.e., orbital cellulitis, preseptal cellulitis) [42, 45]. All B-lactams inhibit bacterial cell wall synthesis by inhibiting high-molecular-weight penicillin-binding proteins (PBPs) [46]. Vancomycin is a tricyclic glycopeptide that works by binding to the D-alanyl-D-alanine part of a cell wall precursor and thus inhibiting the late stages of bacterial cell wall synthesis [47]. Linezolid is one of the oxazolidinones that works by inhibiting protein synthesis. It binds to the 50S ribosome within the 30S unit to prevent 70S complex formation [48]. B-lactam antibiotics (penicillins, cephalosporins, and carbapenems), vancomycin, and linezolid may be added to cover gram-positive and gram-negative organisms depending on the culture result (Table 9.3).

Invasive ocular infections caused by fungi are rare but associated with poor response rate; thus the treatment consists of systemic antifungal agents in combination with surgery, intravitreal injections, or both. Amphotericin B has been most studied and experienced in treating intraocular fungal infection to date [43]. It is a fungicidal agent that works by binding to ergosterol in the cell membrane of susceptible fungi and changes membrane permeability, which results in the leakage of intracellular potassium and other molecules and cell death [49]. Currently there are four different amphotericin B formulations: amphotericin B deoxycholate, amphotericin B colloidal dispersion, amphotericin B lipid complex, and liposomal amphotericin B. It is a broad-spectrum antifungal agent that has activity against most *Candida* species except for *C. lusitaniae*; dimorphic fungi such as *Histoplasma capsulatum*, *Blastomyces dermatitidis*, and *Coccidioides immitis*; and filamentous fungi such as *Aspergillus* spp. and the *Mucorales* group [50]. Spectrum of activity is not influenced by different amphotericin B products.

Flucytosine is often used with amphotericin B as it is synergistic against *Candida* spp. and *Cryptococcus neoformans*. It is a fluorinated pyrimidine that works by disrupting RNA and DNA synthesis [43]. Flucytosine lacks activity against the dimorphic fungi and filamentous fungi, and it should not be used as monotherapy due to rapid development of resistance for the treatment of candidiasis [49].

Azoles are ergosterol synthesis inhibitors, and each azole has slight variation in its spectrum of activities. Fluconazole is mainly active against *Candida* species, *C. neoformans*, and dimorphic fungi such as *C. immitis*, *H. capsulatum*, and *B. dermatitidis*. Although most *Candida albicans* are susceptible to fluconazole, fluconazole-resistant *C. albicans* has been reported. Resistance in other *Candida* species such as *Candida glabrata* has been noted [43]. Fluconazole is not active against *Candida krusei*, *Aspergillus* spp., *Fusarium* spp., *Scedosporium* spp., and *Mucorales* [50]. Itraconazole is active against some *Candida* species, dimorphic fungi, and *Aspergillus* species; however, it does not penetrate the ocular structure well [49]. Similarly, posaconazole has poor ocular penetration. It has a broad-spectrum coverage including *Candida* species, *C. neoformans*, *Aspergillus* species, *Fusarium* species, and *Zygomycetes* [49, 51]. Voriconazole is a broad-spectrum azole that is the drug of choice for treatment of invasive aspergillosis. It also has activity against *Candida* species, *C. neoformans*, *Scedosporium* species, and *Curvularia* species [49, 51]. Unlike posaconazole and itraconazole, voriconazole penetrates the eye and can adjust the dose based on the trough goal level of 2–5 mg/L [52, 53]. The newest addition to the class of azole is isavuconazonium sulfate. It is a prodrug of isavuconazole with broad spectrum of activity including most *Candida* species, dimorphic fungi, *C. neoformans*, *Aspergillus* species, and *Mucorales* [54]. To date, no data are available regarding ocular penetration of this new agent.

Echinocandins work by inhibiting the synthesis of 1, 3-β-D-glucan, which is the predominant component of the fungal cell wall. Currently there are three echinocandins on the market: caspofungin, micafungin, and anidulafungin. In general, echinocandins are active against *Candida* species and *Aspergillus* species, but lack activity for *Fusarium*, *Scedosporium*, and *Zygomycetes* [49, 51]. Furthermore, echinocandins do not penetrate the ocular structure; therefore, it is not widely used to treat invasive ocular infections.

Viral conjunctivitis can be caused by HSV and adenovirus [55]. Although no effective treatment is available for viral conjunctivitis caused by adenovirus, oral antivirals are used to shorten the course of HSV conjunctivitis [55]. Acyclovir and valacyclovir work by blocking viral DNA synthesis and are much more potent against HSV type 1 and 2 compared to cytomegalovirus [40]. Ganciclovir and valganciclovir are potent against CMV and have better activity against herpes B virus compared to acyclovir [40].

Table 9.4 Factors to improve corneal absorption

Nonionic surfactants
Polymers
Viscous preparations
Solvents
Improving drug stability

Data are from McCloskey [2]

Mode of Administration and Pharmacokinetics

Delivering a therapeutic concentration of antibiotic at the site of infection is a challenge. Important factors that could influence the intraocular penetration of antibiotics are the charge of the drug, corneal epithelium status, drug formulation, drug concentration, and the dosage regimen [1]. Natural barriers such as eyelids, iris, tears, and cornea prevent diffusion of antibiotics into intraocular tissue. In order to promote corneal absorption, certain formulation factors should be considered (Table 9.4) [2]. Furthermore, the corneal area can only contain about 30 μl; therefore, topical solutions are given more frequently to ensure adequate absorption of medication [2]. Ophthalmic medications that have both lipid- and water-soluble properties will help enhance overall drug absorption [4]. Due to these challenges of the topical application method, infections involving vitreous humor, sclera, or cornea may require additional strategies to administer drug therapy.

Unlike topical antibiotic application, subconjunctival injection can reach high antibiotic concentration in sclera and cornea. This mode of administration is used to treat intraocular infection as it gains access to the episcleral and conjunctival vessels [4]. However, subconjunctival injection does not provide adequate antibiotic penetration into the vitreous humor [42].

Intravitreal injection of air has been practiced by ophthalmologists to repair retinal detachments since 1911 [56]. Intravitreal injection is used to treat endophthalmitis, cytomegalovirus (CMV) retinitis, and more. This method provides direct exposure of antibiotic to the infected site for a prolonged period with minimal systemic absorption [57]. Thus, bypassing the blood-retinal barrier ensures immediate high concentration of antibiotic in the vitreous cavity [42].

Systemic antibiotic therapy is used as an adjunctive strategy to intravitreal injection, subconjunctival injection, and/or topical administration. This mode of administration is added when treating ocular infections that involve the posterior segment of the eye or the orbit (i.e., endophthalmitis, orbital cellulitis, or chorioretinitis), where topical antibiotics will provide negligible drug penetration [4]. Limited data concerning systemic antibiotics and ocular penetration are available; however, linezolid and fluoroquinolones such as levofloxacin and moxifloxacin have been shown to achieve good ocular penetration [42].

Antibiotic Toxicity

Antibiotics can cause serious side effects if not used appropriately. Topical antibiotics are concentrated locally; therefore, systemic side effects should not occur. However, topical antibiotic formulations can cause some serious tissue side effects. Tissue side effects could be due to the antibiotic or the preservatives and vehicles used in the formulation [1]. Topical chloramphenicol is no longer used, but this drug had been known to cause idiosyncratic bone marrow suppression, aplastic anemia, and death [1, 4]. Topical neomycin is in multiple combination products such as Polytrim® and Neosporin®. Neomycin has been associated with punctate staining of the cornea [1]; therefore, patients should be informed about this undesirable side effect. Fluoroquinolones are one of the commonly used topical antibiotics, yet these agents also have side effects. One study found that moxifloxacin had the least cytotoxic effects against corneal and/or conjunctival epithelial cells compared to other fluoroquinolones, while all caused thinning of the corneal epithelial layer after 7 days of treatment [58]; however, other studies have not shown the same effects [59, 60]. The conflicting data on moxifloxacin was explained by the absence of preservatives such as 0.005 % or 0.006 % benzalkonium chloride, whereas other fluoroquinolones have preservatives which have been associated with tissue toxicity [61].

The preservatives or vehicles in the ophthalmic formulation can cause additive side effects such as hypersensitivity reaction or reduction in antimicrobial activity, which are mainly known from experience with thimerosal (a common preservative in contact lens solution) [1, 4]. As previously mentioned, benzalkonium chloride may inhibit epithelial adhesion, cause a loss of superficial epithelial cells, and delay healing of the epithelium [1].

Antibiotic toxicity could also occur due to the mode of administration. Retinal toxicity has been reported from intravitreal injection as well as subconjunctival injection of aminoglycosides. These modes of antibiotic administration will reach high concentration in the intraocular site; however, it increases the exposure of high drug concentration near the retina which could cause chemical damage. Multiple case series have shown that retinal toxicity and macular ischemia can occur with intravitreal injection of aminoglycosides such as amikacin or gentamicin [62, 63]. When using intravitreal injection, these medications should be administered close to the anterior part of the vitreous cavity to help avoid retinal side effects [42]. Another mode of administration is intracameral antibiotic injection which can be done after cataract surgery to prevent postoperative bacterial endophthalmitis [64]. This is often completed with cefuroxime, and multiple cases have been reported with retinal toxicity and hemorrhagic retinal infarction [65, 66].

Parenteral antibiotics are known to have numerous adverse side effects. Penicillin derivatives are most commonly associated with hypersensitivity reactions that range from minor drug rash to life-threatening reactions such as Stevens-Johnson syndrome or anaphylaxis [4, 46]. Patients may also develop serum sickness with fever, urticaria, joint pains, and angioneurotic edema; however, this syndrome is very rare.

Penicillin and penicillin derivatives can also cause renal toxicity such as allergic angiitis or interstitial nephritis. Antistaphylococcal penicillins (i.e., methicillin or nafcillin) have been highly associated with interstitial nephritis which presents with fever, macular rash, eosinophilia, proteinuria, eosinophiluria, and hematuria [46]. Penicillin and penicillin derivatives can lower the seizure threshold; however, this effect is more common with large doses and in patient with renal dysfunction. When prescribing penicillin derivatives to treat ocular infections, it is important to obtain the patient's allergy history to ensure that these antibiotics are appropriate for the specific patient.

Cephalosporins have adverse reactions that are similar to those encountered with penicillin and penicillin derivatives, but these medications are generally well tolerated. Hypersensitivity reactions can occur, although not as commonly as with the penicillins [67]. Adverse reactions between the different generations of cephalosporins include gastrointestinal, hematologic, and central nervous system effects that are mostly similar. However, the third-generation cephalosporin, ceftriaxone, has been specifically associated with obstructive biliary toxicity [68, 69]. This syndrome is reversible after antibiotic cessation [67], but the ophthalmologist should consider an alternative therapy in patients with known hepatic diseases and neonates younger than 28 days. Elevation of serum creatinine has been reported; however, renal toxicity is not as common as is seen with the penicillins [70]. Although cephalosporins may not play a significant role in renal toxicity, cefepime should be used with caution as encephalopathy and seizures have been reported in patients with renal insufficiency [71–73].

Carbapenems do not have major adverse effects and are generally well tolerated. The most serious side effect that requires monitoring is seizure activity, as all carbapenems possess a structural similarity to γ-aminobutyric acid (GABA) and can have an antagonistic effect on the action of this neurotransmitter [74]. Cross-reactivity with the penicillins has been documented as between 0 and 11 %; however, carbapenem use is considered safe if the penicillin skin test is negative [75].

Fluoroquinolones can cause severe adverse effects that need close monitoring. Although not generally severe or serious, gastrointestinal-related symptoms are the most common side effects. Similar to carbapenems, adverse events involving the central nervous system such as headache, dizziness, insomnia, and seizures can manifest with fluoroquinolone [13]. Cardiovascular effects, especially QT interval prolongation, are well known with the older quinolones; the newer generations also possess these side effects but with a lesser intensity [76–78]. Although tendinitis and joint toxicity have been reported with fluoroquinolones, these side effects are not as common. One adverse event of concern in ophthalmology patients is the potential for retinal detachment with fluoroquinolones. Due to their ability to achieve high concentration in the ocular tissue and cause collagen and connective tissue damage, the patients in one study who were prescribed fluoroquinolones carried a 4.5-fold increased risk for retinal detachment [79]. Another study has shown a similar result when fluoroquinolones were compared to amoxicillin [80]; however, a third study did not show the same effect [81]. Ophthalmologists should use caution when prescribing oral fluoroquinolones, especially in patients with high risk for retinal detachment.

As resistance has been increasing, more broad-spectrum antibiotics such as vancomycin and linezolid have been used to treat intraocular infection with methicillin-resistant *Staphylococcus aureus* (MRSA). Vancomycin has been used for the past 50 years, and its adverse effects have been studied extensively. The most common side effect of vancomycin is related to medication infusion rate, also known as red man syndrome. This can be minimized with reduction of infusion rate or premedication with antihistamines. Numerous studies have been done to find the risk factors for vancomycin-associated nephrotoxicity. Such risk factors are large total daily dose (≥4 g/day), obesity (weight ≥ 101.4 kg) [82], higher vancomycin trough levels (≥15 μg/mL), concomitant use of nephrotoxic medications, and prolonged duration of therapy [83, 84]. Other adverse events such as drug rash, drug-related fever, thrombocytopenia, and neutropenia can occur, but these effects are not as common [47].

Thrombocytopenia with linezolid has been well documented in the literature. The decrease in platelet count occurs with longer duration of therapy, at least 2 weeks; however, it can occur earlier and thus requires close monitoring [85]. Another serious side effect associated with linezolid is a potential drug interaction with serotonergic agents and serotonin syndrome with fever, agitation, mental status changes, and tremor [85]. Therefore, caution should be practiced when prescribing linezolid to a patient who is already taking other serotonergic agents. Although not as common, peripheral neuropathy and optic neuropathy can occur when taking linezolid [86]. Optic neuropathy is another consequence of its enhanced ability to penetrate the eye which can cause vision loss [48]. Therefore, patients who are taking linezolid for a prolonged duration should follow up with an ophthalmologist for early detection of any vision changes to prevent visual loss.

One of the serious side effects associated with amphotericin B is nephrotoxicity. It damages renal tubular cells, which disrupts tubular basement membrane and causes functioning nephron loss [49]. It also leads to electrolyte wasting, especially of potassium, magnesium, and bicarbonate [49]. This is associated with all four formulations; however, amphotericin B deoxycholate is associated with acute infusion-related reactions such as chills, fever, and tachycardia. Nausea, vomiting, and liver enzyme elevations have been associated with amphotericin B. Similarly, flucytosine should be used with caution in patients with renal dysfunction. It can cause fatal bone marrow toxicity such as leukopenia and thrombocytopenia [49]. Therapeutic drug monitoring is recommended for flucytosine twice weekly. It is also teratogenic, therefore, contraindicated in pregnancy. Azoles are generally well tolerated with minimal side effects such as gastrointestinal and hepatic toxicity. Voriconazole has been known to cause visual disturbances, hallucination, and confusion [49]. For patients who are intolerant to voriconazole due to visual disturbances, the newest azole, isavuconazonium sulfate, could be an alternative option if broad-spectrum coverage is necessary. Echinocandins infrequently cause adverse reactions. Occasionally histamine-mediated symptoms such as rash, pruritus, dyspnea, and hypotension may occur, but echinocandins are not hepatotoxic or nephrotoxic [49].

Intravenous acyclovir can cause reversible renal dysfunction and neurotoxicity. Clinical manifestations such as lethargy, confusion, hallucinations, seizures, or coma could occur, and patients can experience neurotoxicity within 1–3 days of treatment [40]. This is more common with valacyclovir. Oral acyclovir is generally well tolerated but could cause diarrhea, rash, and headache. Ganciclovir and valganciclovir cause myelosuppression and CNS toxicity. The most common reasons for early discontinuation of these agents are severe neutropenia and thrombocytopenia [40].

Summary

Ocular infections can be treated with topical antibiotic agents, subconjunctival or intravitreal antibiotic injections, or systemic antibiotics depending on the type of infection and the depth of intraocular eye involvement. Each mode of administration has advantages and disadvantages with regard to delivery of an appropriate drug concentration at the site of infection and the potential for antibiotic toxicity. Choosing the right therapy with appropriate bacterial, fungal, and/or viral coverage, mode of administration, and pharmacologic activity is critical when treating ocular infections.

References

1. Snyder RW, Glasser DB. Antibiotic therapy for ocular infection. West J Med. 1994;161:579–84.
2. McCloskey R. Topical antimicrobial agents and antibiotics for the eye. Med Clin North Am. 1988;72:717–22.
3. Baum J. Infections of the eye. Clin Infect Dis. 1995;21:479–86.
4. Stein HA, Stein RM, Freeman MI. Pharmacology. In: The ophthalmic assistant. A text for allied and associated ophthalmic personnel. 9th ed. Philadelphia: Saunders; 2012. p. 49–66.
5. Besivance®. DailyMed, Bethesda. 2013. http://dailymed.nlm.nih.gov/dailymed/drugInfo.cfm?setid=a3e6d688-7e5e-4ca3-b27e-79756c322a32&audience=consumer. Accessed 30 Aug 2015.
6. Ciloxan® ointment. DailyMed, Bethesda. 2013. http://dailymed.nlm.nih.gov/dailymed/drugInfo.cfm?setid=1c292706-a900-4d6f-979e-9c42d6ff2fb2&audience=consumer. Accessed 30 Aug 2015.
7. Ciloxan® solution. DailyMed, Bethesda. 2013. http://dailymed.nlm.nih.gov/dailymed/drugInfo.cfm?setid=614af481-f9ef-44ac-9cb8-f421660d9cdd&audience=consumer. Accessed 30 Aug 2015.
8. Gatifloxacin. DailyMed, Bethesda. 2013. http://dailymed.nlm.nih.gov/dailymed/drugInfo.cfm?setid=1160b16c-929a-4e85-9c0b-1d8c96a7678b&audience=consumer. Accessed 30 Aug 2015.
9. Quixin®. DailyMed, Bethesda. 2013. http://dailymed.nlm.nih.gov/dailymed/drugInfo.cfm?setid=09b3a912-97f9-45ae-a162-9f45c860dc22&audience=consumer. Accessed 30 Aug 2015.
10. Iquix®. DailyMed, Bethesda. 2013. http://dailymed.nlm.nih.gov/dailymed/drugInfo.cfm?setid=067ea8ec-99a3-4a0b-9116-4ffd6160b24b&audience=consumer. Accessed 30 Aug 2015.

11. Vigamox®. DailyMed, Bethesda. 2013. http://dailymed.nlm.nih.gov/dailymed/drugInfo.cfm?setid=0e6ab6ba-5eeb-4faf-ba80-4bf21a74228a&audience=consumer. Accessed 30 Aug 2015.
12. Ocuflox®. DailyMed, Bethesda. 2013. http://dailymed.nlm.nih.gov/dailymed/drugInfo.cfm?setid=7aab4449-3dda-4e2c-8e40-b3244a548bf5&audience=consumer. Accessed 30 Aug 2015.
13. Hooper D, Strahilevitz J. Quinolones. In: Bennett JE, Dolin R, Blaser MJ, editors. Mandell, Douglas, and Bennett's principles and practice of infectious diseases. 8th ed. Philadelphia: Saunders; 2015. p. 419–39.
14. Hass W, Pillar CM, Torres M, Morris TW, Sahm DF. Monitoring antibiotic resistance in ocular microorganisms: results from the Antibiotic Resistance Monitoring in Ocular micRorganisms (ARMOR) 2009 surveillance study. Am J Ophthalmol. 2011;152:567–74.e3. doi:10.1016/j.ajo.2011.03.010. Epub 2011 Jun 8.
15. Sivapalasingam S, Steigbigel NH. Macrolides, clindamycin, and ketolides. In: Bennett JE, Dolin R, Blaser MJ, editors. Mandell, Douglas, and Bennett's principles and practice of infectious diseases. 8th ed. Philadelphia: Saunders; 2015. p. 358–76.e6.
16. Azasite™. DailyMed, Bethesda. 2013. http://dailymed.nlm.nih.gov/dailymed/drugInfo.cfm?setid=5dc0f75a-1e14-469f-af4f-c668a32f2328&audience=consumer. Accessed 30 Aug 2015.
17. Erythromycin ointment. DailyMed, Bethesda. 2013. http://dailymed.nlm.nih.gov/dailymed/drugInfo.cfm?setid=f4b57b8a-089e-4bbc-bcc7-3a9b9b600930&audience=consumer. Accessed 30 Aug 2015.
18. Neu HC. Clinical microbiology of azithromycin. Am J Med. 1991;91:12S–8.
19. Thornsberry C, Sahm DF, Kelly LJ, Critchley IA, Jones ME, Evangelista AT, et al. Regional trends in antimicrobial resistance among clinical isolates of *Streptococcus pneumoniae*, *Haemophilus influenzae*, and *Moraxella catarrhalis* in the United States: results from the TRUST Surveillance Program, 1999–2000. Clin Infect Dis. 2002;34 Suppl 1:S4–16.
20. Hsueh PR, Liu CY, Luh KT. Current status of antimicrobial resistance in Taiwan. Emerg Infect Dis. 2002;8:132–7.
21. Farrell DJ, File TM, Jenkins SG. Prevalence and antibacterial susceptibility of mef(A)-positive macrolide-resistant *Streptococcus pneumoniae* over 4 years (2000–2004) of the PROTEKT US Study. J Clin Microbiol. 2007;45:290–3.
22. Green MD, Beall B, Marcon MJ, Allen CH, Bradley JS, Dashefsky B, et al. Multicentre surveillance of the prevalence and molecular epidemiology of macrolide resistance among pharyngeal isolates of group A streptococci in the USA. J Antimicrob Chemother. 2006;57:1240–3.
23. Villaseñor-Sierra A, Katahira E, Jaramillo-Valdivia AN, de los Angeles Barajas-Garćia M, Bryant A, Morfin-Otero R, et al. Phenotypes and genotypes of erythromycin-resistant *Streptococcus pyogenes* strains isolated from invasive and non-invasive infections from Mexico and the USA during 1999–2010. Int J Infect Dis. 2012;16:e178–81.
24. Gordon KA, Beach ML, Biedenbach DJ, Jones RN, Rhomberg PR, Mutnick AH. Antimicrobial susceptibility patterns of beta-hemolytic and viridans group streptococci: report from the SENTRY Antimicrobial Surveillance Program (1997–2000). Diagn Microbiol Infect Dis. 2002;43:157–62.
25. Gentak®. DailyMed, Bethesda. 2013. http://dailymed.nlm.nih.gov/dailymed/drugInfo.cfm?setid=561cf436-74b8-452c-9fd2-e42f859c87dd&audience=consumer. Accessed 30 Aug 2015.
26. Tobrex®. DailyMed, Bethesda.2013. http://dailymed.nlm.nih.gov/dailymed/drugInfo.cfm?setid=cdd423c5-a231-47d4-bf51-00b5c29e6a60&audience=consumer. Accessed 30 Aug 2015.
27. Egger SF, Ruckhofer J, Alzner E, Hell W, Hitzl W, Huber-Spitzy V, et al. In vitro susceptibilities to topical antibiotics of bacteria isolated from the surface of clinically symptomatic eyes. Ophthalmic Res. 2001;33:117–20.
28. Leggett JE. Aminoglycosides. In: Bennett JE, Dolin R, Blaser MJ, editors. Mandell, Douglas, and Bennett's principles and practice of infectious diseases. 8th ed. Philadelphia: Saunders; 2015. p. 310–21.e7.

29. Robert PY, Adenis JP. Comparative review of topical ophthalmic antibacterial preparations. Drugs. 2001;61:175–85.
30. Kaye KS, Pogue JM, Kaye D. Polymyxins (polymyxin B and colistin). In: Bennett JE, Dolin R, Blaser MJ, editors. Mandell, Douglas, and Bennett's principles and practice of infectious diseases. 8th ed. Philadelphia: Saunders; 2015. p. 401–405.e1.
31. Bacitracin. DailyMed, Bethesda. 2013. http://dailymed.nlm.nih.gov/dailymed/drugInfo.cfm?setid=6ed2f2bd-9d2f-46af-a44c-95a02ca034de&audience=consumer. Accessed 30 Aug 2015.
32. Polycin®. DailyMed, Bethesda. 2013. http://dailymed.nlm.nih.gov/dailymed/drugInfo.cfm?setid=3abbfb58-26d1-460d-a60f-db63c0193a0d. Accessed 29 Aug 2015.
33. Polytrim®. DailyMed, Bethesda. 2013. http://dailymed.nlm.nih.gov/dailymed/drugInfo.cfm?setid=5ce95658-d2eb-4d35-b387-ded0d7e4a122. Accessed 29 Aug 2015.
34. Neosporin®. DailyMed, Bethesda. 2013. http://dailymed.nlm.nih.gov/dailymed/drugInfo.cfm?setid=33e9b6d3-2b2b-4036-dd89-47177e23fcfe. Accessed 30 Aug 2015.
35. Zinner S, Myer KH. Sulfonamides and trimethoprim. In: Bennett JE, Dolin R, Blaser MJ, editors. Mandell, Douglas, and Bennett's principles and practice of infectious diseases. 8th ed. Philadelphia: Saunders; 2015. p. 410–8.e2.
36. Bleph®-10. DailyMed, Bethesda. 2013. http://dailymed.nlm.nih.gov/dailymed/drugInfo.cfm?setid=27c8bd30-89ec-464c-b7ac-ca2dbe27e861. Accessed 29 Aug 2015.
37. Natamycin®. DailyMed, Bethesda. 2013. https://dailymed.nlm.nih.gov/dailymed/drugInfo.cfm?setid=d262661c-860d-482e-aa8d-3cf1f252b32a. Accessed 13 Mar 2016.
38. Behrens-Baumann W. Topical antimycotics in ophthalmology. Ophthalmolgica. 1997;211 Suppl 1:33–8.
39. Klotz SA, Penn CC, Negvesky GJ, Butrus SI. Fungal and parasitic infections of the eye. Clin Microbiol Rev. 2000;13:662–85.
40. Aoki FY. Antivirals against herpes viruses. In: Bennett JE, Dolin R, Blaser MJ, editors. Mandell, Douglas, and Bennett's principles and practice of infectious diseases. 8th ed. Philadelphia: Saunders; 2015. p. 546–62.e7.
41. Zirgan (ganciclovir ophthalmic gel 0.15%) [prescribing information]. Tampa: Bausch & Lomb Inc; 2014.
44. Pappas PG, Kauffman CA, Andes DR, Clancy CJ, Marr KA, Ostrosky-Zeichner L, et al. Clinical practice guideline for the management of candidiasis: 2016 update by the Infectious Diseases Society of America. Clin Infect Dis. 2016. doi:10.1093/cid/civ933.
42. Lopez-Carbezas C, Muner DS, Massa MR, Mensa Puevo JM. Antibiotics in endophthalmitis: microbiological and pharmacokinetic considerations. Curr Clin Pharmacol. 2010;5:47–54.
43. Riddell 4th J, Comer GM, Kauffman CA. Treatment of endogenous fungal endophthalmitis: focus on new antifungal agents. Clin Infect Dis. 2011;52:648–53.
45. Thielen TL, Castle SS, Terry JE. Anterior ocular infections: an overview of pathophysiology and treatment. Ann Pharmacother. 2000;34:235–46.
46. Doi Y, Chambers HF. Penicillins and beta lactamase inhibitors. In: Bennett JE, Dolin R, Blaser MJ, editors. Mandell, Douglas, and Bennett's principles and practice of infectious diseases. 8th ed. Philadelphia: Saunders; 2015. p. 263–77.e3.
47. Murray BE, Arias CA, Nannini EC. Glycopeptides (vancomycin and teicoplanin), streptogramins (quinupristin-dalfopristin), lipopeptides (daptomycin), and lipoglycopeptides (telavancin). In: Bennett JE, Dolin R, Blaser MJ, editors. Mandell, Douglas, and Bennett's principles and practice of infectious diseases. 8th ed. Philadelphia: Saunders; 2015. p. 377–400.e4.
48. Cox HL, Donowitz GR. Linezolid and other oxazolidinones. In: Bennett JE, Dolin R, Blaser MJ, editors. Mandell, Douglas, and Bennett's principles and practice of infectious diseases. 8th ed. Philadelphia: Saunders; 2015. p. 406–9.e2.
49. Rex JH, Stevens DA. Drugs active against fungi, pneumocystis, and microsporidia. In: Bennett JE, Dolin R, Blaser MJ, editors. Mandell, Douglas, and Bennett's principles and practice of infectious diseases. 8th ed. Philadelphia: Saunders; 2015. p. 479–94.e4.
50. Nett JE, Andes DR. Antifungal agents: spectrum of activity, pharmacology, and clinical indications. Infect Dis Clin North Am. 2016. doi:10.1016/j.idc.2015.10.012.
51. Chhablani J. Fungal endophthalmitis. Expert Rev Anti Infect Ther. 2011;9:1991–201.

52. Smith J, Safdar N, Knasinski V, Simmons W, Bhavnani SM, Ambrose PG, et al. Voriconazole therapeutic drug monitoring. Antimicrob Agents Chemother. 2006;50:1570–2.
53. Pascual A, Calandra T, Bolay S, Buclin T, Bille J, Marchetti O. Voriconazole therapeutic drug monitoring in patients with invasive mycoses improves efficacy and safety outcomes. Clin Infect Dis. 2008;46:201–11.
54. Cresemba (isavuconazonium) [prescribing information]. Northbrook: Astellas Pharma US Inc; 2015.
55. Azari AA, Barney NP. Conjunctivitis: a systemic review of diagnosis and treatment. JAMA. 2013;310:1721–9.
56. Jager RD, Aiello LP, Patel SC, Cunningham Jr ET. Risks of intravitreous injection: a comprehensive review. Retina. 2004;24:676–98.
57. Intravitreal Injections. In: American academy of ophthalmology. 2015. http://www.aao.org/clinical-statement/intravitreal-injections--november-2008. Accessed 20 Aug 2015.
58. Sosa AB, Epstein SP, Asbell PA. Evaluation of toxicity of commercial ophthalmic fluoroquinolone antibiotics as assessed on immortalized corneal and conjunctival epithelial cells. Cornea. 2008;27:930–4. doi:10.1097/ICO.0b013e31816f27ab.
59. Tsai T-H, Chen WL, Hu FR. Comparison of fluoroquinolones: cytotoxicity on human corneal epithelial cells. Eye (Lond). 2010;24:909–17. doi:10.1038/eye.2009.179. Epub 2009 Jul 24.
60. Kim SY, Lim JA, Choi JS, Choi EC, Joo CK. Comparison of antibiotic effect and corneal epithelial toxicity of levofloxacin and moxifloxacin in vitro. Cornea. 2007;26:720–5.
61. Alfonso E, Crider J. Ophthalmic infections and their anti-infective challenges. Surv Ophthalmol. 2005;50 Suppl 1:S1–6.
62. Campochiaro PA, Lim JI. Aminoglycoside toxicity in the treatment of endophthalmitis. The Aminoglycoside Toxicity Study Group. Arch Ophthalmol. 1994;112:48–53.
63. Seawright AA, Bourke RD, Cooling RJ. Macula toxicity after intravitreal amikacin. Aust N Z J Ophthalmol. 1996;24:143–6.
64. Braga-Mele R, Chang DF, Henderson BA, Mamalis N, Talley-Rostov A, Vasavada A. Intracameral antibiotics: safety, efficacy, and preparation. J Cataract Refract Surg. 2014;40:2134–42.
65. Faure C, Perreira D, Audo I. Retinal toxicity after intracameral use of a standard dose of cefuroxime during cataract surgery. Doc Ophthalmol. 2015;130:57–63. doi:10.1007/s10633-014-9465-7. Epub 2014 Oct 16.
66. Ciftci S, Ciftci L, Daq U. Hemorrhagic retinal infarction due to inadvertent overdose of cefuroxime in cases of complicated cataract surgery: retrospective case series. Am J Ophthalmol. 2014;157:421–5.e2. doi:10.1016/j.ajo.2013.10.018. Epub 2013 Nov 6.
67. Craig W, Andes DR. Cephalosporins. In: Bennett JE, Dolin R, Blaser MJ, editors. Mandell, Douglas, and Bennett's principles and practice of infectious diseases. 8th ed. Philadelphia: Saunders; 2015. p. 278–292.e4.
68. Heim-Duthoy KL, Caperton EM, Pollock R, Matzke GR, Enthoven D, Peterson PK. Apparent biliary pseudolithiasis during ceftriaxone therapy. Antimicrob Agents Chemother. 1990;34:1146–9.
69. Park HZ, Lee SP, Schy AL. Ceftriaxone-associated gallbladder sludge. Identification of calcium-ceftriaxone salt as a major component of gallbladder precipitate. Gastroenterology. 1991;100:1665–70.
70. Letellier G, Desjarlais F. Analytical interference of drugs in clinical chemistry: II. The interference of three cephalosporins with the determination of serum creatinine concentration by the Jaffe reaction. Clin Biochem. 1985;18:352–6.
71. Grill MF, Maganti R. Cephalosporin-induced neurotoxicity: clinical manifestations, potential pathogenic mechanisms, and the role of electroencephalographic monitoring. Ann Pharmacol. 2008;42:1843–50.
72. Martinez-Rodriguez JE, Barriga FJ, Santamaria J, Iranzo A, Pareja JA, Revilla M, et al. Nonconvulsive status epilepticus associated with cephalosporins in patients with renal failure. Am J Med. 2001;111:115–9.

73. Lamoth F, Buclin T, Pascual A, Vora S, Bolay S, Decosterd LA, et al. High cefepime plasma concentrations and neurological toxicity in febrile neutropenic patients with mild impairment of renal function. Antimicrob Agents Chemother. 2010;54:4360–7.
74. Miller AD, Ball AM, Bookstaver PB, Dornblaser EK, Bennett CL. Epileptogenic potential of carbapenem agents: mechanism of action, seizure rates, and clinical considerations. Pharmacotherapy. 2011;31:408–23.
75. Doi Y, Chambers HF. Other beta-lactam antibiotics. In: Bennett JE, Dolin R, Blaser MJ, editors. Mandell, Douglas, and Bennett's principles and practice of infectious diseases. 8th ed. Philadelphia: Saunders; 2015. p. 293–7.e2.
76. Noel GJ, Natarajan J, Chien S, Hunt TL, Goodman DB, Abels R. Effects of three fluoroquinolones on QT interval in healthy adults after single doses. Clin Pharmacol Ther. 2003;73:292–303.
77. Morganroth J, Dimarco JP, Anzueto A, Niederman MS, Choudhri S, CAPRIE Study Group. A randomized trial comparing the cardiac rhythm safety of moxifloxacin vs levofloxacin in elderly patients hospitalized with community-acquired pneumonia. Chest. 2005;128:3398–406.
78. Briasoulis A, Agarwal V, Pierce WJ. QT prolongation and torsade de pointes induced by fluoroquinolones: infrequent side effects from commonly used medications. Cardiology. 2011;120:103–10.
79. Etminan M, Forooghian F, Brophy JM, Bird ST, Maberley D. Oral fluoroquinolones and the risk of retinal detachment. JAMA. 2012;307:1414–9.
80. Kuo SC, Chen YT, Lee YT, Fan NW, Chen SJ, Li SY, et al. Association between recent use of fluoroquinolones and rhegmatogenous retinal detachment: a population-based cohort study. Clin Infect Dis. 2014;58:197–203.
81. Pasternak B, Svanström H, Melbye M, Hviid A. Association between oral fluoroquinolone use and retinal detachment. JAMA. 2013;310:2184–90.
82. Lodise TP, Lomaestro B, Graves J, Drusano GL. Larger vancomycin doses (at least four grams per day) are associated with an increased incidence of nephrotoxicity. Antimicrob Agents Chemother. 2008;52:1330–6.
83. Hidayat LK, Hsu DI, Quist R, Shriner KA, Wong-Beringer A. High-dose vancomycin therapy for methicillin-resistant *Staphylococcus aureus* infections: efficacy and toxicity. Arch Intern Med. 2006;166:2138–44.
84. Jeffres MN, Isakow W, Doherty JA, McKinnon PS, Ritchie DJ, Micek ST, et al. Predictors of mortality for methicillin-resistant *Staphylococcus aureus* health-care-associated pneumonia: specific evaluation of vancomycin pharmacokinetic indices. Chest. 2006;130:947–55.
85. Zyvox® (linezolid) [package insert]. New York: Pharmacia and Upjohn Company; 2012.
86. Narita M, Tsuji BT, Yu VL. Linezolid-associated peripheral and optic neuropathy, lactic acidosis, and serotonin syndrome. Pharmacotherapy. 2007;27:1189–97.

Chapter 10
Role of the Clinical Microbiology Laboratory

David W. Craft and Wallace H. Greene

The microbiology laboratory offers a variety of procedures and diagnostic technologies to assist in the diagnosis of ocular infection. Laboratory procedures that support the identification of ocular pathogens include smear and microscopy, conventional culture, serological assays, and a number of specific molecular assays to include nucleic acid amplification and DNA sequencing. As many organisms cause eye infection, the specimen site and specific comments concerning a potential etiology should be communicated to the laboratory so that appropriate methods can be applied.

Recommendations for the laboratory diagnosis of ocular infection are often based on studies where only small numbers of clinical specimens were examined, so the evidence base for many recommendations is limited [1]. Frequently, pretreatment with topical antimicrobial agents further complicates laboratory diagnosis of both bacterial conjunctivitis and keratitis [2].

Specimen Collection and Transport

Specimens may be collected from the surface of the eye or from the intraocular tissues. It is important to select the appropriate specimen for a particular ocular infection, collect it properly, and label it accurately. If a certain pathogen is suspected, the laboratory should be notified to ensure that pathogen-specific protocols are followed. If acceptable to the microbiology laboratory used by the ophthalmologists in a given medical practice, specimens can be inoculated to primary culture media at the bedside or in the clinic and then sent for evaluation in the laboratory. Fresh

D.W. Craft, PhD, D(ABMM) (✉) • W.H. Greene, PhD, D(ABMM)
Department of Pathology, Penn State College of Medicine, Penn State Health-Milton S. Hershey Medical Center, 500 University Drive, Hershey, PA 17033, USA
e-mail: dcraft1@hmc.psu.edu; whg2@psu.edu

N.V. Laver, C.S. Specht (eds.), *The Infected Eye*,
DOI 10.1007/978-3-319-42840-6_10

Table 10.1 Types of ocular specimens

Types of ocular specimens
Conjunctival swab
Corneal scrapings
Aqueous and vitreous fluid aspirates
Aspirate from an abscess or wound
Periocular tissue
Corneal donor ring in storage media
Contact lens solutions

unexpired media must be made available to clinical areas that routinely collect ocular cultures. Ideally a separate set of primary media should be used for each specimen site. The types of specimens that may be taken for ocular infection are found in Table 10.1.

Conjunctival specimens collected by swab, spatula scrapings from the cornea, and aspirated samples of intraocular fluids or pus may be planted to agar plates and then sent to the laboratory, or they may be sent directly to the laboratory for processing. Specimens should be collected before topical anesthetics are instilled. When a swab is used for specimen collection, premoistening the swab in sterile broth lessens trauma and increases the yield of growth in culture. If conjunctival swabs are collected from both eyes, always use a separate swab for each eye. If planted in the clinic to the same culture plates, ensure that the swabs are streaked in distinctly different areas of the plates and marked as such. It is important to remember that the conjunctiva is home to various bacteria from the environment and the ocular adnexa and that these organisms can sometimes contaminate cultures taken from within the ocular globe or orbital tissues. Specimens from the conjunctiva may be collected as a control to compare with specimens collected by more invasive techniques [3].

For specimens such as intraocular fluids or suppurative material from an abscess that are aspirated by needle and syringe, it is important that the needle is removed and the syringe capped before transport to the laboratory. Tissue fragments or foreign bodies should be collected into sterile containers and transported to the laboratory for processing.

Specimens for culture of anaerobic bacteria should be sent to the laboratory in anaerobic transport media, chlamydial and viral culture samples should be taken using Dacron swabs with non-wood shafts. Ideally, flocked swabs should be used as they collect more cells for release into the transport medium. Some fluids used for storage or transport in ophthalmology, such as contact lens solution and the storage media used for corneal rims, include antibiotics or other chemical components that can alter the growth characteristics of microorganisms. The value of routinely submitting corneal donor rims for microbiological testing at the time of keratoplasty is unclear; however, culture-positive results are related to increased risk of ocular infection [4]. Corneal donor rings are often submitted to the laboratory for culture in storage media that contain antibiotics, and the predictive value of negative culture results is uncertain. It is thus important to communicate with the laboratory about the type of transport fluid being sent, as this can impact the interpretation of culture results.

Immediate transportation of microbiological specimens or inoculated media to the laboratory is important. Once microbiological media is inoculated with a specimen for culture, best results are obtained if the culture is incubated in appropriate environmental conditions. If incubators are not available and transport is delayed, then inoculated media should be maintained at room temperature until delivery to the laboratory. However, microbiology specimens should be maintained at room temperature for no longer than 24 h. Collection and transport devices, including transport media such as Amies, have compared favorably to direct inoculation [2]. Inoculated culture media do not require additional processing once received in the laboratory and can proceed immediately to microscopic examination, culture incubation, or molecular assay protocols.

It is not uncommon for a microbiology facility to receive extremely small tissue specimens that may be hidden or difficult to recognize in the container. These specimens are also at risk for dehydration that can affect the viability of the organisms. Communication with the laboratory and the use of a sterile fluid to humidify the containers during transport may help to mitigate these transportation and processing challenges.

Handling of Specimens for the Diagnosis of Ocular Infections

For common types of ocular infection, primary pathogens and recommended isolation media are summarized in Tables 10.2, 10.3, 10.4, 10.5, 10.6, and 10.7.

Processing Specimens for Culture

When spatula scrapings, biopsy tissue specimens, fluid samples, or swabs in transport media are received by the laboratory for culture of bacteria, fungi, or acid-fast bacilli (AFB), they are inoculated to primary agar plates and broths that are appropriate for the organisms of interest as indicated by the clinician [5]. The agar plates are planted with specimen and streaked for quantitation or isolation, while broth cultures are inoculated using at least 100 μls of fluid or minced tissue. In addition, smears are prepared; stained for bacteria, fungi, or AFB; and evaluated with microscopy; this can yield a rapid morphological diagnosis when positive.

Conjunctival specimens collected by swab are planted and streaked across agar plates. For spatula scrapings of corneal tissue, three to five scrapings per cornea are planted to agar plates. Intraocular fluids or pus may be planted to agar plates and broth as indicated. In all cases, microscopic evaluation of a smeared specimen on a glass slide is part of the regular evaluation of these specimens. Vitrectomy specimens are diluted and require centrifugation in the laboratory. The resulting concentrated

Table 10.2 Handling of specimens for the diagnosis of ocular infection[a]

Clinical condition	Primary isolation media[b]	Primary pathogen(s)	Comments
Blepharitis *Nasolacrimal duct obstruction* including Canaliculitis Dacryocystitis Dacryoadenitis	SBA CHOC MAC AnaeBA (if secondary to trauma) Fungal media[c] Viral media: Universal transport medium[d]	*Staphylococcus aureus* Coagulase-negative staphylococci (CNS) *S. pneumoniae* *Streptococcus* spp. *Actinomyces* spp. Gram-negative bacteria (including *E. coli* and *H. influenzae*) are rare	Bacterial culture includes morphological evaluation with a Gram stain *Actinomyces* spp. are often associated with canaliculitis Fungal culture includes morphological evaluation with a calcofluor white stain Mites that infest lid margins may be found by histopathology

[a]Handling of specimens for the diagnosis of ocular infection (Adapted from *Clinical Microbiology Procedures Handbook*, 3rd ed. Table 3.10-2)
[b]Bacterial media: sheep blood agar (SBA), chocolate agar (CHOC), MacConkey agar (MAC), and anaerobic blood agar (AnaeBA). These media are adequate for the growth of yeast
[c]Fungal media may include inhibitory mold agar (IMA), brain heart infusion (BHI), or potato flake agar (PFA)
[d]Universal transport medium (UTM) is a standardized transport solution for optimal preservation of viruses and *Chlamydia* and may be used with molecular amplification assays

pellet is harvested for smears and culture. In addition to culture, vitreous fluids may be used for molecular amplification, liquid-based cytology, and cell blocks if enough tissue is available [6, 7].

Upon receipt in the laboratory, corneal rim tissue is removed from the storage medium with sterile forceps and plated to media that support the growth of bacteria and yeast. Smears are prepared and may be stained for bacteria, fungi, and AFB. The storage medium may then be concentrated by centrifugation, using the sediment to make smears. For small volumes of fluid, a cytospin slide may be prepared for staining.

Additional organisms that cause ocular infections and that may be associated with travel outside the United States require laboratory testing beyond the routine protocols found in the clinical microbiology laboratory. These pathogens include *Corynebacterium diphtheriae*, *Leptospira interrogans*, *Trypanosoma* spp., *Leishmania* spp., *Loa loa*, *Onchocerca volvulus*, *Microsporidia* spp., and *Mycobacterium leprae*. Postinfectious uveitis can develop in patients who have had Ebola virus disease, and this syndrome may be emerging in survivors of the recent outbreak in sub-Saharan West Africa [8].

Specimen collection and processing requirements for viral and chlamydial pathogens are very similar to those for bacteria and fungi. Specimens are often collected with swabs or corneal scrapings which are best transported to the laboratory in universal transport media, a standardized liquid media formulated for optimal preservation of viruses and *Chlamydia*. Antibiotics are included to suppress

Table 10.3 Handling of specimens for the diagnosis of ocular infection[a]

Clinical condition	Primary isolation media[b]	Primary pathogen(s)	Comments
Cellulitis	SBA CHOC MAC AnaeBA (if secondary to trauma) Fungal media[c] Viral media: Universal transport medium[d]	*S. aureus* *S. pneumoniae* Viridans group streptococci (including the Anginosus group) *S. pyogenes* (Group A *Streptococcus*) *H. influenzae* *Moraxella catarrhalis* Gram negatives including *P. aeruginosa* Anaerobes	*Periorbital* Localized soft tissue infection around the eye *H. influenzae* may be recovered in infants and young children *Orbital* Mixed aerobic and anaerobic infection secondary to trauma or sinusitis Blood cultures should be obtained Fungi, including *Aspergillus* spp. and *Mucor* spp., may be important in diabetic or other immune-compromised patients

[a]Handling of specimens for the diagnosis of ocular infection (Adapted from *Clinical Microbiology Procedures Handbook*, 3rd ed. Table 3.10-2)

[b]Bacterial media: sheep blood agar (SBA), chocolate agar (CHOC), MacConkey agar (MAC), and anaerobic blood agar (AnaeBA). These media are adequate for the growth of yeast

[c]Fungal media may include inhibitory mold agar (IMA), brain heart infusion (BHI), or potato flake agar (PFA)

[d]Universal transport medium (UTM) is a standardized transport solution for optimal preservation of viruses and *Chlamydia* and may be used with molecular amplification assays

the growth of bacteria and fungi. Samples taken in this way are also suitable for the application of molecular amplification assays. Corneal scrapings may be placed on glass microscope slides and stained with immunofluorescence methods for specific viruses [2, 9]. If anesthetics or dyes have been used prior to collecting a specimen, the eye should be thoroughly rinsed with sterile saline or water before obtaining the specimen. These substances may interfere with molecular amplification assays.

Smears and Histology

Smears for microscopic examination may be prepared in the laboratory from swabs, tissue scrapings, or fluids. Materials are placed or smeared onto a cleaned microscope slide, fixed appropriately, and stained. Slides may be stained for bacteria with the Gram stain method; for acid-fast bacilli (AFB) with the Kinyoun, Ziehl-Neelsen, or fluorochrome methods; for fungi (yeasts; molds) or *Acanthamoeba* with the calcofluor white/KOH method; or for *C. trachomatis* using direct fluorescent antibody (DFA) methods. Fluids may be cytospun to increase the sensitivity of stained smears for identification of microorganisms.

Table 10.4 Handling of specimens for the diagnosis of ocular infection[a]

Clinical condition	Primary isolation media[b]	Primary pathogen(s)	Comments
Conjunctivitis	SBA CHOC MAC AnaeBA (if secondary to trauma) Fungal media[c] Viral media: Universal transport medium[d]	*Staphylococcus* spp. *Haemophilus influenzae* *Streptococcus pneumoniae* *Streptococcus pyogenes* *Moraxella* spp. *Pseudomonas aeruginosa* Enteric Gram-negative rods (rare) *Neisseria gonorrhoeae* *C. trachomatis* Picornavirus Rubella Rubeola Mumps Influenza EBV Papillomavirus Molluscum contagiosum HIV West Nile virus Zika virus Vaccinia virus (postvaccination)	*Enterobacteriaceae* and *P. aeruginosa* may be important in children, hospitalized, and/or immunocompromised patients DFA[e] for *Chlamydia trachomatis* in neonates. Commensal skin flora such as CNS and *Corynebacterium* spp. can be pathogens Parasites and fungi (rare) may be detected by histopathology

[a]Handling of specimens for the diagnosis of ocular infection (Adapted from *Clinical Microbiology Procedures Handbook*, 3rd ed. Table 3.10-2)

[b]Bacterial media: sheep blood agar (SBA), chocolate agar (CHOC), MacConkey agar (MAC), and anaerobic blood agar (AnaeBA). These media are adequate for the growth of yeast

[c]Fungal media may include inhibitory mold agar (IMA), brain heart infusion (BHI), or potato flake agar (PFA)

[d]Universal transport medium (UTM) is a standardized transport solution for optimal preservation of viruses and *Chlamydia* and may be used with molecular amplification assays

[e]*DFA*, direct fluorescent antibody testing

For surgical pathology tissue that has been fixed and prepared as histological slides in the histopathology laboratory, staining with tissue modifications of the Gram stain for bacteria, the Grocott methenamine silver stain for fungi and *Acanthamoeba*, or the Ziehl-Neelsen stain for AFB may allow identification of an infectious pathogen. Nonspecific stains such as Giemsa can also be used to reveal microorganisms in histological slides.

In the case of AFB and fungi, this histological identification can be made before culture results are available. In all cases, however, morphological identification only provides information about the general type of organism involved in an infection. Although this can be clinically useful, only microbiological culture methods or molecular assays provide information that allows for definitive classification of the organism with genus and species.

Table 10.5 Handling of specimens for the diagnosis of ocular infection[a]

Clinical condition	Primary isolation media[b]	Primary pathogen(s)	Comments
Keratitis	SBA CHOC MAC AnaeBA (if secondary to trauma) Fungal media[c] AFB media[d] Viral: Universal transport medium[e]	*Corneal trauma/ulcer* *Pseudomonas aeruginosa* *S. aureus* CNS *S. pneumoniae* *S. pyogenes* (Group A *Streptococcus*) Viridans group streptococci *Propionibacterium* spp. *Enterobacteriaceae* *Moraxella* spp. Anaerobes AFB *Nocardia* spp. HSV VZV Adenovirus Vaccinia virus (postvaccination) *Contact lens associated* Gram-negative bacteria, including *P. aeruginosa*, *Serratia* spp. *Acanthamoeba* spp. *Fusarium* spp. *Candida* spp. *Aspergillus* spp. AFB – rapid growers *Bacillus* spp.	Keratitis is caused by a variety of organisms, depending upon the mechanism of corneal injury Fungal, AFB and, nocardial keratitis should be ruled out in chronic infection or following refractive surgery Additional serologic tests are required for some parasitic and all syphilitic or Lyme-associated keratitis Corneal ulcers may be examined by a molecular amplification assay or viral culture, particularly for patients with trigeminal herpes zoster infection

[a]Handling of specimens for the diagnosis of ocular infection (Adapted from *Clinical Microbiology Procedures Handbook*, 3rd ed. Table 3.10-2)

[b]Bacterial media: sheep blood agar (SBA), chocolate agar (CHOC), MacConkey agar (MAC), and anaerobic blood agar (AnaeBA). These media are adequate for the growth of yeast

[c]Fungal media may include inhibitory mold agar (IMA), brain heart infusion (BHI), or potato flake agar (PFA)

[d]AFB media: AFB (mycobacterial) media may include Löwenstein-Jensen (LJ) or Middlebrook agar and broth culture

[e]Universal transport medium (UTM) is a standardized transport solution for optimal preservation of viruses and *Chlamydia* and may be used with molecular amplification assays

Bacterial Culture and Antimicrobial Susceptibility Testing

When received in the laboratory, smears are Gram stained, specimens are planted to primary agar media, and broth is inoculated for aerobic culture and anaerobic culture (if requested by the clinician). Primary media generally include sheep blood

Table 10.6 Handling of specimens for the diagnosis of ocular infection[a]

Clinical condition	Primary isolation media[b]	Primary pathogen(s)	Comments
Endophthalmitis	SBA CHOC MAC AnaeBA (if secondary to trauma) Fungal media[c] AFB media[d] Viral: Universal transport medium[e]	*Candida* spp. CNS *S. aureus* *S. pneumoniae* Viridans group streptococci *Bacillus* spp. *P. aeruginosa* *Acinetobacter* spp. *P. acnes* *H. influenzae* *Neisseria* spp. Anaerobes Gram-negative bacteria Molds (*Aspergillus*, *Fusarium*) HSV	Endophthalmitis is caused by a variety of organisms, depending upon the mechanism of infection Fungal, AFB, and nocardial endophthalmitis should be ruled out in chronic postsurgical and traumatic infections *Bacillus cereus* is the most common and fulminant of the *Bacillus* spp. Viral cultures should be considered, particularly for patients with trigeminal herpes zoster infection The inner eye chambers may be seeded by any bacteria or fungi that cause bacteremia or fungemia, so blood cultures should be obtained

[a]Handling of specimens for the diagnosis of ocular infection (Adapted from *Clinical Microbiology Procedures Handbook*, 3rd ed. Table 3.10-2)
[b]Bacterial media: sheep blood agar (SBA), chocolate agar (CHOC), MacConkey agar (MAC), and anaerobic blood agar (AnaeBA). These media are adequate for the growth of yeast
[c]Fungal media may include inhibitory mold agar (IMA), brain heart infusion (BHI), or potato flake agar (PFA)
[d]AFB media: AFB (mycobacterial) media may include Löwenstein-Jensen (LJ) or Middlebrook agar and broth culture
[e]Universal transport medium (UTM) is a standardized transport solution for optimal preservation of viruses and *Chlamydia* and may be used with molecular amplification assays

agar (SBA), chocolate agar (CHOC), and MacConkey agar (MAC); these cultures are incubated with 5% CO_2 at 37 °C for 3 days. If anaerobic culture has been requested, anaerobic media such as thioglycolate broth or CDC anaerobic blood agar (AnaeBA) plates can be added. These cultures are maintained in an anaerobic environment at 37 °C for 4 days. Incubation of broth cultures for *Propionibacterium acnes* in invasively collected ocular specimens may be extended to 7 days.

In order to produce clinically relevant results, the laboratory may not fully identify commensal or skin flora, and antimicrobial susceptibility testing (AST) may be limited. Culture growth of clinically insignificant bacteria, especially from conjunctival specimens, may result from contamination of the specimen by organisms from the surrounding skin. Commensal or normal flora of the skin surrounding the eye includes coagulase-negative staphylococci (CNS), viridans group streptococci, diphtheroids such as *Corynebacterium* spp., *Propionibacterium* spp., *Moraxella* spp., and *Peptostreptococcus* spp.

Table 10.7 Handling of specimens for the diagnosis of ocular infection[a]

Clinical condition	Primary isolation media[b]	Primary pathogen(s)	Comments
Uveitis	SBA CHOC MAC AnaeBA (if secondary to trauma) AFB media[c] Viral: Universal transport medium[d]	*M. tuberculosis* *Spirochetes* (syphilis, Lyme) *Toxoplasma gondii* *Toxocara* spp. *Candida* spp. HSV VZV CMV *Onchocerca volvulus*	Most uveitis infections are not diagnosed by conventional culture methods Serological assays are used for spirochetal and parasitic disease Uncommon ocular diseases include cat scratch disease (*Bartonella* spp.), West Nile virus, brucellosis, Whipple's disease, leprosy, leptospirosis, and Ebola virus disease

[a]Handling of specimens for the diagnosis of ocular infection (Adapted from *Clinical Microbiology Procedures Handbook*, 3rd ed. Table 3.10-2)
[b]Bacterial media: sheep blood agar (SBA), chocolate agar (CHOC), MacConkey agar (MAC), and anaerobic blood agar (AnaeBA). These media are adequate for the growth of yeast
[c]AFB media: AFB (mycobacterial) media may include Löwenstein-Jensen (LJ) or Middlebrook agar and broth culture
[d]Universal transport medium (UTM) is a standardized transport solution for optimal preservation of viruses and *Chlamydia* and may be used with molecular amplification assays

Chlamydia may be identified using direct immunofluorescence (DFA), through growth in cell culture, or with molecular methods [2]. Detection by DFA is rapid and was widely used in the past. However, this is much less sensitive than molecular methods and is no longer readily available in most laboratories. Growth in cell cultures was once commonly used to detect *Chlamydia* in ocular samples, but this has been widely replaced by molecular assays. Cell culture methods have fallen out of favor due to the time required for *Chlamydia* to grow and because maintaining the viability of these organisms in cell culture can be difficult. In current practice, the use of molecular assays including the polymerase chain reaction (PCR) is recommended to detect chlamydial infections. This has the advantage of superior sensitivity and yields a more rapid test result than culture. The use of molecular testing also eliminates the problem of decreased viability that may occur when culture specimens are sent to reference laboratories for detection.

Close coordination between the clinician and the laboratory in developing culture protocols and result reporting is essential for proper interpretation of results and therapeutic management of the patient. *Neisseria gonorrhoeae* or *C. trachomatis* in a conjunctival culture, *P. aeruginosa* in a corneal culture, or *Bacillus* spp. in a vitreous aspirate or anterior chamber tap are considered critical reports, and the clinician should be notified immediately [2].

Antimicrobial susceptibility testing (AST) yielding minimum inhibitory concentration (MIC) values with breakpoint interpretations is useful for therapeutic decision-making on patients requiring systemic therapy. MIC breakpoint interpretations are not defined for drugs that are applied topically or that are injected into the anterior or posterior segments of the eye, as concentrations achievable through direct administration can be significantly greater than those measured in serum after oral or parenteral administration.

Culture for Acid-Fast Bacilli (AFB)

For AFB (including mycobacteria), smears of material submitted to the laboratory should be stained with a fluorochrome stain such as auramine-rhodamine for maximum sensitivity. Primary media generally include a Löwenstein-Jensen (LJ) slant, a Middlebrook (7H11) agar plate, and a Middlebrook (7H9) broth; these are incubated in 5 % CO_2 at 35 °C for up to 42 days. Growth on culture plates may be confirmed as AFB by evaluation with the Kinyoun or Ziehl-Neelsen staining methods. *Nocardia* spp. are gram-positive beaded rods and weakly acid-fast. When received in the laboratory, smears of the submitted material should be stained using a modified acid-fast staining procedure. The organisms can be cultured on chocolate plates incubated in 5 % CO_2 at 35 °C for 5 days.

Culture for Fungal Organisms

Smears of material submitted to the laboratory should be evaluated with a fluorescent stain such as calcofluor white with KOH. For common yeasts such as *Candida* spp. and *Cryptococcus* spp., the organisms can be cultured on SBA and chocolate agar for 3 days. Fungal media for molds such as *Aspergillus* spp. and *Fusarium* spp. may include inhibitory mold agar (IMA), brain heart infusion (BHI), or potato flake agar (PFA). For fungal dimorphs that can grow as either molds or as yeast forms, such as *Blastomyces* spp. and *Histoplasma* spp., cultures can be plated on brain heart infusion (BHI) with blood agar and Sabouraud (SAB) agar and grown at 30 °C for 4 weeks. Special blood cultures for dimorphic fungi may also be obtained, and this should be coordinated with the laboratory prior to collection. Growth on culture plates can be microscopically examined for final morphological identification using smears stained with lactophenol cotton blue/KOH.

Detection of Parasitic Organisms

When present as the cyst form, *Acanthamoeba* spp. may be readily detected in smears using the calcofluor white stain; however, the sensitivity of this method is dependent on the number of cysts in the sample, and the method requires a fluorescent microscope equipped with an appropriate UV filter in order to visualize the organism [2, 10]. The amoebic form of *Acanthamoeba* may be grown on non-nutrient agar that has been overlaid with *E. coli* to serve as a food source [11]. Cultures are usually positive in 2–5 days, depending on the number of organisms in the sample. Suitable sample types include corneal scrapings, contact lens, and the contact lens case.

Toxoplasma gondii can cause acute or congenital ocular infections, including chorioretinitis. Although the organism has been grown in cell culture, this technique is rarely used and has been replaced by detecting the DNA of the organism or the local production of specific antibody in the aqueous humor [12].

While not endemic in the United States, infection with the filarial parasite *Onchocerca volvulus* is occasionally found in travelers from countries where it is common. The microfilariae may be directly observed in the cornea and the anterior chamber of the eye. They may also be detected by collecting a small skin biopsy from the nape of the neck or shoulders and placing it in normal saline. If present, the microfilariae will emerge within a few hours or up to 24 h later and can be easily seen with a microscope [13]. Serologic assays to detect IgG antibodies to the organism are also available from reference laboratories.

Detection of Viral Organisms

Numerous viruses can cause ocular disease [2]. Viral conjunctivitis is most frequently caused by adenovirus; however, *Herpes simplex* virus (HSV), *Varicella zoster* virus (VZV), picornaviruses, and other less common viruses may also produce this condition [14]. Keratitis can be caused by HSV, VZV, adenovirus, Epstein-Barr virus (EBV), and various enteroviruses [15]. HSV, VZV, and *Cytomegalovirus* (CMV) can cause infection of the intraocular tissues with involvement of the retina and uvea [16]. A variety of methods has been used in the past to detect these viruses, but there is overwhelming evidence that molecular amplification assays such as PCR are superior as they provide increased sensitivity and have the ability to detect viruses that do not grow in cell culture [16].

Members of the herpes family that infect humans and produce ocular infections include HSV, CMV, VZV, and EBV. Primary HSV infection and recurrent outbreaks with significant symptoms can be detected in smears of corneal scrapings using an immunofluorescent stain; this method also allows the differentiation of HSV-1 and HSV-2 infections [2, 9, 14, 17]. Cell culture or molecular assays are often used to further evaluate negative specimens. However, to obtain antiviral sensitivities, a viral isolate from cell culture is required.

CMV infection produces characteristic intranuclear inclusions in tissue that can be detected with immunohistochemical or direct fluorescent antibody (DFA) stains, although molecular assays are more sensitive [16]. VZV is very difficult to culture but may be detected by immunohistochemical or DFA stains. Negative results should be confirmed by a sensitive molecular assay [16]. EBV does not grow in cell culture; therefore, molecular assays are recommended for detection of this virus. The presence of EBV in histological tissue sections can be demonstrated with in situ hybridization for EBV-encoded RNA (EBER) [16].

Adenovirus and picornaviruses can infect the eye, usually causing conjunctivitis. With acute adenoviral conjunctivitis (epidemic conjunctivitis; "pink eye"), a high concentration of virus is often present that can be detected with DFA staining of smears. This method provides a rapid result when positive. Most strains of adenovirus will grow in cell culture, but this often requires several days. Molecular assays are recommended as the best way to detect. Many strains of picornavirus are difficult to grow in culture but are readily detected with molecular assays.

Numerous other viruses such as respiratory viruses, rubella, rubeola, mumps, Zika virus, papillomavirus, and molluscum contagiosum that can produce a variety of different disease syndromes may also cause conjunctivitis as a symptom [14]. Infection with these viruses can often be identified based on clinical presentation. However, when it is necessary to do laboratory testing to confirm a diagnosis, serologic assay for specific IgM or IgG antibodies is the most reliable method. An adequate period of time between the onset of symptoms and collection of the serum sample must be allowed for the immune response to develop.

References

1. Baron EJ, Miller JM, Weinstein MP, Richter SS, Gilligan PH, Thomson Jr RB, et al. A guide to utilization of the microbiology laboratory for diagnosis of infectious diseases: 2013 recommendations by the IDSA and the ASM. Clin Infect Dis. 2013;57:1–100.
2. Gray LD, Gilligan PH, Fowler WC. Laboratory diagnosis of ocular infections. In: Snyder JW, editor. Cumitech 13B. Washington, DC: ASM Press; 2011. p. 5–20.
3. Hall GS, York MK, Church DL. Ocular cultures. In: Garcia LS, Isenberg HD, editors. Clinical microbiology procedures handbook. 3rd ed. Washington, DC: ASM Press; 2010. p. 3.10.1–9.
4. Wilhemus KR, Hassan SS. The prognostic role of donor corneoscleral rim cultures. Corneal Transplant Ophthalmol. 2007;114:440–5.
5. Baron EJ. Specimen collection, transport, and processing: bacteriology. In: Jorgensen JH, Pfaller MA, Carroll KC, Funke G, Landry ML, Richter SS, et al., editors. Manual of clinical microbiology. 11th ed. Washington, DC: ASM Press; 2015. p. 270–315.
6. Metha M, Rasheed R, Duker J, Reichel E, Feinberg E, Husain D, et al. Vitreous cytology: a diagnostic challenge. Ophthalmology. 2015;122:531–7.
7. Laver NMV. Ocular cytopathology. A primer for the generalist. Semin Diagn Pathol. 2015;32: 311–22.
8. Varkey JB, Shantha JG, Crozier I, Kraft CS, Lyon GM, Mehta AK, et al. Persistence of Ebola virus in ocular fluid during convalescence. N Engl J Med. 2015;18:2423–7.
9. Dunn J. Specimen collection, transport, and processing: virology. In: Jorgensen JH, Pfaller MA, Carroll KC, Funke G, Landry ML, Richter SS, et al., editors. Manual of clinical microbiology. 11th ed. Washington, DC: ASM Press; 2015. p. 1405–21.
10. Visvesvara GS. Parasite culture: *Acanthamoeba* and *Naegleria* spp. In: Garcia LS, Isenberg HD, editors. Clinical microbiology procedures handbook. 3rd ed. Washington, DC: ASM Press; 2010. p. 9.9.2.1–8.
11. Visvesvara G. Pathogenic and opportunistic free-living amebae. In: Jorgensen JH, Pfaller MA, Carroll KC, Funke G, Landry ML, Richter SS, et al., editors. Manual of clinical microbiology. 11th ed. Washington, DC: ASM Press; 2015. p. 2387–98.

12. McAuley JB, Jones JL, Singh K. Toxoplasma. In: Jorgensen JH, Pfaller MA, Carroll KC, Funke G, Landry ML, Richter SS, et al., editors. Manual of clinical microbiology. 11th ed. Washington, DC: ASM Press; 2015. p. 2373–86.
13. Chatterjee S, Nutman TB. Filarial nematodes. In: Jorgensen JH, Pfaller MA, Carroll KC, Funke G, Landry ML, Richter SS, et al., editors. Manual of clinical microbiology. 11th ed. Washington, DC: ASM Press; 2015. p. 2461–70.
14. Barnes SD, Kumar NM, Pavan-Langston P, Azar DT. Microbial conjunctivitis. In: Bennett JE, Dolin R, Blaser MJ, editors. Principles and practice of infectious diseases. 18th ed. Philadelphia: Elsevier Saunders; 2015. p. 1392–401.
15. Barnes SD, Hallak J, Pavan-Langston D, Azar DT. Microbial keratitis. In: Bennett JE, Dolin R, Blaser MJ, editors. Principles and practice of infectious diseases. 18th ed. Philadelphia: Elsevier Saunders; 2015. p. 1402–14.
16. Durand ML. Infectious causes of uveitis. In: Bennett JE, Dolin R, Blaser MJ, editors. Principles and practice of infectious diseases. 18th ed. Philadelphia: Elsevier Saunders; 2015. p. 1423–31.
17. Landry ML, Caliendo AM, Ginocchio CC, Tang YW, Valsamakis A. Algorithms for detection and identification of viruses. In: Jorgensen JH, Pfaller MA, Carroll KC, Funke G, Landry ML, Richter SS, et al., editors. Manual of clinical microbiology. 11th ed. Washington, DC: ASM Press; 2015. p. 1432–5.

Index

N.V. Laver, C.S. Specht (eds.), *The Infected Eye*,
DOI 10.1007/978-3-319-42840-6

D

P

MIX
Papier aus verantwortungsvollen Quellen
Paper from responsible sources
FSC® C105338

If you have any concerns about our products,
you can contact us on
ProductSafety@springernature.com

In case Publisher is established outside the EU,
the EU authorized representative is:
Springer Nature Customer Service Center GmbH
Europaplatz 3, 69115 Heidelberg, Germany

Printed by Libri Plureos GmbH
in Hamburg, Germany